MEDICAL DEPARTMENT, UNITED STATES ARMY

UNITED STATES ARMY DENTAL SERVICE IN WORLD WAR II

By

GEORGE F. JEFFCOTT
Colonel, DC, USA

OFFICE OF THE SURGEON GENERAL

DEPARTMENT OF THE ARMY

WASHINGTON, D. C., 1955

The volumes comprising the history of the Medical Department of the U. S. Army in World War II are divided into two series: (1) The Administrative and Operational series which constitutes a part of the general series of the history of the *U. S. Army in World War II*, published under the direction of the Office of the Chief of Military History, and (2) the Professional, or clinical and technical, series published as *The Medical Department of the United States Army* under the direction of the Office of The Surgeon General. Both series are being prepared by the Historical Unit, Army Medical Service. This is one of a number of volumes to be published in the latter series.

JOHN BOYD COATES, JR.
Colonel, MC, USA
Editor in Chief

For sale by the Superintendent of Documents, U. S. Government Printing Office
Washington 25, D. C. - Price $3.25

THE MEDICAL DEPARTMENT OF THE UNITED STATES ARMY

A History of the United States Army Dental Service
in World War II

By

George F. Jeffcott, D. M. D., F. A. C. D.
Colonel, DC, USA

This volume was prepared by the Historical Unit, Army Medical Service, under the direction of Colonel Calvin H. Goddard, MC, AUS, formerly Editor in Chief; Associate Editor for this volume, Rebecca L. Duberstein.

Preface

In the preparation of this volume free use has been made of the published and unpublished works of earlier authors, among which the contributions of Colonel Walter D. Vail, DC, Colonel Pearson W. Brown, DC, and Colonel John C. Brauer, DC, are particularly significant. In addition, the author has had the benefit of advice and assistance from a large number of individuals who filled key positions in the Office of The Surgeon General during and following World War II, whose wide experience and personal understanding of the problems of operating a wartime dental service enabled them to provide invaluable information not available in official files.

It is regretted that the necessary screening and destruction of obsolete Army files has resulted in the loss of a considerable number of the documents from which information in this volume was compiled. Though these documents are no longer available for study, they have not been removed as references since identification of source material may enable the reader to assess the validity of the information. Documents which are no longer available are specifically identified in the footnotes by a [D] symbol.

While this volume is primarily concerned with the Army Dental Service during World War II, some discussion of problems and events preceding that conflict has been included. The inclusion of some of this material is justified on the ground that it involves problems or policies which later affected the operation of the Dental Service in wartime. Other material concerning the initiation and early development of the Army Dental Service has been included because of its general interest and the fact that very little information on this subject is available in standard publications to date.

GEORGE F. JEFFCOTT
Colonel, DC, U. S. Army.

Foreword

The techniques of dentistry as practiced in the United States Army do not differ significantly from those in civilian life. The task and problems, however, involved in applying these techniques in providing dental care to some 8,000,000 men and women, under such trying conditions as existed in a global war, stand unique and unparalleled.

The Dental Corps expanded from its strength at the end of 1939 of approximately 250 dental officers to over 15,000 during the World War II period of hostilities. The Dental Service was constantly confronted with the perplexities concerned with personnel procurement, training, assignment, utilization, and administration. In addition, equipment, supplies, and ancillary dental facilities had to be obtained, distributed, and maintained throughout the world in support of American troops. Further, as the result of increased manpower requirements on the part of the Army, and the necessary concurrent lowering of dental standards for individuals entering the military service, the Dental Service was called upon and expected to accomplish a mission of Herculean magnitude—that of restoring and maintaining the dental health of the Army.

This record, so admirably presented by Colonel George F. Jeffcott, Dental Corps, relates how such dental care was provided. The lessons learned and experiences gained by those concerned primarily with that care should be studied by all who are now, or may be in the future, confronted with similar responsibilities.

Finally, this portion of the History of the Medical Department is a tribute to the dental profession and to the men and women who faithfully, with outstanding success, served with the Army Dental Service during World War II.

GEORGE E. ARMSTRONG
Major General, United States Army
The Surgeon General

CHAPTER I

Development of the United States Army Dental Service

ORGANIZATION OF THE ARMY DENTAL CORPS PRIOR TO WORLD WAR II

Dentistry, during the pioneer days of the profession in the United States, had no military status; and there exist only a few unofficial references to dental treatment in the accounts of the first wars in which the country was engaged. A notable exception, however, was the dental treatment accomplished for General George Washington, who experienced dental difficulties during the time he served as Commander in Chief of the Colonial Army and later during his terms as President. Records reveal that Washington had several dentures made by civilian dentists and that he was very much pleased with his dental service.[1]

Almost one hundred years passed after the Revolutionary War before there was any official Army recognition of dentistry or legislative action to initiate the organization of an Army Dental Corps. During these hundred years the profession continued to develop and to broaden its scope.

The first organized effort to secure dentists for an army was the conscription of these to serve in the Confederate Army in 1864.[2] The soldiers of the Confederate armies could not pay for dental treatment in the depreciated currency of the Confederacy since the fee for one gold filling was more than 6 months' pay of a private. Consequently, the Confederate States Congress passed a law for the conscription of dentists who were to have the rank, pay, and allowances to which their position in the Army entitled them, and in addition extra duty pay for extraordinary skill as allowed by The Surgeon General. The rank and pay offered the Confederate dental officers is not recorded. Each dentist furnished his own instruments, but other equipment and supplies were purchased from hospital funds.

After the Civil War, a number of years passed before there developed another wave of concerted interest in making dental service available to the Armed Forces. Members of the dental profession and the National Dental Association initiated and sponsored legislative measures to provide for the appointment of dental surgeons for service in the United States Army. The

---

[1] Robinson, J. B.: The foundations of professional dentistry. *In* Maryland State Dental Assoc., and Am. Dent. A.: Proceedings Dental Centenary Celebration, 1840–1940. Baltimore, Waverly Press, Inc., 1940.
[2] Burton, W. Leigh: Dental surgery as applied in the armies of late Confederate States. Am. J. Dent. Sc. vol. I, 3d series, No. 4. Baltimore, Snowden and Cowman, August 1867, p. 180–189. SG: 39611.

first such legislation approved by The Surgeon General and the War Department was enacted 2 February 1901. This bill authorized the employment of a maximum of 30 dental surgeons, on a contract basis, to serve the officers and enlisted men of the Regular and Volunteer Army.[3]

One of the first dentists so appointed was Dr. John S. Marshall who formulated the plans for the organization of the dental service.[4] Dr. Marshall, who was one of the most active, versatile, and forward-looking men in the new service, served as senior dentist until 1911. His continual efforts to promote a better dental service for the Army and to effect a more favorable status for the contract dental surgeon are reflected in the legislative acts and Army regulations which have appeared in the years since 1901. These are tributes to Dr. Marshall and the small group of original dental surgeons who were willing to sacrifice position, pride, and income to demonstrate the real value of dentistry to the military service.

Initially, the contract dental surgeons were *attached* to the Medical Department and assigned to duty by The Surgeon General or chief surgeon of a military department. In 1908, they were authorized by law to become a part of the Medical Department,[5] and finally, in 1911, a bill which included a provision for the commissioning of dentists was enacted into law. That part of the act of 3 March 1911 (36 Stat. 1054), pertaining to dentistry, reads:[6]

> Hereafter there shall be attached to the Medical Department a dental corps, which shall be composed of dental surgeons and acting dental surgeons, the total number of which shall not exceed the proportion of one to each thousand of actual enlisted strength of the Army; the number of dental surgeons shall not exceed sixty, and the number of acting dental surgeons shall be such as may, from time to time, be authorized by law. All original appointments to the dental corps shall be as acting dental surgeons, who shall have the same official status, pay, and allowances as the contract dental surgeons now authorized by law. Acting dental surgeons who have served three years in a manner satisfactory to the Secretary of War shall be eligible for appointment as dental surgeons, and, after passsing in a satisfactory manner an examination which may be prescribed by the Secretary of War, may be commissioned with the rank of first lieutenant in the dental corps to fill the vacancies existing therein. Officers of the dental corps shall have rank in such corps according to date of their commissions therein and shall rank next below officers of the Medical Reserve Corps. Their right to command shall be limited to the dental corps. The pay and allowances of dental surgeons shall be those of first lieutenants, including the right to retirement on account of age or disability, as in the case of other officers: *Provided*, That the time served by dental surgeons as acting dental or contract dental surgeons shall be reckoned in computing the increased service pay of such as are commissioned under this Act. The appointees as acting dental surgeons must be citizens of the United States between twenty-one and twenty-seven years of age, graduates of a standard

---

[3] GOs and Cirs 1901, Hq of the Army, GO 9, 6 Feb 1901, sec 18, p. 8. SG : 1027.

[4] Marshall, John S.: Organization of the Dental Corps of the U. S. Army, with suggestions upon the educational requirements for military dental practice. *In* Transactions of the National Dental Association, Dental Digest. Chicago, J. N. Crouse, 1902, p. 32–46.

[5] GOs and Cirs 1908, vol I, WD, GO, 67, 2 May 1908, Washington, Government Printing Office, 1909, p. 1. SG : 1036.

[6] U. S. Statutes at Large, 61st Congress, Washington, Government Printing Office, 1911, Pt I, 26 : 1054–1055.

Contents

	Page
FOREWORD	v
PREFACE	vii

Chapter

		Page
I.	DEVELOPMENT OF THE UNITED STATES ARMY DENTAL SERVICE	1
II.	ADMINISTRATION OF THE DENTAL SERVICE	22
III.	THE PROCUREMENT OF DENTAL OFFICERS	35
IV.	PERSONNEL AND TRAINING	105
V.	DENTAL EQUIPMENT AND SUPPLY	165
VI.	OPERATION OF THE DENTAL SERVICE—GENERAL CONSIDERATIONS	199
VII.	DENTAL SERVICE IN ZONE OF INTERIOR	257
VIII.	DENTAL SERVICE IN A THEATER OF OPERATIONS	287
IX.	DEMOBILIZATION OF DENTAL PERSONNEL	332
	INDEX	344

dental college, of good moral character and good professional education, and they shall be required to pass the usual physical examination required for appointment in the Medical Corps, and a professional examination which shall include tests of skill in practical dentistry and of proficiency in the usual subjects of a standard dental college course: *Provided,* That the contract dental surgeons attached to the Medical Department at the time of the passage of this Act may be eligible for appointment as first lieutenants, dental corps, without limitation as to age: *and provided further,* That the professional examination for such appointment may be waived in the case of contract dental surgeons in the service at the time of the passage of this Act whose efficiency reports and entrance examinations are satisfactory. The Secretary of War is authorized to appoint boards of three examiners to conduct the examinations herein prescribed, one of whom shall be a surgeon in the Army and two of whom shall be selected by the Secretary of War from the commissioned dental surgeons.

The following were appointed dental surgeons with the rank of first lieutenant, after the act of 3 March 1911:[7]

1. John R. Ames
2. Julien R. Bernheim
3. Siebert D. Boak
4. Alden Carpenter
5. George H. Casaday
6. William H. Chambers
7. George D. Graham
8. George I. Gunckel
9. John H. Hess
10. Raymond E. Ingalls
11. Frank K. Laflamme
12. Clarence E. Lauderdale
13. Samuel H. Leslie
14. Charles J. Long
15. John A. McAlister
16. John S. Marshall
17. George L. Mason
18. Robert H. Mills [8]
19. Robert T. Oliver [9]
20. Robert F. Patterson
21. Rex H. Rhoades
22. Edward P. R. Ryan
23. Harold O. Scott
24. Minot E. Scott
25. George E. Stallman
26. Frank P. Stone
27. Edwin P. Tignor
28. Hugh G. Voorhies
29. Franklin F. Wing
30. Frank H. Wolven

A number of the men among this group played important roles in the further development of the Corps and participated actively in both the First and Second World Wars.

Forty-seven dental surgeons entered into contract with The Surgeon General during the period from 1901 to 1911. Contracts of 3 were terminated as a result of death and 15 were annulled, 10 at the dentists' own request and 5 for miscellaneous reasons.[10]

---

[7] Memo, SG for CofS, 8 Feb 11, Dental surgeons in the U. S. Army, with list of dental surgeons, and their years of service, attached. Natl Archives, SG: 106047.

[8] Lt Robert H. Mills was destined to become the first major general in the Army Dental Corps some 30 years later. WD SOs, 1943, vol IV, Nos. 276–363, WD SO 280, 7 Oct 43, sec 1.

[9] In 1942 the general hospital located at Augusta, Ga., was designated as the Oliver General Hospital in honor of Col Robert T. Oliver, Dental Corps, U. S. Army. WD GO 64, 24 Nov 42.

[10] The Dental Corps. The Dental Bulletin Supplement to The Army Medical Bulletin 6: 18, Jan 1935.

Early in 1915, the Association of Military Dental Surgeons submitted to The Surgeon General a "Bill to Increase the Efficiency of the Dental Corps, U. S. Army."[11] The Adjutant General informed The Surgeon General 5 February 1915 that the Secretary of War did not approve of any legislation for the Dental Corps.

However, the Legislative Committee, National Dental Association, whose chairman was Dr. Homer C. Brown, continued to initiate and support legislative measures which would increase the efficiency of the Dental Corps. Late in 1915, recommendations which provided for the organization of a Dental Reserve Corps, and for the increase in rank in the Dental Corps to captains, majors, and one chief with the rank of colonel, were submitted to The Secretary of War and to The Surgeon General.

The Surgeon General, in response to the recommendations made by the Legislative Committee, directed a memorandum to the Chief of Staff in which he declared that the Dental Corps as organized then did not attract the best men graduating from the various dental colleges, and that he was in favor of the various grades with the exception of colonel. The Surgeon General believed that the grade of colonel and a chief of the Dental Corps was unnecessary. The organization of a Dental Reserve Corps, however, was deemed advisable.

The next development was the receipt by The Surgeon General on 20 February 1916 of the following telegram:[12]

> The National Dental Association of nearly 20,000 members and an equal number in other dental organizations must vigorously oppose the contract status and the relative rank for dental corps as proposed in your recently published bill. We consider this discrimination as unnecessary and humiliating and must insist that our representatives in Army be accorded dignified recognition and actual rank in keeping with importance of service rendered. We prefer to cooperate with you and will greatly appreciate your support but under herein mentioned conditions we have no choice. Wire collect if your attitude is misunderstood or any change in situation.

In his reply to Dr. Brown, The Surgeon General stated that: "My desire is to increase the efficiency of the Dental Corps and provide a proper flow of promotion. The question of titles given to the various grades is, I believe, a matter of secondary importance. There is no objection upon my part to the same provision regarding rank as is now authorized for the Medical Corps."[13]

Finally, after much activity on the part of the National Dental Association, the Association of Military Dental Surgeons, state, and city societies, legislation was enacted on 3 June 1916[14] which provided for the organization

---

[11] Ltr, Pres, Assoc of Mil Dent Surgs, to SG, 12 Jan 15. Natl Archives, SG : 90384–I.
[12] Telegram, Dr. Homer C. Brown, Chairman, Legislative Committee, Natl Dent Assoc, to SG, 20 Feb 16. Natl Archives, SG : 106047, Pt II–65.
[13] Telegram, SG to Dr. Homer C. Brown, Chairman, Legislative Committee, Natl Dent Assoc, 21 Feb 16. Natl Archives, SG : 106047, Pt II–65.
[14] H. R. 12766, National Defense Act approved 3 Jun 16, sec 10.

of a Dental Corps in the National Guard, and for the establishment of an Officers' Reserve Corps. Included in this legislation was the following section which gave further advantages to the Army Dental Corps:

> The President is hereby authorized to appoint and commission, by and with the advice and consent of the Senate, dental surgeons, who are citizens of the United States between the ages of 21 and 27 years, at the rate of one for each 1,000 enlisted men of the line of the Army. Dental surgeons shall have the rank, pay, and allowances of first lieutenants until they have completed 8 years' service. Dental surgeons of more than 8 but less than 24 years' service shall, subject to such examinations as the President may prescribe, have the rank, pay, and allowances of captains. Dental surgeons of more than 24 years' service shall, subject to such examinations as the President may prescribe, have the rank, pay and allowances of major; *Provided*, That the total number of dental surgeons with rank, pay, and allowances of major shall not at any time exceed 15: *and provided further*, That all laws relating to the examination of officers of the Medical Corps for promotion shall be applicable to dental surgeons.

The act of 3 June 1916 authorized the President through the governors of States and Territories and the Commanding General of the District of Columbia to appoint and commission dental surgeons as first lieutenants at the rate of one for each thousand enlisted men of the line of the National Guard. However, only the President was authorized to appoint and commission reserve officers in the various sections of the Officers' Reserve Corps. The act provided that the proportion of officers in any section of the Officers' Reserve Corps should not exceed the proportion for the same grade in the corresponding army, corps, or department of the Regular Army, except that the number commissioned in the lowest authorized grade in any section was not to be limited.

According to The Surgeon General's annual report to the Secretary of War, 30 June 1918, the National Guard included 249 dental officers on 5 August 1917. By 30 June 1918 the number had increased only to 253, of whom 251 were first lieutenants. There were only two who were promoted to the rank of captain, and this was not accomplished until March 1918.[15]

The same report indicated that by 31 July 1917 there were 598 commissioned in the Reserve Corps, while on 30 June 1918 there were 5,372. The distribution of rank in the total number of dental reserve officers commissioned and on duty on the latter date was as follows: majors—36, captains—244, and first lieutenants—5,092.[16]

With the advent of World War I,[17] the rapid mobilization of the Army and with it the Dental Corps led to many additional responsibilities for the dental surgeons. The National Dental Association, various state dental societies, as well as individual officers of the Dental Corps made requests for increased rank

---

[15] Annual Report of The Surgeon General, U. S. Army, 1918, Washington, Government Printing Office, 1918 (cited hereafter as Annual Report . . . Surgeon General).
[16] Ibid.
[17] Annual Report . . . Surgeon General, 1917.

and privileges commensurate with these responsibilities.[18] [19] The Surgeon General was favorable to the request that the Dental Corps be given equal status with that of the Medical Corps, and this status was achieved by the passage of H. R. 4897, the act of 6 October 1917, which provided that:

> Hereafter the Dental Corps of the Army shall consist of commissioned officers of the same grade and proportionally distributed among such grades as are now or may be hereafter provided by law for the Medical Corps, who shall have the rank, pay, promotion, and allowances of officers of corresponding grades in the Medical Corps, including the right to retirement as in the case of other officers, and there shall be one dental officer for every thousand of the total strength of the Regular Army authorized from time to time by law: *Provided further*, That dental examining and review boards shall consist of one officer of the Medical Corps and two officers of the Dental Corps: *Provided further*, That immediately following the approval of this Act all dental surgeons then in active service shall be recommissioned in the Dental Corps in the grades herein authorized in the order of their seniority and without loss of pay or allowances or of relative rank in the Army: *Provided further*, That no dental surgeon shall be recommissioned who has not been confirmed by the Senate.

Much credit for the passage of this bill was reflected upon Dr. Homer C. Brown, chairman of the Legislative Committee of the National Dental Association [20] for his untiring efforts to place dentistry on a plane equal to that of medicine in public service. The Journal of the Association of Military Dental Surgeons of the United States in commenting on the splendid work of Dr. Brown said:

> In regard to credit, much credit for wholehearted, unselfish, untiring devotion to this cause is due to several of a small coterie of men. Some of these have been laboring to this end for years; others for months only, but for once in the history of dental politics all had a hold on the same end of the rope in the final tug of war, and by pulling together achieved the result.[21]

In the period between the two World Wars, enactment of various legislative measures [22] did not significantly change the status of the Dental Corps. It was not until the United States was actively engaged in the hostilities of World War II that attempts were again initiated to enact legislation specifically designed to accomplish this. The primary basis for such action was the increasingly frequent charge that the morale of dental officers and the efficiency of the Dental Service suffered from the so-called "domination" of the Dental

---

[18] Ltr, Hon Ambrose Kennedy, Cong from R. I. to SecWar, 12 Apr 17 with incl R. I. Dental Society Resolutions. Natl Archives, SG: 106047, Pt II–84.

[19] Telegram, Dr. Homer C. Brown, Chairman, Legislative Committee, Natl Dent Assoc, to SecWar, 30 Jul 17. Natl Archives, SG: 106047. Pt. II–85.

[20] Hereinafter referred to as the American Dental Association, ADA.

[21] Our new status. J. A. Mil. Dent. Surgs. of the United States 2: 10–13, January 1918.

[22] Act of 4 June 1920 authorized a quota of 298 dental officers which allowed 1 dental officer for every 1,000 strength of the Regular Army Establishment; established exact peacetime promotion schedule. Acts of 30 June 1921 and 20 June 1922, reduced strength of Dental Corps to 180 and 158, respectively. Acts of May 1936, through 29 Jan 1938, and 3 April 1939 increased Dental Corps strength to 183, 208, 258, and finally 316. Act of 29 January 1938 also credited to the officers of the Dental Corps, for the purposes of retirement, any service as Contract Dental Surgeon and Acting Dental Surgeon.

Corps by medical officers.[23][24] Since such charges were made by responsible persons, and since they received wide publicity, a discussion of medicodental relations, as reflected in the subsequent legislative proposals, is necessary in spite of its highly controversial nature.

MEDICODENTAL RELATIONS [25]

A certain amount of friction between the professions concerned with health care is, of course, nothing new. By nature the professional man is usually independent, and the long years of training necessary to master his subject fosters the attitude that no outsider can understand his particular problems or be competent to exercise control over his treatment of patients. Historically, both medicine and dentistry were originally practiced by persons of low standing in the community, but medicine attained professional status much earlier than dentistry, which remained largely a mechanical art to the end of the 19th century. As the health implications of dentistry were recognized, and as the educational background of dentists improved, the latter began a rapid climb toward professional, social, and economic equality. Nevertheless, relations with medicine were occasionally marred by the physician's conservative tendency to regard dentists as upstarts in the health field, and by the dentist, as a member of a profession fighting for recognition, to suspect discrimination where none was intended. Also, the physician irritated the dentist by telling his patients that they should have their teeth extracted, and the dentist reciprocated by advising that dental treatment would cure general medical conditions.

As both professions gained experience they realized that their patients would receive better care if the physician and the dentist cooperated to use their special skills to the utmost, and such teamwork has become routine. But in the process of adjustment dentistry has rigidly maintained its independence and has fully shared medicine's traditional objection to control from outside the profession. As late as 1945 the Committee on Dental Education of the American Dental Association (ADA) withdrew its approval of a large and respected dental school because it had been integrated with a medical school and placed under the general supervision of a medical educator, justifying

---

[23] Articles on this subject appeared in the dental press almost continuously after 1943. The following were typical: (1) Rank without authority. Oral Hyg. 33: 932–937, July 1943; (2) Freedom for the Dental Corps. Ibid. 33: 960–961, July 1943; (3) The score of discrimination. Ibid. 33: 1230, September 1943.

[24] (1) The Army Dental Corps. J. Am. Dent. A. 32: 487–488, April 1, 1945. (2) The right to gripe. Ibid 33: 118–122, January 1, 1946.

[25] By the very nature of the subject, documentation of this discussion must be very imperfect. Dentists who felt that the dental service suffered from the unwise interference of medical officers were naturally slow to put their complaints in official reports which had to pass through the hands of those same officers. They wrote instead to the American Dental Association, to their congressmen, or to the editors of professional journals. In the absence of official sources, the author has had to rely heavily on information gleaned personally from dental officers in three foreign theaters and in several major installations in the U. S., realizing fully the difficulties of an attempt to evaluate opinions, which were by no means unanimous, on such a controversial matter.

this action with the statement that any interference by medicine in the field of dental education was considered dangerous.[26]

In the Armed Forces the position of both the professional services has necessarily been less independent than in civilian practice. All activities of a military organization must be directed toward a common objective and subject to the orders of a commander responsible for the results achieved. At some level both medicine and dentistry must come under lay control since the highest staff positions must be filled by combat officers. So far as the dental service was concerned, therefore, the question at issue was not: "Were dental officers under the supervision of nondentists?" but: "Was the nature of the supervision such as to hamper their activities unnecessarily?"

On the basis of Army regulations and directives alone, the dental officer certainly exercised less control over the dental service than officers of most other branches did over their respective activities. This situation resulted from the two following circumstances: (1) As a staff officer the dental surgeon did not enjoy the usual privilege of presenting his views and recommendations directly to the executive authority; (2) while all medical treatment was given in installations under the direct command of medical officers, dentists did not command dental installations.[27]

As a subordinate of the surgeon, the dental surgeon was limited to submitting recommendations only to that officer; if they were approved they were submitted to the commander secondhand by an officer who might be neither completely familiar with the matter under discussion nor personally interested in supporting the dentist's views against opposition from other staff members. If the surgeon did not approve the dentist's proposals they could be dropped without formality, and if he chose to substitute his own recommendations the lay commander did not necessarily know that they were not the views of the dental surgeon.

The practical effect of this situation of course depended upon the attitude of the surgeon. Many surgeons with long experience as staff officers gave loyal and effective support to their dental surgeons, and in some cases their reputation and standing even enabled them to get more consideration for the dental service than the dental surgeon could have himself obtained, especially when the latter was a junior officer. It was also held by some that the medical officer would generally show more understanding and sympathy toward dental problems than would a line officer. On the other hand, it could not be denied that the dentist was one step removed from the authority which made decisions, and this fact inevitably resulted in some delay even when action was favorable; the dental surgeon's proposals had to be approved by two officials rather than one. The more severe critics of the dental surgeon's status held

---

[26] Dental Education at Columbia University. J. Am. Dent. A. 32 : 1150, 1 Sep 45.

[27] In the latter part of the war certain minor units, such as the mobile prosthetic teams, were commanded by dental officers, but these were a negligible exception to the general rule that dental officers did not command.

that medical officers could not have a full understanding of dental problems and requirements, and that at times they were actually in competition with the dental service for personnel and funds. The fact that lack of direct staff representation did entail some disadvantage was pointed out by The Surgeon General in 1943 when he protested that service command surgeons were being hampered in their duties by the necessity for presenting their recommendations to the commanding general through a subordinate staff officer. At that time he noted that: [28]

> ... the Medical Department has continued to function in the service commands and to produce excellent results as a whole. I feel, however, that these results have been obtained from extra efforts and personal contacts rather than from that at which we are aiming; namely, simplified procedure and efficiency.

Officially, the dental surgeon was an adviser to the surgeon, without formal authority even within the dental clinic. Here again, the actual status of the dental surgeon depended upon the attitude of the surgeon. Many medical officers routinely consulted the dentist on matters concerning the dental service and accepted his advice in the absence of important reasons to the contrary. On the other hand, it cannot be denied that a determined surgeon could, by invoking his authority to make out efficiency reports, completely dominate the dental service, even in respect to determining treatment or assigning personnel within the dental clinic, matters which were specifically reserved to the dental officer by regulation.[29] The dentist was not inclined to demand even his legal rights if he could expect, as a result, to receive a poor efficiency rating and be transferred to an undesirable post because he was "uncooperative."

The mere fact that the dental service functioned with reasonable efficiency during the war is strong evidence that medical officers generally showed considerable restraint and good judgment in their supervision of dental activities. The editor of Oral Hygiene, who was a constant critic of the status of the Army and Navy Dental Corps, conceded this when he wrote:

> It is true that the relationship between many individual dental officers and medical officers is characterized by cordiality, understanding, and faithful cooperation in caring for the soldiers and sailors of the United States. It is the exceptional case in which the medical officer actually attempts to dominate or exert authority over the dental officer.[30]

However, it was too much to expect that all of the 45,000 medical officers in the Army would have the necessary experience and judgment to administer the dental service wisely. Some of them were junior officers who had been promoted rapidly to important positions in connection with the expansion of the defense forces; others were former civilian physicians who did not understand that staff supervision did not imply detailed interference in routine matters of internal administration. When medical officers of these types felt

---
[28] Rpt. Conference of CGs, SvCs, ASF, 22–24 Jul 43. HD: 337.
[29] AR 40–510, par 1, 31 Jul 42.
[30] See footnote 23 (1), p. 7.

called upon to "run" the dental service the results could only be unhappy. The Surgeon General himself pointed out that "special problems related to the professional dental service as well as to the special skills and techniques common only to dentistry are best understood and administered by those trained in that field." [31]

Some of the more specific aspects of the problem of medicodental relations are discussed in the following paragraphs.

Effect of the Administrative Status of the Dental Service on Morale

The fact that the morale of dental officers at the end of the war left much to be desired is discussed in chapter IV. This situation is significant here because it was widely blamed on unsatisfactory relations with medical officers. This subject covers a wide field, however, and it is necessary to consider complaints on a more specific basis.

One of the common causes of criticism was lack of opportunity for promotion in the Dental Corps compared with the Medical Corps. In April 1945 the proportion of medical and dental officers in each grade was as follows: [32]

Grade	Percentage Distribution	
	Medical Corps	Dental Corps
Colonel	2.3	0.8
Lieutenant Colonel	7.3	2.7
Major	21.6	10.4
Captain	56.6	67.3
Lieutenant	12.2	18.8

It is clear that the dental officer had much less chance to reach field grades, but the extent to which this was the fault of the Medical Department is not so clear. The Surgeon General had only advisory authority over the allotment of grades within the service commands, in the Air Force, in tactical units, or in theaters, leaving a negligible part of the Army in which his influence was decisive. Also, the War Department itself was slow to approve increases in ratings for dental officers in table-of-organization units due to the tradition that high grades should go only with the command of large numbers of troops. Common sense had of course forced many modifications of this principle; the chief of staff of an army was at least a major general though he did not command any soldiers, and the chief of the surgical service of a large hospital was likewise a colonel, while the commander of a collecting company, with a hundred men, was only a captain. Obviously, responsibility should be the criterion for the allotment of grades, not mere numbers of troops commanded. Nevertheless, this attitude cropped up whenever advanced rank

---

[31] Ltr, Col Robert J. Carpenter to CG ASF, 12 Apr 45, sub: Revision of AR 40-15. SG: 300.3.
[32] Strength of the Army, 1 May 45.

for staff positions was mentioned. The Surgeon General supported successful efforts to speed the promotion of dental lieutenants in tactical outfits; he recommended the promotion of the chief of the Dental Division to the grade of major general; and he made a sincere and fairly successful effort to obtain the same grades for the chiefs of hospital dental services as were held by the corresponding chiefs of the medical or surgical services.[33] Occasionally, however, the Medical Department appeared to foster the view that dental officers had no responsibilities beyond the rendering of treatment at the chair on an individual basis. Thus, when a representative of the Surgeon General's Office testified against legislation to provide additional general officers in the Dental Corps by stating that so far as he knew no dentist ever commanded more than one man (his dental assistant), he ignored the fact that a colonel of the Dental Corps would have been held directly responsible for any defects of the dental treatment rendered by more than 4,000 dental officers in Europe alone.[34] It is pertinent to note, in this connection, that the Medical Corps had itself carried on a similar fight for increased rank for medical officers during World War I, claiming that line officers ignored the advice of junior medical officers, and that such increases had been opposed by line officers on the ground that physicians had no command responsibilities![35]

Dental officers also complained of discrimination when they were held for 36 months of total service following the war, while medical officers were released after only 30 months. The president of the ADA wrote:[36]

> From time to time during the war period, there has been considerable resentment from the dental officers due to the present Army regulations. These complaints were minor and few compared to the protests that are arriving now. These men have developed a bitterness toward the American Dental Association, threatening to resign and form a new association. They are also bitter in their condemnation of the Government and the several branches of the service.

Basically, the need to hold dentists arose from a single action: the termination of the dental Army Specialized Training Program (ASTP) in July 1944. The War Department decided to discontinue the dental ASTP in spite of opposition by The Surgeon General who had supported the recommendation of the Dental Division that the ASTP be continued and that sufficient older officers be released to create the necessary vacancies for younger graduates.[37] Nor does this decision indicate any conscious discrimination on the part of the War Department itself. At the time it was taken the Dental Corps was at maximum authorized strength, while the Medical Corps was desperately scrambling for manpower. The General Staff felt that in view of the critical need

---

[33] Final Rpt for ASF, Logistics in World War II. HD: 319.1-2 (Dental Division).
[34] Testimony Brig Gen Guy B. Denit on the Army Promotion Bill, H. R. 2536. J. Am. Dent. A. 35: 447, 15 Sep 47.
[35] Army Medical Corps Legislation. J. Am. Dent. A. 5: 635, June 1918; also Authority and Rank for Surgeons. Ibid. 5: 323, March 1918.
[36] Ltr, Dr. W. H. Scherer, Pres ADA to SG, 17 May 46. SG: 210.8.
[37] See discussion of the Dental ASTP in the chapter on Personnel and Training.

for men to carry the war to an end, the dental ASTP could no longer be justified, while the need for the continuance of the medical ASTP was obvious. It may or may not be held that a mistake was made, but there is no evidence of any intent to treat the Dental Corps unfairly in this instance.

Evidence is more definite that, justifiably or not, the morale of the dental officers suffered from the belief that the Dental Service was unnecessarily subordinate to the will of medical officers. A senior dental officer who conducted an official investigation of the Dental Service in Europe reported that:[38]

> With the exception of one or two dental officers interviewed, all were either Reserve or AUS. The majority of these officers were very bitter as to the treatment or discrimination towards the Dental Corps by medical officers. Most of them stated that they would take action through their local dental societies on return to the states. As one officer expressed it, they were "damned sick of being kicked around by medical officers."

The editor of Oral Hygiene reported that the number of dentists who blamed the ADA for not taking more vigorous corrective action was so large that it threatened the future of that organization.[39] The dean of one of the larger dental schools warned that returning officers were advising young dentists to stay out of the armed services Dental Corps,[40] and the ADA charged that personnel troubles encountered after the war were largely due to the resentment of dentists at their status during hostilities.[41] This latter claim appears exaggerated since the unusually large income to be made in private practice during the period of postwar inflation was also an important factor, but it is significant that such a charge should be made by a reputable organization.

It is difficult to determine the exact extent to which this widespread feeling of resentment was justified. Wartime conditions inevitably led to some confusion and injustices, and even the ADA admitted that some of the instances of failure to assign officers to duty for which they felt they were fitted, or of failure to provide warranted promotions, were probably unavoidable.[42]

Presumably some dentists failed to understand the need for more supervision in the Army than in private practice and suspected discrimination where it did not exist. It is further possible that many criticisms arose over relatively minor incidents. Such was the case when a captain of the Dental Corps and a lieutenant of the Medical Corps started for a supply center in a jeep; the captain climbed into the front seat and was promptly ordered into the back seat by the lieutenant because the latter, as surgeon, was the dentist's commanding officer.[43] Such instances were merely exhibitions of bad judgment on the

---

[38] Pers ltr, Col James B. Mockbee to Lt Col George F. Jeffcott, 8 Sep 46.
[39] They cannot speak for themselves. Oral Hyg. 33 : 1244–1245, September 1943.
[40] Pers ltr, Dr. Charles W. Freeman, Dean, Northwestern Univ Dent Sch to Maj Maurice E. Washburn, 21 May 46. SG : 322.0531.
[41] Dental officers pay again. J. Am. Dent. A. 33 : 755, 1 Jun 46.
[42] Present status of dentistry in the Armed Forces : A report from the Committee on Legislation. J. Am. Dent. A. 31 : 270–277, 1 Feb 44.
[43] See footnote 38.

part of inexperienced officers but they inevitably received considerable publicity and tended to create resentment even on the part of officers who had never known such treatment personally.

But after discounting many claims of arbitrary treatment at the hands of medical officers, it must be admitted that surgeons possessed the authority to dominate the dental service if they so desired, and it seems probable that this authority was exercised unwisely in some cases. Responsible members of the organized dental profession denied categorically that the letters they received came from any minority group of malcontents.[44] The fact that both the Director of the Dental Division, SGO, and The Surgeon General recommended certain administrative changes designed to give dental officers increased authority supports the belief that discontent was based on something more than emotional and groundless resentment.

Effect of the Status of the Dental Service on Efficiency

Failure to Consult Dental Surgeons on Matters Affecting Their Dental Service. In December 1944 the Director of the Dental Division reported the following situation to The Surgeon General:[45]

> Information continues to reach this office that there are some stations where the Post Surgeon does not give proper consideration to the Dental Service and, instead of coordinating the Dental Service with the Medical Service, he places it in a subordinate position and in many instances ignores the chief of the Dental Service and his recommendations, even to the extent of recommending dental officers for promotion without consulting the Camp Dental Surgeon. Such conditions as this should not and would not exist if the Service Command Surgeons concerned would not condone such action by their Post or Station Surgeons.
>
> The Dental Corps is an integral part of the Medical Department and should always remain as such. It is unfortunate that there are still some medical officers, who, apparently, do not realize this and that the Dental Corps desires to assist in every way possible and assume its share of the responsibility in carrying out the mission of the Medical Department.
>
> The attitude of some few medical officers, who apparently are determined to subordinate the Dental Corps, tends to offset the wonderful attitude of comradeship and friendliness exhibited by the majority of Medical Corps officers. These acts of subordinating the Dental Corps by the few officers reach the civilian profession through dental officers on duty, and have caused much agitation by a certain group for a complete separation from the Medical Department. I am entirely opposed to any such action as it would lessen the efficiency of both the Medical and Dental Corps.
>
> I am sure The Surgeon General desires that Service Command Surgeons correct any subordinated status of the Dental Corps which may exist at their headquarters, and in their taking steps to pass this on down to the lower echelons.

The Surgeon General's disapproval of this undesirable situation which did exist in some cases was confirmed by the Director of the Dental Division

---

[44] See footnote 24 (2), p. 7.
[45] Memo, Maj Gen R. H. Mills for Exec Off SGO, 5 Dec 44, sub: Agenda for the Service Command Surgeons' Conference, 11 December through 15 December. SG: 337.

in his remark that "General Kirk is fully cognizant of the administrative problems in some of the lower echelons of command and accordingly plans for a change in Army regulations are now under way."[46] He also stated that The Surgeon General had "offered every assistance and approval for more administrative control of dental affairs by dental officers in the lower echelons,"[47] and further, that "General Kirk . . . has given the Dental Division a free hand in the direction of its policies and personnel. . . . If a comparable relationship could be obtained throughout all the channels of command, the primary objections now raised by many . . . would be erased. . . ."[48]

Lack of Effective Control of Dental Personnel. One of the most frequent causes of complaint by dental officers was their inability to control dental personnel. Under unfavorable conditions the surgeon could, and did, take the following actions detrimental to the morale and efficiency of dental officers:

1. Failed to allot sufficient dental officers to the dental clinic.[49]

2. Failed to provide adequate grades for the dental service so as to make possible reasonable promotion.[50]

3. Used dental officers in unimportant nonprofessional duties.[51] At times this latter abuse was carried to fantastic lengths. Thus when the surgeon of a service command was directed to send 12 Medical Department officers to the Medical Field Service School he sent 12 dental officers because he held that medical officers could not be spared, and on their return these dentists were used in administrative functions because they alone had the necessary training.[52] Even worse, the same dentist was occasionally sent to the Medical Field Service School twice to avoid losing the services of a medical officer.[53] These were, admittedly, extreme examples, and the misuse of dental officers was largely eliminated in the United States by the determined efforts of The Surgeon General. Overseas, however, it continued to exist to some degree until the end of hostilities.

4. Granted leaves of absence to dental personnel without consulting the dental surgeon.

5. Promoted dental personnel against the advice of the dental surgeon.[54]

6. Rendered efficiency reports on dental officers without consulting the dental surgeon.[55]

---

[46] Major General Mills prefers changes in regulations to legislation to correct inequalities in the Dental Corps. J. Am. Dent. A. 32: 489, 1 Apr 45.

[47] Ltr, Maj Gen R. H. Mills to Dr. Edward J. Ryan, 17 Mar 45. [D]

[48] See footnote 46.

[49] See discussion in the chapter of this history on Personnel and Training.

[50] Ibid.

[51] See discussion in the chapter of this history on The Procurement of Dental Officers.

[52] Proceedings of The Surgeon General's Conference with Corps Area and Army Dental Surgeons, 8–9 Jul 42. HD: 337.

[53] Ibid.

[54] Testimony before the House Naval Affairs Committee on bill to improve the efficiency of the Dental Corps. J. Am. Dent. A. 32: 364: 374, 1 Mar 45.

[55] Ibid.

7. Failed to assign enlisted assistants in sufficient numbers and in appropriate grades. Dental enlisted assistants were assigned to the dental clinic by the surgeon, they were promoted by the surgeon, and they could be withdrawn at any time. Lack of a permanent corps of enlisted men, with adequate ratings, was one of the most serious deficiencies noted by the Director of the Dental Division after the war.[56]

8. Removed enlisted assistants from the dental clinic for outside duties on short notice. This situation was of course unavoidable in an emergency, but practically paralyzed the dental service when it occurred.[57]

Professional Interference. It was reported that surgeons sometimes prohibited dental surgeons from committing patients to the hospital, using general anesthetics, or prescribing certain drugs legally used by dentists.[58] It is believed, however, that this difficulty was more commonly encountered in the Navy; it appears to have been a matter of minor concern to Army dentists.

Extent of Medical Interference in Dental Administration

The extent to which the efficiency of the Dental Service actually suffered from medical supervision, if at all, is extremely hard to determine. Wartime conditions varied so much from camp to camp that it is impossible to compare the actual output of clinics operating under different degrees of medical control, and neither medical nor dental officers were impartial enough to render completely unbiased opinions in the matter. Editorials in the dental press would indicate that medical interference was almost universal, but closer contact with individual dentists revealed that many of them were angry at injustices they had heard about rather than experienced. Further, while almost every dental officer felt that some interference had occurred, some of them were not sure that they would not have encountered equal restrictions under line officers. It is certain, however, that most dental officers, from the Chief of the Dental Division down, felt that a clearer definition of the responsibilities and rights of dental officers was imperative.[59] [60] [61]

LEGISLATIVE AND ADMINISTRATIVE ACTION REGARDING THE ARMY DENTAL CORPS

One of the first moves to improve the status of the Dental Service was the campaign of the ADA to get advanced rank for the Director of the Dental

---

[56] See footnote 33, p. 11.
[57] Ibid.
[58] Ibid.
[59] See footnotes 31, p. 10, 45, p. 13, 46, p. 14.
[60] Ltr, Maj Gen R. H. Mills to Ed, J. Am. Dent. A., 23 May 47, quoted in "General Mills Expresses His Opinion Regarding Army Dental Corps Regulations." J. Am. Dent. A. 35 : 231–232, 1 Aug 47.
[61] Report of Activities to Change the Status of the Army Dental Corps. J. Am. Dent. A. 33 : 1030–1040, 1 Aug 46.

Division who was then (April 1943) a brigadier general. When The Surgeon General of that period stated that "the Dental Corps had all the representation in the higher brackets to which it was entitled," [62] bills were introduced in Congress to provide that the Director of the Dental Division should have the grade of major general and that the Dental Corps should be allotted brigadier generals in the same ratio as the Medical Corps.[63] Before these bills could be acted upon a new Surgeon General had taken office and the ADA made new efforts to get action informally, without legislation. The new Surgeon General was apparently somewhat lukewarm to certain aspects of the idea, but he agreed to make the Director of the Dental Division a major general and to consider the possibility of appointing one or more brigadier generals in the Dental Corps.[64] Attempts to pass legislation were then dropped. The promotion of the Director of the Dental Division was announced shortly, but no brigadier generals were appointed until 4 January 1945, and the single officer so promoted was again reduced to the grade of colonel on 1 December 1945. (A bill to provide for a rear admiral in the Dental Corps of the Navy had become law in December 1942.)[65]

About the same time The Surgeon General personally initiated efforts to get more administrative authority for dental officers within the framework of the existing Medical Department organization. In July 1943 he sent the following letter to the commanding generals of all service commands: [66]

> 1. The Dental Corps is an integral part of the Medical Department, and must function as such. But dentistry, being a specialty of which few medical officers have ample knowledge, can function more efficiently if members of the Dental Corps are consulted and their advice sought on all matters pertaining to the Dental Service.
>
> 2. The chief of the medical branch of a service command is responsible to the service commander for the efficient functioning of all branches of the Medical Department, but due to the increased responsibility it has been considered advisable and necessary, for obvious reasons, in order to maintain a highly efficient dental service to assign an experienced dental officer as an assistant to the chief of the medical branch. His duties are clearly defined in par. 5, AR 40–15, December 28, 1942. This Regulation will be complied with, and the duties prescribed therein will not be delegated to any other assistant. By so doing a more efficient service will be maintained and dissatisfaction and misunderstanding obviated.
>
> 3. An efficient medical service requires the complete cooperation of every branch of the Medical Department. The efficiency of any one branch reflects credit on the entire department.

Results of this action were not too encouraging. Protests in the dental press grew in volume and the Director of the Dental Division reported at the end of 1944 that conditions in the field were far from satisfactory.[67]

---

[62] See footnote 42, p. 12.
[63] H. R. 2442, 78th Cong. introduced by Mr. Sparkman on 8 Apr 43; S. 1007, introduced by Mr. Hill on 16 Apr 43.
[64] See footnote 42, p. 12.
[65] Flagstad, C. O.: Wartime Legislation. J. Am. Dent. A. 33 : 63–65, 1 Jan 46.
[66] Ltr, SG to CG 3d SvC, 14 Jul 43, sub: Dental Service. SG : 703.–1.
[67] See footnote 45, p. 13.

Early in 1944 the ADA began to consider seriously the introduction of legislation to change the status of the Dental Service. Its Committee on Legislation finally advised against such action, however, for the following reasons:

1. It was believed that the new Surgeon General should be given a chance to bring about the desired changes through administrative procedures.[68]

2. The Director of the Dental Division advised against legislative action because he felt that administrative correction was preferable and possible, and because he felt that the introduction of permanent legislation in the middle of the war was neither appropriate nor likely to receive favorable action.[69]

The attitude of the Committee was expressed as follows in February 1944: [70]

> He [The Surgeon General] has been very cooperative with the members of the Dental Corps and [he has] stated that beneficial changes will be made.
>
> With such cooperation, the Committee on Legislation will grant every opportunity for the correction of inadequacies by the department itself before seeking correction by legislation. The Surgeon General of the Army and the chief of the Army Dental Corps are in agreement that no legislation should be sought at the present time. This Committee is satisfied to place this responsibility for adjustment in their hands.

The aims of the ADA at this time were stated in very general terms, but they appear to have included two principal objectives:

1. The right of the dental surgeon to take his problems and recommendations directly to the commander of any installation. It was desired that:

> ... dental officers be permitted to present their cases and problems, without lesser intervention, to the officer generally responsible for the activity. In a hospital, this would be the medical officer in charge. In a line organization, this would be the commanding officer. These officers, by virtue of their position and wider responsibility, would bring to their decisions the impartial viewpoint that now does not always characterize such decisions.[71]

2. "Autonomy" for the Dental Service. This word was of course open to many interpretations and it undoubtedly meant different things to different persons. It was defined by the Committee on Legislation of the ADA as "the power, right or condition of self-government, or, in its secondary meaning, as practical independence with nominal subordination." [72]

The condition of "practical independence with nominal subordination" was the one already envisaged in Army regulations. The surgeon of an installation had "nominal" authority, but it was hopefully expected that he would use it principally to arbitrate in matters where the interests of the Dental Service touched those of other activities, leaving the dental surgeon free to handle all routine administration. The fault in this conception was expressed

---
[68] See footnote 42, p. 12.
[69] See footnote 60, p. 15.
[70] See footnote 42, p. 12.
[71] Medicodental relations in the armed services. J. Am. Dent. A. 31: 696–697, 1 May 44.
[72] See footnote 42, p. 12.

by the chef who said "there is no such thing as a little garlic." In view of the accepted military tradition that responsibility must be matched by authority there is no such thing as "nominal subordination" in the Army. As long as the surgeon was in command of dental activities and responsible for their success the War Department rightly objected to any efforts to diminish his final control over those activities. It might recommend very strongly that the surgeon consult the dental officer, but it could not logically direct him to accept the latter's advice; nor could the surgeon excuse his errors by stating that he had taken the dentist's recommendations, for if he felt that the dental surgeon's views were faulty he was not only allowed, but expected, to reject them. Even the authority to go directly to the commanding officer when the surgeon disapproved the proposals of the dental officer would have been a precedent-shattering departure from accepted staff procedure. On the other hand, to give the occasional authoritarian type of officer "nominal authority" is to give him a powerful weapon with instructions not to use it; sooner or later the temptation to "show who is boss" becomes overpowering. It would seem, therefore, that attempts to give the Dental Service actual independence while keeping it under nominal supervision could not be expected to prove uniformly successful.

The "power of self-government" was more definite, although further qualification was needed even here. The Committee on Legislation, ADA, generally agreed, as did the Director of the Dental Division and The Surgeon General, that a completely independent Dental Corps was not necessary or desirable. It was stated that "The profession of dentistry, as a unit, has no hesitation in serving under a surgeon general who is a member of the profession of medicine. This plan, dictated by the close association of dentistry and medicine in the interests of general health, is satisfactory."[73] Again, "From some quarters, there is an insistent demand for a separate Dental Corps. Since the work of the Medical Corps and that of the Dental Corps is so closely allied, it is felt by those who have made a close study of the problem that a complete separation of the Dental Corps from the Medical Department in both the Army and the Navy would hinder the effectiveness of both corps."[74] On the other hand, the Committee on Legislation did not agree with those who felt that authority to go to the commanding officer with dental problems would be sufficient.[75] It also wanted to be assured that local surgeons would not intervene in purely dental affairs. This attitude was expressed as follows by the head of the Canadian Dental Service, which was completely independent, under the Adjutant General of the Canadian Defense Forces:[76]

> We all admire the Medical Service for what it knows and what it does, but there are two great reasons why it is difficult to understand why it should retain control

---

[73] Ibid.
[74] Ibid.
[75] See footnote 61, p. 15.
[76] Lott, F. M.: Wartime functioning of the Canadian Dental Corps. Oral Hyg. 33: 1388–1391, Oct 1943.

of the Dental Service. First, it has a tremendous job on its hands to deal efficiently with the great number of medical problems of the Forces. For this reason alone it is imperative that the Dental Service should carry its own burdens. Second, most Medical Officers admit that they are not trained as Dental Officers and are not qualified to "run the dental show" as is often stated.

Probably the clearest statement of the objective of the ADA was the following:[77]

> We can agree that The Surgeon General must be the final and overall authority in regard to all matters having to do with the health of the soldier. However, as regards dentistry, once certain fundamental policies have been agreed upon, the Dental Corps, under its own chief, should be free to carry out those policies. This is our conception of autonomy in the Dental Corps.

Apparently the aim of the ADA was subordination to The Surgeon General at the major policy-making level, with administrative independence at all lower echelons. The application of such a plan involved some administrative difficulties since the dentist had to commit patients to the hospital, he used clinic space which was generally within the area controlled by the surgeon, and his activities could not altogether be divorced from those of the Medical Corps in the operating installations. Also, the dental surgeon might find himself responsible for personnel administration, the procurement of supplies, and other matters which had previously been handled by the surgeon and his assistants. Such separation of functions was administratively possible, however, and it was later actually carried out in the Navy.

Efforts to secure changes in Army regulations progressed slowly. In April 1945 the ADA stated that unless action was soon taken it would sponsor legislation to bring about the desired modifications.[78] At about the same time The Surgeon General submitted the draft of a revised Army regulation which represented his views on the matter of increased responsibility for dental surgeons.[79] This draft was amended several times before it was submitted, apparently on the basis of informal consultations with ASF, and it is possible that it already represented some compromise between what The Surgeon General wanted and what he thought he could get. As submitted by The Surgeon General this tentative regulation provided that matters affecting the Dental Service as a whole would be administered by The Surgeon General, with the assistance of the Director of the Dental Division. In lower echelons, however, dental affairs were to be administered by the dental surgeon, though the latter was bound to consult the surgeon and seek his concurrence before action was taken. Any matter on which an agreement could not be reached was to be referred to The Surgeon General, though this provision was changed in subsequent drafts to allow settlement of conflicts by the local commanding officer.

---

[77] See footnote 42, p. 12.
[78] See footnote 24 (1), p. 7.
[79] See footnote 31, p. 10.

The War Department, in turn, eliminated some desired features [80] before the regulation was finally published in August 1945.[81]

In its published form the regulation provided that "matters relating to the dental service as a whole are administered by the Director, Dental Division, an assistant to The Surgeon General, through The Surgeon General," giving at least the appearance of greater authority for the Director of the Dental Division than had been implied in the original phrase "by The Surgeon General with the assistance of the Director of the Dental Division." Similar wording was used to describe the authority of subordinate dental surgeons, as follows: "In a theater, service command, or any other headquarters, matters relating to the dental service are administered by the dental surgeon, through the surgeon." All recommendations initiated by the dental surgeon were to be routed through the surgeon, who was required to forward them to the commanding officer with his comments. The dental surgeon was also given authority to render efficiency reports on his own personnel.

The ADA claimed that the new regulation did not make any substantial change in existing relations, asserting that "the causes of frequent complaints by dental officers have been wrapped up with new words but considerable care has been exercised not to remove them. The domination of the Dental Corps by the Medical Corps may have been gently disturbed but, by and large, it remains complete and unshaken." [82] General Mills admitted that he had "had to make some concessions," [83] but he maintained that the new regulations were a great improvement over the old and that they provided "more for our Corps than we could get if we were a small, separate branch." It would appear that there was some truth in each of these statements. The new regulations gave official approval to a general principle for which the ADA was working, but their practical effect was likely to be negligible. The right to present dental problems to the commanding officer, for instance, meant little as long as the surgeon had to be consulted and as long as the latter initiated efficiency reports on the dental surgeon. (The dental surgeon made out the reports for his officers, but his own efficiency report was made out by his immediate superior, the surgeon.) Only a very intrepid dental surgeon would insist on taking a recommendation to the post commander against the expressed opposition of the surgeon when the latter would subsequently report on the dental surgeon's efficiency, including his "cooperativeness," during the year.

At the end of hostilities it appeared that the ADA and the Army would not be able to come to a voluntary agreement concerning changes to be made in the status of the Dental Corps, and the former went ahead with its earlier plan to attain the desired objective through legislation.[84]

---

[80] See footnote 60, p. 15.

[81] AR 40–15, 8 Aug 45.

[82] Editorial: New regulations for the Army Dental Corps. J. Am. Dent. A. 32: 1290–1291, 1 Oct 45.

[83] See footnote 61, p. 15.

[84] The legislation sponsored by the ADA in the postwar years of 1946–48 designed to change the status of the Dental Service failed of enactment. On 27 September 1948, however, a revision of AR

During the above period, however, other legislation which proposed the removal of the command restriction provision of the law of 1911,[85] a limitation which had not been placed on the Medical Administrative, Pharmacy, Veterinary, or Sanitary Corps, was approved by The Surgeon General and The Adjutant General. On 29 June 1945, an act was passed to grant dental officers the same command privileges enjoyed by other officers of the Medical Department.[86] While passage of this legislation did not affect the provision of Army regulations that only Medical Corps officers might command organizations dealing with the treatment, hospitalization, or transportation of the sick or wounded,[87] it did make dental officers eligible for administrative positions which had previously been closed to them for what seemed to be inadequate reasons.

40–15 authorized many of the modifications which had been recommended by the ADA and by dental officers. This revision promised much for long-term improvement in the operation of the Dental Service.—Ed.

[85] See footnote 6, p. 2.
[86] Public Law 94, 79th Cong., 29 June 1945.
[87] AR 40–10, par 2, 17 Nov 41.

CHAPTER II

Administration of the Dental Service

WORLD WAR I

Until World War I, no representative of the Dental Corps had been assigned for duty in The Surgeon General's Office (SGO). The affairs of the Dental Corps prior to this time had been administered as part of the routine work of the Personnel Division, SGO. However, on 9 August 1917 the Dental Section of the Personnel Division was organized, and Major William H. G. Logan, MC, was appointed as its first chief. Major Logan, who later became colonel, had both the D.D.S. and M.D. degrees. The Dental Section became the Dental Division on 24 November 1919.[1][2]

The following dental officers have served as Chief of the Dental Section or Director of the Dental Division, SGO, from 1917 to 1942:

Colonel W. H. G. LOGAN	1917–1919
Lieutenant Colonel F. L. K. LAFLAMME	1919
Colonel ROBERT T. OLIVER	1919–1924
Colonel R. H. RHOADES	1924–1928
Colonel J. R. BERNHEIM	1928–1932
Colonel R. H. RHOADES	1932–1934
Colonel FRANK P. STONE	1934–1938
Brigadier General LEIGH C. FAIRBANK [3]	1938–1942

WORLD WAR II

Dental Division, SGO

During World War II, Army regulations prescribed that "matters relating to the dental service as a whole are administered by The Surgeon General with the advice and assistance of the Dental Corps assistant to The Surgeon General." In 1939 the duties of the Director of the Dental Division were described as follows:[4]

> The Dental Corps assistant to The Surgeon General will serve as the Chief of the Dental Division of The Surgeon General's Office and will be responsible to that officer

---

[1] Lynch, C., et al.: The Medical Department of the U. S. Army in the World War. Washington, Government Printing Office, 1923, vol I, p. 191.

[2] Logan, W. H. G.: The development of the dental service of the United States Army in this country from 8 Apr 17 to 12 Feb 19. J. Am. Dent. A. 20: 1951–1959, Nov 1933.

[3] The rank of brigadier general in the Dental Corps was authorized by Public Act 423, 75th Congress, 29 Jun 38.

[4] AR 40–15, 20 Apr 39.

for the recommendation of plans and policies for the progressive development of the dental service, with special reference to measures for the preservation of the general health of the Army by the prevention and control of dento-oral diseases and deficiencies among persons subject to military control; for advising measures to place approved plans and policies into effect; and for giving technical advice to The Surgeon General on all matters pertaining to the dental service.

The Director of the Dental Division,[5] as an adviser to The Surgeon General, thus had no formal authority in his own right. His recommendations were subject to The Surgeon General's approval and he could not present his views directly to higher officers. But while the Director of the Dental Division exercised very little legal authority over the operation of the Dental Service, his advice on purely dental questions was accepted so routinely that from a practical point of view he enjoyed a substantial measure of actual control over the Dental Corps and its activities (figs. 1, 2, and 3).

The decision of the Director of the Dental Division was therefore generally accepted on the following matters which were of little concern to other agencies:[6]

1. The assignment of individual dental personnel to subordinate major commands. [He could not, however, control the assignment of dentists to specific posts or duties within those commands except in the few installations directly under the control of The Surgeon General.]

2. The selection of items of dental supply for listing in the medical supply catalog.

3. The development of courses of training for dental personnel, within time limits prescribed by higher authority.

4. The establishment of professional standards of dental treatment.

5. Professional requirements for commission in the Dental Corps.

6. Types of treatment to be authorized.

However, as a subordinate of The Surgeon General the Director of the Dental Division could exercise no powers not enjoyed by The Surgeon General himself, and the latter's authority was by no means unlimited. The Surgeon General exerted great influence in those matters which concerned the Medical Department, but he had to defend his proposals against opposition from other interested officials, and the right of final decision remained with the executive branch in the person of the Commanding General, Army Service Forces; the Chief of Staff; or the Secretary of War. Thus when The Surgeon General

---

[5] The Director of the Dental Division at the start of the war and during the early mobilization period was Brig Gen Leigh C. Fairbank. At the end of his tour of duty on 17 Mar 42, General Fairbank was succeeded by Brig Gen Robert H. Mills. The latter was promoted major general on 7 Oct 43, becoming the first dental officer to hold that rank. When General Mills retired on 17 Mar 46 his responsibilities for postwar policies and development were assumed by Brig Gen Thomas L. Smith (later Maj Gen) who had been dental surgeon of the European theater during the combat period.

[6] The practical authority of the Director of the Dental Division was based on custom rather than upon statute, and its extent is therefore a matter of opinion, not subject to documentation. The statements made here are based on personal conferences with Major General Mills and with most of the other senior dental officers who served in the Dental Division during the war.

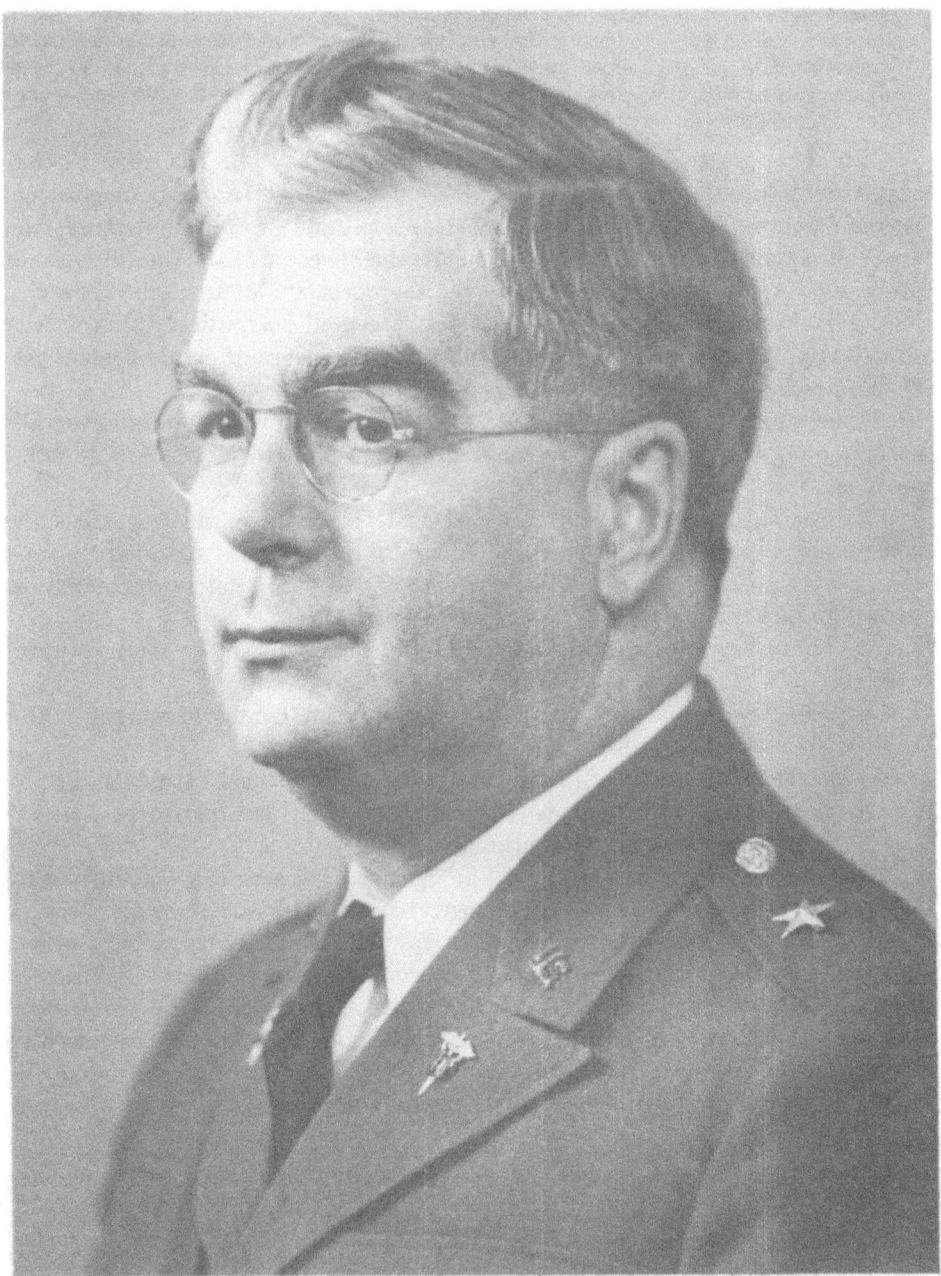

Figure 1. Brig. Gen. Leigh C. Fairbank, Director, Dental Division, 17 March 1938–16 March 1942.

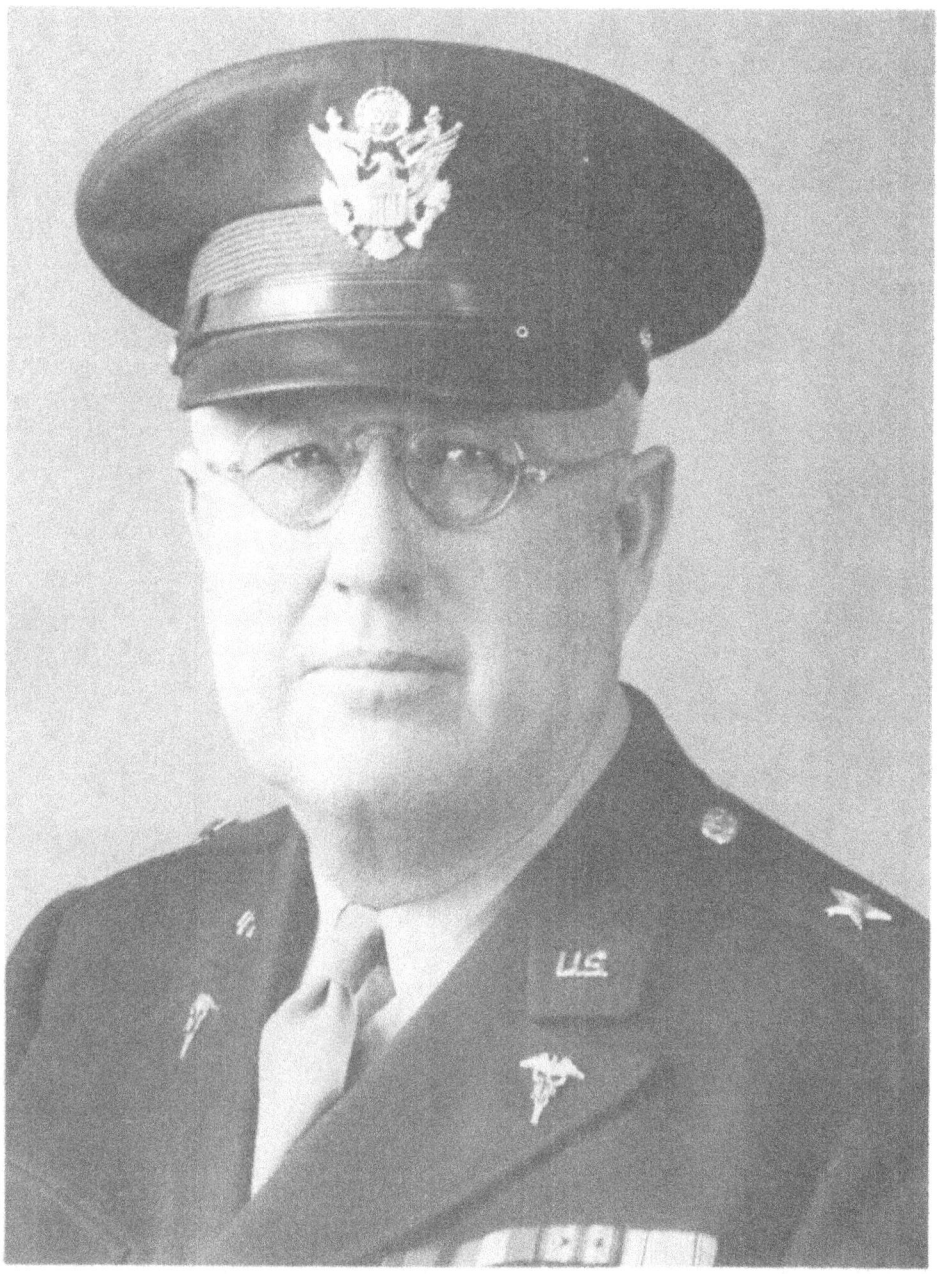

Figure 2. Maj. Gen. Robert H. Mills, Director, Dental Division, 17 March 1942–16 March 1946.

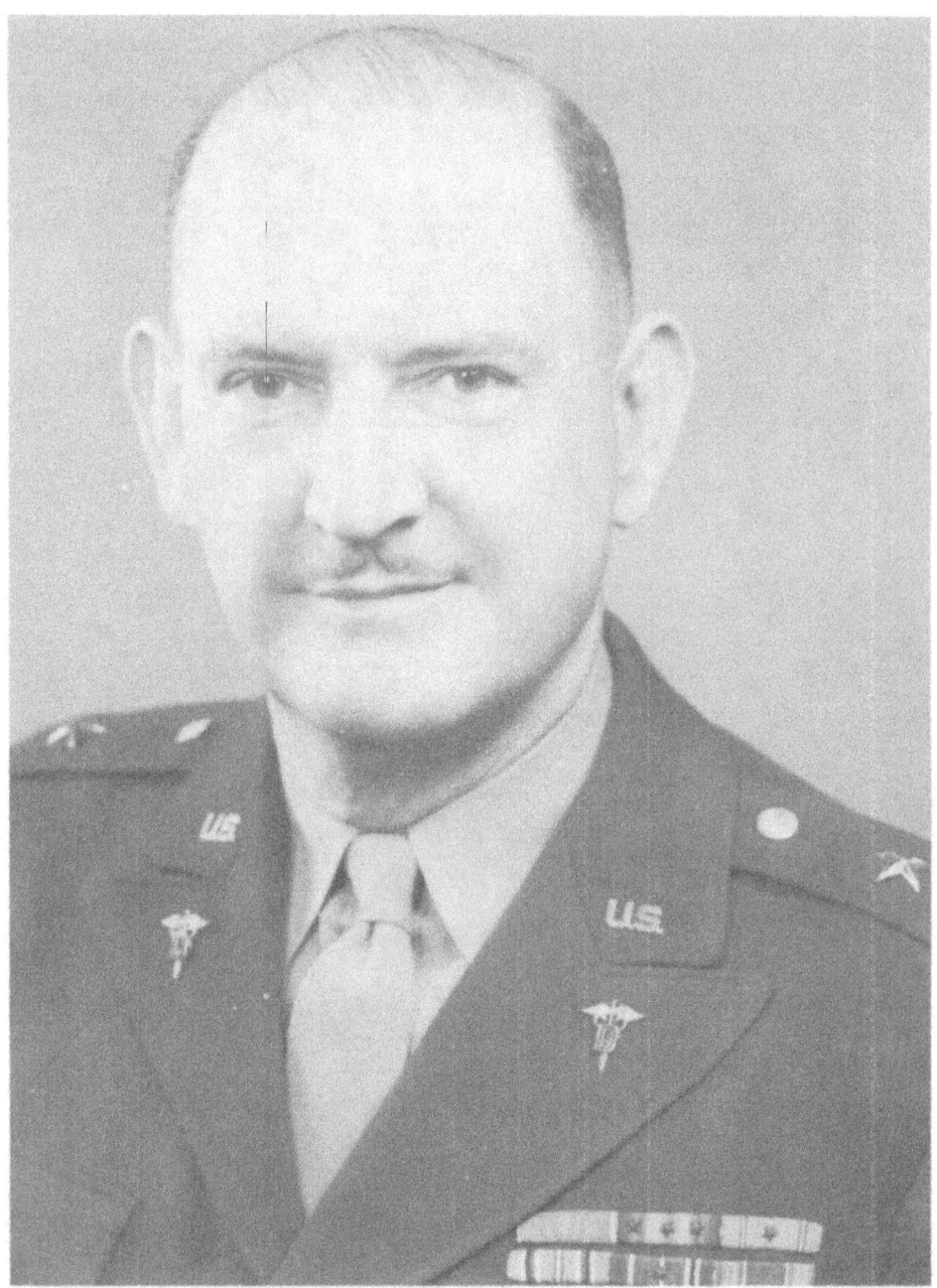

Figure 3. Brig. Gen. Thomas L. Smith, Director, Dental Division, 17 March 1946–20 April 1950.

recommended, on the advice of the Director of the Dental Division, that dental officers be furnished tactical units in a ratio of 1 officer for each 1,000 men, he was overruled when tactical officers convinced the Chief of Staff that such action would add too much to the noncombat overhead of the fighting commands. Similarly, the recommendations of the Director of the Dental Division were given serious consideration, though not always accepted, on the following matters which affected the Dental Service:

1. Dental standards for military service.
2. Personnel requirements for the Dental Service.
3. Tables of organization and equipment for dental installations.
4. Dental reports and records.
5. Plans for dental installations.
6. Personnel authorized to receive dental care.

When the United States entered the war, the Director of the Dental Division, then a brigadier general, was responsible directly to The Surgeon General. He was assisted by a staff of 5 officers and 8 civilian employees. The Dental Division was divided into sections for Finance and Supply, Military Personnel, Plans and Training, and Statistics, with the following assigned responsibilities:[7]

Executive Officer:

 a. Supervision of mail and records.

 b. Review and recommendations of action on inspection reports.

 c. Selection and assignment of dental interns.

 d. Coordination of subdivisions of the Dental Division.

Finance and Supply:

 a. Recommendations on selection and distribution of dental equipment and supplies.

 b. Recommendations on matters pertaining to construction and alteration of dental installations.

 c. Recommendations on claims for dental attendance.

Military Personnel:

 a. Initiation of recommendations to the Personnel Division, SGO, for assignment and transfer of dental personnel.

 b. Transcription and review of efficiency reports.

 c. Classification of personnel.

 d. Review of applications for commission in the Dental Reserve Corps.

 e. Examination of models of teeth and decisions as to dental qualifications.

---

[7] Organization of the Dental Division during the war was very informal and subject to change on short notice in accordance with the number and experience of the assigned personnel. Three days after this organization was outlined Brig Gen Leigh C. Fairbank described five sections in the Dental Division: (1) Personnel, (2) Professional Service, (3) Plans and Training, (4) Statistical, (5) Miscellaneous.

Plans and Training:

    a. Preparation of manuals and films for training dental service personnel.

    b. Preparation of administrative regulations pertaining to the Dental Service.

Statistics:

    a. Collection of historical data on organization and functioning of the Dental Service.

    b. Review of articles for publication and editing of Army Dental Bulletin.

    c. Review of professional reports.

    d. Tabulation of statistical data.

By 30 June 1942 the staff of the Dental Division had reached its maximum strength of 7 officers (including the Director) and 13 civilian employees. The internal organization of the Division underwent several changes during the war, but they were of a minor nature.[8]

With the reorganization of the Army in March 1942 [9] all service and supply branches were placed under a newly formed "Services of Supply" (SOS), later called "Army Service Forces" (ASF). Under this plan The Surgeon General was made responsible to the Commanding General, SOS, rather than to the Chief of Staff, and medical affairs had to be cleared through ASF headquarters. Major dental policies therefore had to be passed upon by (1) The Surgeon General, (2) the Commanding General, ASF, and (3) the General Staff, before they could be made effective. The formation of ASF also proved to be the first step in a general decentralization of authority to the corps areas (later the service commands), a policy which ultimately affected the operation of the Dental Division to a marked degree. Previously, The Surgeon General had had considerable control over the field performance of medical activities, including the immediate supervision of general hospitals and the privilege of assigning personnel to specific installations. In the Annual Report of Army Service Forces for 1943 it was stated that "With the creation of the Service Commands in July 1942, the Administrative Services, for the most part, ceased to have direct control over the field performance of their particular activity. Instead, responsibility . . . was invested in the hands of Service Commanders." [10] The Surgeon General was thus limited to prescribing general policies for the Medical Department, the application of which became the responsibility of service commanders. The control of general hospitals was delegated to the service commands in August 1942.[11]

---

[8] Final Rpt for ASF, Logistics in World War II. HD: 319.1–2 (Dental Div).

[9] WD Cir 59, 2 Mar 42.

[10] Annual Report of the Army Service Forces for the fiscal year 1943 (cited hereafter as Annual Report . . . Army Service Forces).

[11] AR 170–10, par 6, 10 Aug 42.

The service commands were also given increasing authority over personnel. The system of "bulk allotment," in particular, practically ended any control The Surgeon General or the Dental Division might have exercised over the assignment or promotion of dental officers within the service commands. This system has been described as follows: [12]

> Under the system a . . . Service Commander is allotted a total number of officers, nurses, warrant officers, WAAC officers, enrolled women, and enlisted men, restricted only as to percentage in grade, or in small installations, numbers in grade. . . . It removes restrictions upon the distribution of grades among the personnel of the several arms or services, while preserving the limitations upon the distribution of grades within the total organization.

This policy of decentralizing the control of personnel to the service commands relieved the Dental Division of much routine detail which could be handled more efficiently locally, but it also made the correction of inequities more difficult when these were found to exist.

On 26 March 1942, the Dental Division was redesignated the "Dental Service." [13] This change was mainly a "paper transaction" and had no appreciable effect on the operations of the Dental Corps. On 1 September 1942, however, a modification was announced which had more far-reaching results. Up to this time the Dental Division had been an independent branch of the Office of The Surgeon General, and its director had had direct access to that official. Now the Dental Service was placed, with a number of other medical specialties, under a newly organized Professional Services group. The Director of the Dental Division no longer had direct access to The Surgeon General, and all the many decisions affecting some 15,000 officers had to be passed on by at least three higher officers, and usually four, before they could be put into effect.[14] This was not an altogether new experiment since the Dental Division had been placed under Professional Services in 1931,[15] but it had been found advisable to restore its independent status in 1935.[16] The Director of the Dental Division stated that during the war "The Dental Corps experienced greater administrative difficulties while under Professional Service, since all recommendations and activities had to be cleared through that Service to The Surgeon General. Such clearance through Professional Service required too much time when time was at a premium."[17] The Dental Division was restored to its independent status on 25 August 1944.[18]

The Director of the Dental Division claimed repeatedly that there was great need for representation by dental officers in other divisions of the SGO dealing with matters affecting the Dental Service. He stated that "The

---
[12] ASF Cir 39, 11 Jun 43.
[13] Annual Report . . . Surgeon General, 1942. Washington, Government Printing Office, 1942.
[14] SG OO 340, 1 Sep 42.
[15] Annual Report . . . Surgeon General, 1932. Washington, Government Printing Office, 1932.
[16] Annual Report . . . Surgeon General, 1936. Washington, Government Printing Office, 1936.
[17] See footnote 8, p. 28.
[18] SG OO 175, 25 Aug 44.

Dental Corps . . . is vitally interested in all personnel problems, all supply problems, all operations and planning, as well as all training problems," and he recommended that dental officers be placed in the divisions occupied with these activities.[19] Under the stress and confusion of wartime it was very difficult to keep informed of impending actions or changes of policy unless close liaison were maintained. A dental officer was actually assigned to the Supply Division from November 1942 to March 1943.[20] Later, in May 1943, representation was established in the Military Personnel Division and continued for the duration of the war.

DENTAL ADMINISTRATION IN CORPS AREAS (SERVICE COMMANDS)

The administrative status of the senior dental officer in a corps area (service command after 22 July 1942) was analogous to that of the Director of the Dental Division in the War Department. The corps area commander had full executive authority, while the surgeon was his adviser on matters concerning the Medical Department. The dental surgeon was, in turn, charged with furnishing "advisory and administrative assistance to the corps area surgeon on matters pertaining to the dental service in the corps area."[21] Specifically, he made recommendations concerning allotments and assignment of enlisted men and officers, the proper issue and use of dental supplies, the adequacy of contemplated construction of dental facilities, the training program for dental officers and enlisted personnel, and the publication of orders concerning the Dental Service. The corps area dental surgeon could not issue orders in his own name, but submitted his problems to the corps area commander through the surgeon.

Like the Director of the Dental Division in the SGO, the corps area dental surgeon exercised considerable influence over the actual operation of the Dental Service in spite of formal limitations on his authority. His recommendations were normally accepted without question in respect to:[22]

1. The assignment of officers to subordinate installations, within the authorized total strengths.

2. The authorization of equipment and supplies for dental installations.

3. The operation of central dental laboratories and the dental services of general hospitals.

4. The construction of dental facilities.

---

[19] See footnote 8, p. 28.
[20] WD SO 300, par 10, 4 Nov 42.
[21] See footnote 4, p. 22.
[22] Statements concerning the powers of corps area dental surgeons are of course not applicable to all service commands at all times. Some dental surgeons enjoyed greater authority, some less. The summary given here represents only the combined opinions of many senior dental officers interviewed during the war.

ADMINISTRATION OF THE DENTAL SERVICE 31

 5. Directives concerning clinical treatment.

His advice concerning the following was considered seriously, but not necessarily accepted if opposed by other staff divisions:

 1. Total requirements for enlisted and commissioned personnel.
 2. Allotments of personnel for training.
 3. The promotion of dental officers.

At the start of the war general hospitals were operated directly under The Surgeon General, but after August 1942 they became the responsibility of the service command surgeon, and the service command dental surgeon exercised more or less direct control over their dental services.[23] Central dental laboratories were operated under corps area and later, service command, supervision during the entire war.

Prior to October 1940 the duties of corps area dental surgeons were performed, in addition to their normal functions, by senior dental officers assigned in the vicinity of corps area headquarters,[24] though it was provided that full time officers would be assigned in time of war. Dental surgeons were specifically assigned to the corps areas beginning in October 1940, and a revision of Army regulations in December 1942 provided for routine peacetime assignment of service command dental surgeons.[25]

The Director of the Dental Division believed that service command dental surgeons were somewhat hampered by their lack of direct contact with other staff divisions. They could present their views only through the surgeon, and they received only the information relayed to them by that officer. The Director of the Dental Division reported that service command dental surgeons were limited in their authority and that they had insufficient assistance to enable them to perform their office duties and at the same time maintain the necessary supervision in the field.[26]

DENTAL SECTION OF THE AIR SURGEON'S OFFICE, ARMY AIR FORCES [27]

Prior to 28 January 1942, dental affairs in the Office of the Air Surgeon had been administered by the particular division most concerned, i. e., personnel affairs by the Personnel Division, et cetera. On that date a Dental Section was established and Lieutenant Colonel George R. Kennebeck was assigned as Deputy for Dental Service.[28] The need for dental representation in the Office of the Air Surgeon had been pointed out by the Dental Division in Sep-

---

[23] See footnote 11, p. 28.
[24] See footnote 4, p. 22.
[25] AR 40–15, 28 Dec 42.
[26] See footnote 8, p. 28.
[27] Kennebeck, George R.: Dental service of the U. S. Air Forces. Mil. Surgeon 101: 385–392. Nov 1947. (A more complete history of the Air Force Dental Service was (Jan 48) being written by Lt Col Walter J. Reuter.)
[28] WD SO 2, par 16, 2 Jan 42.

tember 1941 [29] but action was delayed by the opposition of the Air Surgeon himself.[30] The new Dental Section assumed staff functions for that part of the dental service assigned to the Air Forces not in theaters of operations. The Dental Division, SGO, continued to prescribe general policies and procedures applicable to the Army Dental Service as a whole, but it no longer acted on those problems peculiar to the Air Force. The functions of the new division were specifically outlined as follows:

1. Review reports of dental activities with the Army Air Forces.
2. Review articles submitted by dental officers with the Army Air Forces prior to publication in professional journals.
3. Initiate timely recommendations for changes in types and allowances of dental supplies and equipment.
4. Make recommendations to the Officers' Section, Personnel Division, regarding assignment, reassignment, and promotion of dental officers with the Army Air Forces.
5. Exercise professional supervision over dental personnel with the Army Air Forces.

The Air Surgeon's Office did not directly control the dental services with Air Force units in theaters of operation; these were under the supervision of theater chief surgeons. However, Air Force commands in foreign theaters did have dental staff officers who were responsible for the dental service of air units, under the theater chief surgeons. Dental personnel for the Air Force were commissioned by the Army and requisitioned as needed from The Surgeon General.

ADMINISTRATION OF THE DENTAL SERVICE IN CAMPS AND STATIONS

In subordinate installations in the Zone of Interior the senior medical officer retained his status as adviser to the commanding officer, but he usually became commander of the hospital or dispensary as well, thus exercising control not only over the making of policies, but over their direct application at the operational level. The dental surgeon, on the other hand, did not become commanding officer of the dental clinic, and legally he continued to enjoy only the right to make recommendations to the surgeon concerning the dental service. In practice he might be delegated almost complete authority by the latter, but such authority was a privilege, not a right, and it varied widely in different installations.

The dental surgeon of a camp or station generally had reasonably effective control over the following activities:

---

[29] Memo, Brig Gen Leigh C. Fairbank for SG, 25 Sep 41, sub: Dental Service for the Air Corps. SG: 703.-1.
[30] Memo, Col David N. W. Grant for Exec Off SGO, 1 Oct 41, sub: Dental Service for the Air Corps. SG: 703-1.

1. The assignment of dental enlisted and commissioned personnel to duties within the dental clinic.

2. The supervision of treatment given. Army regulations provided that "except as otherwise prescribed herein, the selection of professional procedures to be followed in each case, including the use of special dental materials, will be left to the judgment of the dental officer concerned."[31]

3. Initiation of requisitions for supplies for the dental service.

4. The conduct of dental surveys.

5. The technical training of personnel assigned to the dental service.

His recommendations were customarily given serious consideration in respect to the following, but they were not always accepted, and under unfavorable circumstances they might practically be ignored:

1. Requirements for dental personnel or facilities.

2. Promotion of personnel assigned to the dental clinic.

3. Leave or furlough privileges for personnel of the dental service.

4. Efficiency reports on dental personnel.

The dental surgeon often had little to say about the following:

1. The use of clinic personnel for duties outside the dental clinic.

2. Training of dental personnel, outside of training rendered in the dental clinic.

ADMINISTRATION OF THE DENTAL SERVICE, ARMY GROUND FORCES

When the Army Ground Forces (AGF) was established in 1942 as a separate command of the Army no provision was made for a complete medical staff. A small division for Hospitalization and Evacuation was included in Headquarters, AGF, but it was expected that most medical functions would be performed by The Surgeon General. No dental officer was assigned to AGF headquarters. Under The Surgeon General, the Dental Division had authority to prescribe policies for the entire Army, including AGF and Army Air Forces (AAF), but operation of the Dental Service for such a large part of the Armed Forces inevitably involved emergency situations requiring immediate action. Lack of liaison with AGF headquarters delayed solution of some of these problems and increased the difficulty of arriving at decisions based on full and accurate information. An attempt was made to have a dental officer assigned to AGF in the spring of 1945, but it met with no success. The Director of the Dental Division later claimed that lack of liaison with AGF had hampered the Dental Service significantly.[32]

---

[31] AR 40–510, par 1, 19 Feb 40.
[32] See footnote 8, p. 28.

ADMINISTRATION OF THE DENTAL SERVICE IN A THEATER OF OPERATIONS [33]

A theater dental surgeon made recommendations to the theater chief surgeon concerning plans and policies for the dental service of the entire area, including the Air Forces. He advised in respect to requirements for supplies and personnel; he consolidated and forwarded dental reports for the theater; and he made the inspections required to assure a high standard of dental care in compliance with the directives of his own and higher headquarters. The theater dental surgeon was also, very often, the dental surgeon of the communications zone and in that capacity he supervised the operation of the hospital dental services in that communications zone, the dental treatment of service personnel, and the operation of central dental laboratories.

Theaters necessarily enjoyed considerable independence of action, and the theater dental surgeon, under the chief surgeon, had a great deal of freedom in planning for the dental service, as long as personnel allotments were not exceeded and major regulations and policies were not violated. As in other headquarters, however, he was subordinate to the theater chief surgeon and he could act only with the approval of that officer.

---

[33] See chapter VIII.

CHAPTER III

The Procurement of Dental Officers

PROCUREMENT IN WORLD WAR I

At the time of the armistice, World War I, the strength of the Dental Corps totaled 6,284 officers. Not all of these had been called to active duty however, and the maximum number actually functioning with the Corps at any one time was 4,620.[1] As nearly as can be determined, a little over 1,500 additional dentists who did not serve in their professional capacity were in the land forces as enlisted men.[2] The Navy Dental Corps expanded from a total of 30 dental officers at the outbreak of hostilities to over 500 by the end of 1917,[3] but the number of dentists serving as enlisted men in that organization is not known.

The Army, alone, enlisted or inducted 1,789 dental students, and the schools were so depleted that only 906 dentists graduated in 1920 as compared with 3,587 the year before.[4]

At the start of World War I, dentists were provided in an overall ratio of 1 officer for each 1,000 troops, but this figure proved so inadequate that on 30 September 1918 an increase to 2 dentists for each 1,000 men in the continental United States was authorized, and the allowance for hospitals was fixed at 3 officers for each 1,000 beds.[5] The war ended, however, before these ratios could be placed in effect. In 1919 the War Department supported a bill to provide 1 dentist for each 500 men in the peacetime establishment, but in spite of the backing of The Surgeon General and the Secretary of War this legislation failed to pass.[6]

The grades held by Army dentists at the end of the war were as follows:[7]

Colonel _____ 9 (0.2 percent)
Lieutenant colonel _____ 17 (0.4 percent)

---

[1] Annual Report . . . Surgeon General, 1919. Washington, Government Printing Office, 1919, vol. II.
[2] Ibid.
[3] Annual Report of The Surgeon General, U. S. Navy, 1918. Washington, Government Printing Office, 1918.
[4] Horner, Harlan H.: Dental education and dental personnel. J. Am. Dent. A. 33: 872, Jul 1946.
[5] See footnote 2, above.
[6] Colonel Logan's Farewell Letter to the Dental Corps. J. A. Mil. Dent. Surg. U. S. 3: 78–80, Apr. 1919.
[7] See footnote 1, above.

Major _____ 91 (2.0 percent)
Captain _____ 292 (6.5 percent)
Lieutenant _____ 4,101 (90.9 percent)

THE DETERMINATION OF REQUIREMENTS FOR DENTAL OFFICERS, WORLD WAR II

Experience Prior to World War II

In the decade preceding the Second World War, the average civilian dentist was responsible for about 1,800 persons, including infants and the aged who required little or no attention, though the ratio varied from approximately 1:500 in certain urban centers to less than 1:5,000 in some rural districts.[8][9] Dental care for the civilian population was notoriously deficient. It was freely admitted that not over 25 percent of the public received the care needed to preserve dental health,[10][11] and representatives of the dental profession estimated that it would require 1 dentist for each 524 persons just to provide annual maintenance treatment, with no attempt to correct old, accumulated defects. It was further estimated that the fantastic figure of 1 dentist for each 295 persons would be needed to rehabilitate the entire population in one year. These figures had little significance in determining dental officer requirements for a military population for the following reasons:

1. While the average civilian dentist actually saw only about 400 patients a year, many of them received nothing but emergency treatment.[12][13] However, all of the military dentist's patients, regardless of the number, were in the age group needing constant and extensive care.

2. The stresses of military life required that the soldier have a higher level of dental health than his civilian contemporary.

3. The military dentist inevitably lost more time from professional duties than the civilian dentist: he had to devote more time to training for purely military functions, and his work was interrupted by maneuvers and tactical exercises.

Prewar military experience failed equally to provide an answer to the requirement problem. In the years between 1920 and 1939 the inadequate 1:1,000 ratio of World War I was liberalized somewhat, but it never exceeded 1.44 per 1,000 troops, as indicated in the following tabulation:[14]

---

[8] See footnote 4, p. 35.
[9] Bagdonas, Joseph E.: Economic considerations in reestablishing a dental practice. J. Am. Dent. A. 33: 4–20, Jan 1946.
[10] Morey, Lon W.: Dental personnel. J. Am. Dent. A. 32: 131–144, Feb 1945.
[11] Dollar, Melvin L.: Dental needs and the costs of dental care in the United States. Ill. Dent. J. 14: 185–199, May 1945.
[12] See footnote 4, p. 35.
[13] See footnote 9, above.
[14] Memo, Col Albert G. Love for SG, 2 Oct 39, sub: Allowance of medical and dental officers. [D]

Date	Number of officers authorized	Authorized ratio per 1,000
4 June 1920	298	1.00
30 June 1922	158	1.08
15 May 1936	183	1.26
29 January 1938	258	1.44
3 April 1939	*316	1.39

*This authorized strength was not reached prior to the war, and there were only about 269 dentists in the Regular Army Dental Corps in April 1942.

Based on the estimation that a proportion of 1 dentist for each 524 persons would be required just to provide maintenance care, it is not surprising that the cited peacetime authorizations proved inadequate. In 1928, when the ratio was approximately 1 dentist per 1,000 personnel, the Director of the Dental Division, SGO, reported that:[15]

> ... a one to 1,000 proportion of dental officers to total strength is quite insufficient. Dental diseases in our Army have been, and ... are today out of control. There is a limit beyond which it is impossible to go without more personnel. We are today approaching that limit, and about 50 percent remain who are continually in need of dental service.

In 1941, at a hearing before the Committee on Military Affairs, Brig. Gen. Leigh C. Fairbank[16] testified that even under peacetime physical standards a 1:750 ratio had also fallen short of minimum needs.

By the start of the Second World War, therefore, experience had shown that any ratio of less than 1 dental officer for 750 men would be grossly inadequate, but since more liberal ratios had not been tried in practice experience was of little value in predicting the need for dental officers for the defense forces.

Estimates Based on Actual Requirements for Dental Treatment

Had it been known exactly how much work the average wartime inductee would require it would have been possible to calculate the number of dental officers needed at any stage of mobilization. Were it known, for instance, that each new man would require 7.2 hours of treatment for the correction of old, accumulated defects, and 1.8 hours of treatment each year thereafter for regular maintenance care, the needs of a static force of 1,500,000 men, with a yearly turnover of 25 percent, could have been determined as follows:

	Hours
1.8 hours of care for 1,500,000 men (annual maintenance)	2,700,000
7.2 hours of care for 375,000 recruits (rehabilitation)	2,700,000
Total	5,400,000
Number of dentists needed	3,000 (1 per 500 men)

[15] Rhoades, R. H.: The Dental Service of the Army of the United States. J. Am. Dent. A. 15: 257–264, Feb 1928.

[16] Testimony, General Fairbank, 18–20 Mar 41, in U. S. Senate Hearings before Committee on Mil Affairs, S. 783, p. 161.

In this case, which might approximate actual conditions in a peacetime force if dependents received no care, a ratio of 1 dentist for each 500 men would prove adequate.

However, if this hypothetical force were to be increased by nearly 4,000,000 men in one year as occurred in the United States Army in 1942, the situation would be far different. Total needs would then be as follows:

	Hours
1.8 hours of care for 3,500,000 men (average strength during year)	6,300,000
7.2 hours for 4,000,000 men (recruits)	28,800,000
Total	35,100,000
Number of dentists needed	19,500 (1 per 180 men)

In this situation, which also might approximate actual conditions during mobilization, the ratio which was adequate for the static force would provide only about 36 percent of the dentists needed by the expanding Army. Later, however, after this augmented force reached stability, the need for dentists would again be met by the 1:500 proportion, or by an even lower ratio.

Unfortunately, reliable information on which to base actual calculations of requirements for dental personnel was entirely lacking at the start of World War II. The figures used in the preceding illustration are only convenient approximations, useful for the development of a general principle. In chapter VI it is shown that almost no data on the dental condition of males of military age were available when plans for the mobilization of the emergency dental service were being laid.

Even if dental needs were known with considerable accuracy, it would generally be impossible to procure and equip dental officers in strict accordance with calculated needs. In Chart 1 the actual number of dentists on duty each month of World War II is compared with the theoretical requirement for the same period, based on the hypothetical figures used (1.8 hours for maintenance care, 7.2 hours for rehabilitation). The curve on this chart which shows theoretical needs is of course not quantitatively accurate, but the wide fluctuations which are its conspicuous feature would be found on any similar chart, regardless of the exact figures used, as long as the time required for rehabilitation of new men greatly exceeds that required for annual maintenance. By comparison, the slowly rising curve of dental personnel on duty reflects a number of delaying factors which are likely to be operative in any emergency. The two years from 1940 through 1941 represented a training period in which the immediate mobilization of a large force was not anticipated. With the start of actual hostilities considerable time was required to commission the necessary dentists, and through 1942 it was impossible even to equip fully all the dentists actually in uniform.

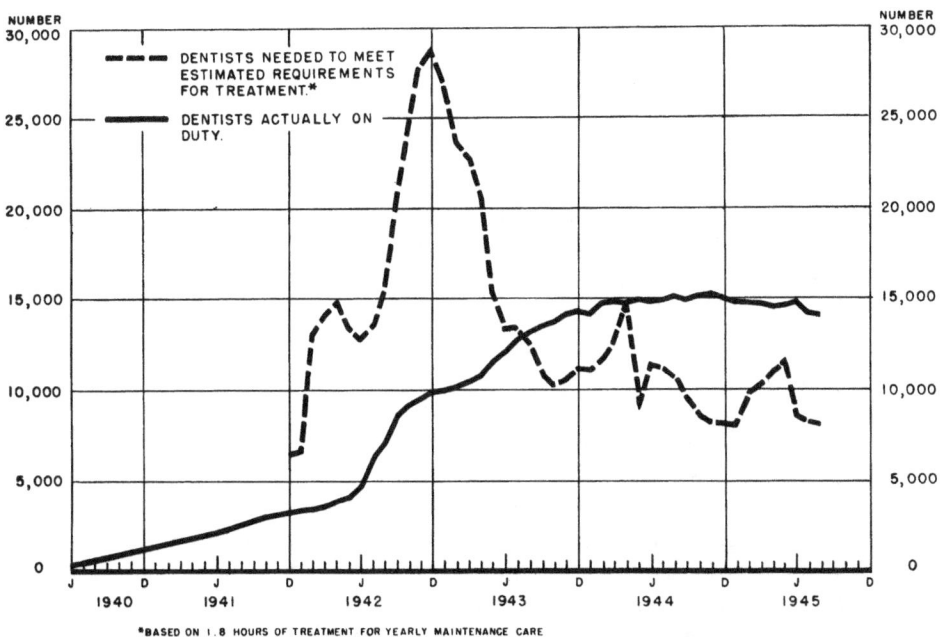

CHART 1. COMPARISON OF THEORETICAL MONTHLY REQUIREMENTS FOR DENTAL OFFICERS DURING WORLD WAR II WITH THE NUMBER ACTUALLY ON ACTIVE DUTY.

In contrast with the gradually rising curve of dental personnel on duty, the curve of theoretical requirements fluctuates rapidly and within wide limits. Nearly 30,000 dentists would have been needed late in 1942, when half a million men were inducted in 1 month, while only 10,000 would have been needed less than a year later, after the tempo of mobilization had slowed. To have procured, trained, and equipped 30,000 dentists in 1942, for only a few months work, would have resulted in a gross waste of manpower and industrial capacity. In most cases it will probably be found impractical or impossible to call to duty, to meet peak requirements, a number of dental officers greatly exceeding the number which will be needed when relative stability has been reached, regardless of calculated needs for short periods.

Nevertheless, reference to calculated requirements, even when based on very incomplete information, may point out possible improvements in the mobilization program. In particular, it will generally emphasize the desirability of building up the Dental Service as rapidly as possible after plans for the augmentation of the Armed Forces are announced, regardless of fixed ratios of dentists to total strength. In many respects the position of the Dental Service is comparable to that of a training activity. If several hundred thousand men are to be "processed" each month the necessary training centers must be established *in advance* of the influx, not built up gradually on the basis of some fixed ratio of training personnel to the number of troops already in uniform. Similarly, the Dental Service should be in maximum practical operation at the *start* of a period of expansion, ready to care for inductees as they pass through the training camps; if, however, the rate of mobilization of dental facilities is gauged to maintain some fixed ratio of dental officers to total Army strength, the necessary men and equipment will be available only at the end of the influx, after most inductees have already completed their training and have been assigned to tactical units. This situation will occur regardless of how liberal the accepted ratio may be.

It has already been pointed out that it will generally be impracticable to mobilize the full facilities needed to meet temporary peak demands; it is also possible that personnel and supply difficulties will hinder or prevent the early establishment of dental clinics in the future as they have in the past. These facts should not obscure the validity of the general principle that, when a major augmentation of the Armed Forces is imminent, the Dental Service should be built up to the total strength which will ultimately be required, as rapidly as may be possible under the circumstances existing at the time. At the start of World War II, for instance, it was patently impossible and undesirable to provide the 30,000 dental officers who might have been used in 1942. Further, it would have been impossible to equip such a number of dentists even if they could have been obtained. But 15,000 dentists were ultimately mobilized, and 10,000 were on duty by the end of 1942, while the average strength of the Dental Corps for that year of expansion was only about 6,000 officers, and only about 3,000 were available at the start of the year. It must be admitted that no improvement in the rate of mobilization of dentists was possible under conditions existing in 1942, but it is equally true that the 1:500 ratio of dentists to total strength, which was maintained fairly well, fell far short of meeting dental demands during that year. Further, if it had been possible to place on duty in May or June of 1942 the 10,000 dental officers who were working in Army clinics in December, the problems of the Dental Service would have been reduced materially.

Reference to calculated requirements for dental treatment will also reveal not only that the application of a fixed ratio of dentists to total strength tends to delay the mobilization of dental facilities, but that it fails to consider the primary factor in determining how many dentists will be required—the *rate of flow* of inductees. This weakness is of course based on the fact that treatment for old, accumulated dental defects has been, and may be expected to be, greatly in excess of requirements for yearly maintenance care. If only maintenance treatment were needed by inductees the amount of that treatment would be directly proportional to the number of men in the service, and a fixed ratio of dentists to total strength, based on past experience, would be satisfactory. But when several times as many hours are necessary for the dental rehabilitation of an inductee as will be required for annual maintenance each year thereafter, the first consideration is not likely to be "how many troops are in the Army?" but "how many new men will be inducted during the year?" Thus, in the discussed hypothetical illustration, the ratio of dentists which met all needs of a static force broke down completely when applied to an expanding organization. These weaknesses of the method of fixing dental personnel on the basis of an established ratio in a time of emergency do not mean that such a ratio may not represent the maximum number of dentists that may be available, or that it may not be valuable as an indication of how many dentists will be required after stability has been reached. They do indicate, however, the need for a critical evaluation of any proposed ratio in the light of the actual probable demand for treatment whenever a major mobilization is planned.

It is possible, of course, that future developments in methods of waging war may alter the mission and function of the medical services even to the point of placing first emphasis on the care of the civilian population.

Limitations on the Number of Dentists Available From Civilian Practice

During World War I only about 6,700 dentists were taken from private practice and the effect on civilian dental care was scarcely noticed. Prior to World War II very little thought had been given to the possibility that the number of dentists who could be obtained for the Armed Forces was, in fact, strictly limited. Nor did it seem probable that there might not be a sufficient number of personnel left to care for the minimum needs of the civil population.

The first attempt to determine how many dentists could be spared for the Armed Forces was made in April 1941, when the American Dental Association (ADA) estimated that 21,000 dentists would fall within the draft age and that only 6,700 of these would be eligible for induction.[17] However, this figure was based on induction criteria rather than on any survey of civilian needs, and it was therefore subject to change as draft regulations were altered.

In June 1942, local complaints of shortages of dental personnel impelled the Procurement and Assignment Service for Physicians, Dentists, and Veterinarians (PAS), of the War Manpower Commission (WMC), to sponsor a general survey of dental manpower.[18] This survey, which was carried out with the assistance of the U. S. Public Health Service (USPHS), was completed in

---

[17] Report of the Chicago meeting of the Committee on Dental Preparedness. J. Am. Dent. A. 28: 635, Apr 1941.
[18] Minutes of the Directing Board, PAS, 22 Jun 42. On file Natl Archives, PAS, WMC.

February 1943 and revealed the following situation (projected to the end of 1943) :[19]

Dentists listed in the 1940 census	70,417
Graduates, 1940–1943	8,928
Total	79,345
Losses by death and retirement, 1940–1942	3,830
Dentists estimated to be in nonprofessional work with various essential agencies	1,021
Anticipated losses, 1943	1,624
Total	6,475
Remaining effectives, end of 1943	72,870

PAS decided that a minimum of 1 dentist for each 2,500 persons should be reserved for civilian care, or a total of 50,250 dentists for a civil population of 125,625,000. This left 22,620 dentists who could be utilized by the Armed Forces, 11,617 of whom were already on active duty in the Army, Navy, and Public Health Service.

The findings of PAS, that 1 dentist was required for each 2,500 civilians and that 22,620 dentists could be made available to the military, were of course open to question on theoretical grounds. In the absence of specific information on the dental condition of the American public any such estimates were necessarily arbitrary and based on opinion rather than upon factual knowledge. It could be pointed out, for instance, that even in peacetime many communities had never had more than 1 dentist for each 5,000 persons. Further, it was obvious that PAS' ratio could not be applied uniformly since those regions which had never approached the 1:2,500 ratio before the war could hardly expect to receive additional dental personnel in a time of national emergency, to bring them up to the authorized proportion. If these areas merely retained their prewar ratios, and if all other districts were reduced to the recommended quota, considerably more dentists would have been released for military service.

It was more difficult to criticize PAS' findings from the practical point of view. No one could claim that a ratio of 1 dentist for 5,000 persons, or an average per capita expenditure for dentistry of 9 cents a year, was adequate for the maintenance of dental health; the fact that such conditions existed in some unfortunate regions did not justify their extension to the entire nation. And while neither PAS nor any other agency could state with certainty that a given ratio of dentists was actually required for civilians, the Armed Forces would have had equal difficulty in justifying any demand for an increased allotment since the figure set by PAS gave them nearly one-third of the nations' dentists for 12 million men, while only two-thirds were reserved for the remaining 125 million civilians.

---
[19] Minutes of Committee on Dentistry, PAS, 20 Feb 43. On file Natl Archives, PAS, WMC.

Also, while many areas which had had less than 1 dentist for each 2,500 persons prior to the war would certainly have to continue with less than the PAS "minimum" ratio, the number of additional dentists made available to the military by this circumstance was very small due to peculiarities of distribution. Dentists who were "excess" by the PAS definition were concentrated mainly in the larger urban centers, and it was not feasible to take from 50 to 80 percent of the men in practice in such cities as New York or Los Angeles to bring those districts down to the recommended quota. A city of one million persons, for instance, with a ratio of 1 dentist for each 1,000 individuals would have 1,000 dentists; of these, 600 would have to be taken into the Armed Forces to reduce the proportion to 1 dentist for each 2,500 persons. But many of the dentists in such a city would be too old for active duty, or physically disqualified for military life; others would be in essential occupations. The number which would be accepted by the Armed Forces would in most cases be far below the 600 which would theoretically be declared available. The only way in which the remainder could be utilized would be to relocate them in less favored districts to release younger men who would in turn be taken by the Army or Navy. The alternative would be to leave a higher proportion of dentists in centers which had normally enjoyed a high ratio in peacetime, offsetting those regions which could not attain the 1:2,500 ratio.

In view of these considerations, the findings and broad recommendations of PAS in respect to minimum requirements for civilian dental care must be considered reasonable and justifiable, at least until such time as more definite information is available concerning dental needs. When it is noted that the Army and Navy, together, mobilized about 22,318 dental officers in the war it is apparent that they were close to the bottom of the manpower barrel, and that no significant increase in the overall ratio of dental officers to total strength was possible. Any future mobilization plan must certainly recognize that the essential, minimum needs of the civilian population must be met, and that the supply of dental personnel is far from inexhaustible.

ACTUAL BASIS FOR DETERMINING DENTAL MANPOWER REQUIREMENTS, WORLD WAR II

While formal requests for procurement objectives were generally brief, with no discussion of the method of calculation, the ultimate goal of the Chief of the Dental Division, SGO, and The Surgeon General was an overall ratio of 1 dentist for each 500 men. Since information on the dental condition of inductees was too meager to permit an accurate determination of the number of dental officers needed to provide a calculated amount of treatment, it seems probable that the 1:500 ratio was based on one or more of the following considerations:

1. When the 1:1,000 ratio proved grossly inadequate in World War I, the 1:500 proportion was authorized in Zone of Interior installations (except

hospitals). Though this number of dental officers was not obtained before the end of hostilities, the ratio had been approved by the Secretary of War and the Chief of Staff, and it was probably given serious consideration by the officers responsible for organizing the Dental Service in World War II.

2. Ratios of from 1:1,000 to 1:700 had proved inadequate in peacetime and a further increase to 1:500 may have seemed to be the next logical step, especially when dental standards for induction were being drastically lowered.

3. It is possible that a ratio of 1:500 was considered the maximum which would be approved by the General Staff, regardless of demonstrable needs.

While the ratio of 1 dental officer for each 500 troops would ultimately have led to the mobilization of only a little more than the total number of dentists which PAS had decided could be spared for the Armed Forces, there is no evidence that this factor was originally considered in arriving at the figure for the Army Dental Corps. The 1:500 ratio appears to have been generally accepted during the early stages of the expansion of the defense forces, when it was not expected that the Army would reach a strength where its requirements for dentists would seriously threaten civilian practice. Virtual agreement between PAS and the Armed Forces in this case was apparently a happy coincidence.

Col. Robert C. Craven, who was responsible for personnel matters in the Dental Division, SGO, during the early part of the war, stated that the 1:500 ratio was first agreed upon informally between Brig. Gen. Leigh C. Fairbank, Director of the Dental Division, SGO, and Brig. Gen. George F. Lull, Chief of Personnel Services, SGO. When Brig. Gen. Robert H. Mills became Director of the Dental Division, SGO, in March 1942 he attempted to have that ratio officially recognized, but The Surgeon General felt that no definite action should be taken until requirements were more clearly established.[20] General Mills was assured, however, that he could procure all the dentists he might need for corps area service commands, regardless of any fixed ratio, and relying on that promise he relaxed his efforts to obtain formal approval of the desired proportion.[21] No further effort was made to have the 1:500 ratio recognized until near the end of hostilities, when postwar policies were being considered. During the early part of the war, procurement objectives seem to have been determined by informal agreement between the principal personnel officers concerned, with the proportion of 1 officer for each 500 men serving as a convenient, though unofficial, yardstick.[22]

In practice the 1:500 ratio was attained only for very short intervals during the war, and the average ratio over this period was 1 officer for 557

---

[20] Memo, Brig Gen R. H. Mills for SG, 8 Apr 42, no sub. SG: 703.–1.

[21] Proceedings of The Surgeon General's Conference with Corps Area and Army Dental Surgeons, 8–9 July 42. HD: 337.

[22] The highly informal manner in which dental procurement objectives were established during the war has been confirmed in personal correspondence and conversations between the author and Col Robert C. Craven, Dental Div, SGO, and Maj Ernest J. Fedor, dental liaison officer with the Personnel Service during much of the war.

men.[23] Efforts to maintain the 1 : 500 ratio were finally abandoned in September 1943, when ASF placed a ceiling of 15,200 officers on the Dental Corps.[24]

As the war progressed an effort was made to refine estimated requirements for dental officers on a more definite basis than an overall ratio. In a memorandum from the SGO to ASF, dated 5 June 1944, analyzing the dental personnel situation, it was noted that anticipated needs had been calculated as follows: [25]

1. For tactical units in the Zone of Interior and overseas, according to authorized tables of organization.

2. For other Zone of Interior installations, on the basis of 1 dentist for each 500 troops, except for replacement training centers and separation centers, which were authorized 1 dentist for each 300 troops.

3. For general hospitals, according to tables published in War Department Circular No. 209, 26 May 1944.

4. Attrition was estimated at 50 officers monthly.

Tables of organization for tactical units mentioned in item 1 of the cited memorandum were planned to provide an average of 1 dentist for each 1,200 men. Many adjustments were necessary before this general principle could be applied to a host of smaller commands, and the results were sometimes unsatisfactory (see discussion in chapter VIII), but at least these tables of organization provided a means for calculating requirements for projected combat forces on an exact, if arbitrary, basis.

The determination of requirements for dental officers in Zone of Interior installations was more difficult. The following were some of the more important problems involved:

1. While procurement was based on the general ratios outlined in item 2 of the cited memorandum, the number of dentists actually requisitioned by any installations was established by the corps area commander, with the advice of his staff and local officials. As a result, dentist-troop ratios might vary widely, even in commands of the same general type. As early as December 1940, The Surgeon General asked that mandatory tables of organization be set up for the dental services of Zone of Interior camps and stations,[26] but this request was disapproved by The Adjutant General as being contrary to the policy of

---

[23] Calculated by the author from data in the files of the Dental Div, SGO.

[24] The manner in which the ceiling for the Dental Corps was established, and the exact date, is not entirely clear. In a memorandum to the Deputy Surgeon General, of 7 Sep 43, Lt Col D. G. Hall of the Personnel Service, SGO, stated that his office had "that day" been notified of a revised requirement based on changed plans in ASF. (Memo, Lt Col Durward G. Hall to Dep SG, sub: Revised requirements for dental officers in the Army. SG : 322.0531.) Other incidental references indicate that representatives of the Dental Division, the Military Personnel Division, SGO, and of G-1 attended conferences on the matter before a decision was reached. It is also probable that PAS had a hand in the matter, but the extent to which its influence affected ASF is not known.

[25] Memo, Brig Gen R. W. Bliss for CG, ASF, 5 Jun 44, sub: Requirements for Dental Corps officers. SG : 322.053-1.

[26] Ltr, Col Larry B. McAfee to TAG, 10 Dec 40, sub: Personnel table, camp dental clinics. SG : 320.2-1.

decentralizing all possible authority to subordinate facilities.[27] Recommended tables of organization for Zone of Interior installations were published from time to time, but they were merely "suggestions" which could be ignored by subordinate commands. In October 1943, the Director of the Dental Division, SGO, noted that few service commands had requisitioned what was considered an adequate number of dentists, and one service command had only 73 percent of the recommended total.[28]

The first "recommended" allotment of dental officers to Zone of Interior installations, published in December 1940, provided for 18 officers and 26 enlisted men in each DC-1, and 11 officers and 17 enlisted men for each DC-2. These clinics had 25 and 15 chairs, respectively, but it was anticipated that they would be partially manned by tactical units in the Zone of Interior.[29] In May 1944, War Department Circular No. 209 recommended the following manning levels:[30]

DC-1	25 officers	42 enlisted men
DC-2	15 officers	25 enlisted men
DC-3	8 officers	13 enlisted men
DC-4	3 officers	3 enlisted men
DC-5	1 officer	1 enlisted man

This directive also recommended that dental officers be assigned to general hospitals as follows:

1,000 beds	7 officers
1,500 beds	8 officers
1,750 beds	9 officers
2,000 beds	12 officers
2,500 beds	14 officers
3,000 beds	16 officers
3,500 beds	19 officers
4,000 beds	21 officers

However, this publication failed to answer many questions, since it based its recommendations on clinic types rather than on the number of troops served. Thus a DC-1 might be found in a camp with 7,000 men or in a camp with 12,000; obviously the dental needs of the two installations would not be identical.

An ASF circular of 16 October 1945 recommended that dentists be provided Zone of Interior camps on the basis of 2 officers and 3 enlisted men for each 1,000 troops served, plus 1 officer and 1½ enlisted men for each 200 beds in the station hospital.[31] It further suggested specific grades and classifications for both officers and enlisted men, as shown in Tables 1 and 2. The influence of these recommendations on the determination of Zone of Interior dental allotments cannot be determined.

---

[27] (1) 1st ind, TAG, to footnote 26, 30 Dec 40. (2) See footnote 21, p. 44.
[28] Memo, Dir, Dent Div for Chief, Prof Serv, SGO, 1 Oct 43, no sub. SG : 703.-1.
[29] See footnote 27, above.
[30] WD Cir 209, 26 May 44.
[31] ASF Cir 389, 16 Oct 45.

2. It was difficult to predict the extent to which the dentists of tactical units in training in the Zone of Interior could be utilized in camp clinics. For a discussion of this problem see chapter VII.

3. The rate of attrition in the Dental Corps was not constant and it could not be predicted with accuracy. During the early part of the war it was less than had been expected, while later it was necessary to accelerate normal attrition to permit the replacement of older men with ASTP graduates.

TABLE 1. DENTAL OFFICERS RECOMMENDED FOR ZONE OF INTERIOR DENTAL CLINICS BY ASF CIRCULAR No. 389, 16 OCTOBER 1945

Grade	Qualifications	DC-1	DC-2	DC-3	DC-4	DC-5
Lieutenant colonel	Dental staff officer	1				
Lieutenant colonel	General		1			
Major	General		1	1	1	
Major	Oral surgeon	1				
Major	Exodontist	1	1			
Major	Prosthodontist	2	1			
Major	Periodontist	1				
Captain or lieutenant	General	19	11	5	2	1
Captain or lieutenant	Exodontist			1		
Captain or lieutenant	Prosthodontist			1		
Total officers		25	15	8	3	1

TABLE 2. ENLISTED ASSISTANTS RECOMMENDED FOR ZONE OF INTERIOR DENTAL CLINICS BY ASF CIRCULAR No. 389, 16 OCTOBER 1945

Grade	Qualifications	DC-1	DC-2	DC-3	DC-4	DC-5
Technical sergeant	Administrative	1				
Staff sergeant	Administrative		1			
Sergeant	Administrative			1		
Corporal	Clerk	1	1			
Technician, 3d gr	Laboratory technician	2	1	1		
Technician, 4th gr	Laboratory technician	3	2	1		
Technician, 4th gr	X-ray technician	1				
Technician, 4th gr	Chair assistant	9	5	3	1	
Technician, 5th gr	Laboratory technician	5	3	1		
Technician, 5th gr	X-ray technician		1	1		
Technician, 5th gr	Chair assistant	17	9	5	2	1
Private, first class	Supply clerk	1	1			
Private, first class	Basic	1				
Private	Basic	1	1			
Total enlisted men		42	25	13	3	1

CHRONOLOGICAL PROGRESS OF THE MOBILIZATION OF DENTAL OFFICERS

Table 3 shows the monthly procurement of dental officers for the period 1 January 1939 to 28 February 1946.[32]

Though tension in Europe mounted during the late 1930's, staff officers responsible for the Army Dental Service showed little concern over dental personnel problems. It was expected that the fully mobilized ground and air forces would number only about 4,000,000 troops and that a ratio of 1.4 dentists for each 1,000 total strength would be sufficient. This would provide for a Dental Corps of 5,600 men.[33] No difficulty had been experienced in obtaining almost this number of dentists during World War I, even without the benefit of a strong Organized Reserve. Also, in spite of the termination of the dental ROTC in 1932 (see chapter IV), 258 Regular Army dentists, 250 National Guard officers, and 5,197 Reserve officers were enrolled in the Dental Corps in September 1938; thus it appeared that if war came very few additional dentists would be required. It was also the opinion of The Surgeon General that dental officers could be procured rapidly and put on active duty with very little training, and it was frankly stated that no uneasiness need be felt even if the Dental Reserve fell to 50 percent of its authorized strength.[34] At this time it was certainly not foreseen that the Army would reach a strength of over 8 million men, that a drastic lowering of physical standards would be necessary, and that the 1.4 ratio, which had failed to measure up to the lesser needs during and following World War I, would be completely inadequate for this expanded force.

TABLE 3. OFFICERS CALLED TO ACTIVE DUTY IN THE DENTAL CORPS, BY COMPONENT, JANUARY 1939 THROUGH FEBRUARY 1946

Date	Component				Total
	Regular Army	Reserve	National Guard	Army of the United States	
1939					
Total	19	25			44
January					
February		1			1
March					
April					
May					
June					
July	13	2			15
August		2			2

[32] Monthly procurement of dental officers, 1 Jan 39 through Feb 46. Info furnished by Strength Acctg Br, AGO, 3 Jul 46.
[33] Memo, Col James E. Baylis, Tng Div, SGO, for SG, 6 Sep 38. [D]
[34] Ibid.

TABLE 3. OFFICERS CALLED TO ACTIVE DUTY IN THE DENTAL CORPS, BY COMPONENT, JANUARY 1939 THROUGH FEBRUARY 1946—Continued

Date	Component				Total
	Regular Army	Reserve	National Guard	Army of the United States	
1939					
September		3			3
October		1			1
November	6	9			15
December		7			7
1940					
Total	29	408	145		582
January			1		1
February		3	1		4
March		30			30
April		13	1		14
May		2			2
June	17	6			23
July	7	17			24
August		21			21
September		42	62		104
October		100	36		136
November		103	31		134
December	5	71	13		89
1941					
Total	6	1,938	165	48	2,157
January		125	57		182
February		159	71		230
March		202	31		233
April	1	340	3	1	345
May		218	1		219
June		140	1		141
July	4	250	1	1	256
August		150			150
September		120		1	121
October		119		12	131
November		62		23	85
December	1	53		10	64

TABLE 3. OFFICERS CALLED TO ACTIVE DUTY IN THE DENTAL CORPS, BY COMPONENT, JANUARY 1939 THROUGH FEBRUARY 1946—Continued

Date	Component				Total
	Regular Army	Reserve	National Guard	Army of the United States	
1942					
Total	21	1,134	1	5,670	6,826
January	1	126		179	306
February	2	77		97	176
March		85		34	119
April	4	157		149	310
May	1	149		292	442
June	5	95		457	557
July	4	259		966	1,229
August		100	1	1,038	1,139
September	3	56		1,171	1,230
October		13		561	574
November		15		356	371
December	1	2		370	373
1943					
Total		59		4,941	5,000
January		5		162	167
February		9		192	201
March		4		277	281
April		5		374	379
May		4		910	914
June		10		556	566
July		11		679	690
August		4		540	544
September		2		347	349
October		3		266	269
November				364	364
December		2		274	276
1944					
Total		40		1,889	1,929
January		4		346	350
February		14		536	550
March		5		108	113
April		8		129	137
May		1		58	59
June				19	19
July				104	104
August				5	5
September				117	117

TABLE 3. OFFICERS CALLED TO ACTIVE DUTY IN THE DENTAL CORPS, BY COMPONENT, JANUARY 1939 THROUGH FEBRUARY 1946—Continued

Date	Component				Total
	Regular Army	Reserve	National Guard	Army of the United States	
1944					
October		2		233	235
November		6		186	192
December				48	48
1945 Total		2		233	235
January		1		49	50
February				45	45
March		1		47	48
April				85	85
May				1	1
June				4	4
July					
August				1	1
September					
October					
November					
December				1	1
1946 Total				2	2
January				1	1
February				1	1
1939–1946 Aggregate	75	3,606	311	12,783	16,775

In September 1938, when the Dental Reserve had reached a level slightly over its authorized strength,[35] The Surgeon General recommended that all further procurement for that organization be suspended. This recommendation, which reflected the then optimistic attitude of The Surgeon General, was approved by the General Staff and, with a few exceptions (successful candidates for the Regular Army, recent graduates desiring immediate active duty) no new commissions were offered until October 1940.[36] Between 30 June 1938 and 30 June 1941 the Dental Corps Reserve suffered a net loss of 771 officers, in spite of the fact that 722 commissions were given young dentists during fiscal

---
[35] See footnote 33, p. 48.
[36] Ltr, ACofS, G-1 to TAG, 29 Sep 38, sub: Suspension of appointments in the Dental Reserve Corps. [D]

year 1941.[37] On the latter date the Dental Reserve numbered 4,428 officers.

Increases in the number of dentists on active duty were small prior to the inauguration of Selective Service in September 1940. The authorized strength of the Regular Army Dental Corps was raised to 316 officers in April 1939 [38] and about 50 Reserve officers were called to voluntary duty in April and September 1939.[39] On 30 June 1940, 354 dentists, including 101 Reserve officers, were on duty.[40]

By the end of July 1940, 150 Reserve dentists had accepted voluntary active service, but this number was 391 less than the total then required, and it was anticipated that 1,259 dentists would be needed when expansion under the Selective Service Act was started in October.[41] On 27 August 1940 the President was empowered to call to active duty, with or without consent, any member of the Reserve or National Guard.[42] Any officer below the grade of captain, with dependents, could resign, however, and a considerable number of Medical Department officers made use of this privilege.[43] By 26 October 1940 The Surgeon General foresaw an early exhaustion of the Dental Reserve and he recommended that the suspension on new commissions, which had been in effect since September 1938, be lifted without delay.[44] Three days later the ban was lifted to the extent of permitting the corps area commanders to fill existing vacancies.[45] Under current procurement objectives, however, there were very few dental vacancies at this time, and it was found impossible in some cases even to offer commissions to those few dentists who had been inducted as enlisted men.[46]

By 30 April 1941, 35.5 percent of all Dental Reserve officers were on active duty, though the proportion varied from 20 percent to 59 percent in different corps areas.[47]

On 5 May 1941 previous restrictions against new commissions in the Dental Reserve were further modified to permit the acceptance of any qualified dentists who had been inducted as enlisted men, and the corps areas were instructed to

---

[37] Annual Reports . . . Surgeon General, 1938–41. Washington, Government Printing Office, 1938–41.

[38] Sec 8, 53 Stat 558.

[39] See footnote 14, p. 36.

[40] Annual Report . . . Surgeon General, 1940. Washington, Government Printing Office, 1940.

[41] Ltr, SG to TAG, 6 Aug 40, sub: Shortage of Medical Department personnel. SG: 320.2–1.

[42] Annual Report . . . Surgeon General, 1941. Washington, Government Printing Office, 1941.

[43] Ltr, TAG to all CA or Dept Comdrs, 1 Sep 40, sub: Resignation of officers of the Officers' Reserve Corps. SG: 210.83–ORC.

[44] Ltr, Col Larry B. McAfee to TAG, 26 Oct 40, sub: Appointment in the Medical, Dental, and Veterinary Reserve Corps. AG: 210.1.

[45] Ltr, Col Larry B. McAfee to all CA surgs, 29 Oct 40, sub: Extended active duty vacancy required for approval of applicant for commission. [D]

[46] See footnote 16, p. 37.

[47] Ltr, TAG to all CGs, CofS, GHQ, Chiefs of all Arms and Services, 2 Jun 41, sub: Information as to the percentage of eligibile reserve officers who are on extended duty as of April 30, 1941. AG: 210.31–ORC.

encourage applications from persons in this category.[48] By 30 June 1941, 2,111 dental officers, predominantly Reserve, were on active duty.[49]

In October 1941 The Surgeon General reported some concern over the number of resignations and physical disqualifications in the Dental Reserve, and requested authority to reopen procurement in that branch. However, he still recommended against any great increase in the Reserve, since to grant commissions to men who could not be used by the Army would amount to conferring exemption from military service, which was properly the prerogative of the Selective Service System.[50] Apparently it was still believed that the Reserve, augmented with a few inductees and recent graduates, would be sufficient to meet anticipated needs. This optimism was not shared by the Federal Security Administrator, Paul V. McNutt. On 30 October 1941, in his recommendation to the President for the establishment of a Procurement and Assignment Service to insure the most economical use of limited medical personnel, Mr. McNutt also included a tentative plan for a draft of civilian professional men, should such action prove necessary.[51] The attitude of The Surgeon General at this time is probably explained by the fact that 2,905 dental officers were on duty, or only 6 less than the authorized procurement objective, and Pearl Harbor was still in the future.[52]

Three days after entrance of the United States into the war all releases from active duty, except for physical disability or incompetence, were suspended.[53] On 19 December the Medical Department was instructed to establish pools of medical personnel from which replacements could be made without delay. No specific level was prescribed for the Dental Corps, but 1,500 officers were to be maintained in such pools by the Medical Department as a whole.[54]

With the entry of the United States into actual hostilities the need for a rapid expansion of the Medical Department was clear. On 1 January 1942 The Surgeon General requested authority to call to duty 1,350 additional dentists,[55] but The Adjutant General approved an increase of 500 only.[56]

In the latter part of January 1942, it was directed that only a limited num-

---

[48] Rad, TAG to CGs all CAs, 5 May 41. AG : 210.1–ORC.
[49] Officers appointed in the Dental Corps from 1 January 1939 through February 1946. Info furnished by Strength Accounting Branch, AGO, 3 Jul 46. HD : 320.2.
[50] Memo, Lt Col R. C. Craven for TAG, 8 Oct 41. AG : 080 (ADA).
[51] Ltr, Paul V. McNutt, Federal Security Administrator, to the President, 30 Oct 41. [D]
[52] Lt Col Alfred Mordecai : A history of the Procurement and Assignment Service for physicians, dentists, veterinarians, sanitary engineers, and nurses, War Manpower Commission. HD : 314.7–2.
[53] Ltr, TAG to Chief of the Army Air Forces ; Commanding General, Air Force Combat Command ; Chief of Staff, GHQ ; and the Chiefs of all Arms and Services, 10 Dec 41, sub : Suspension of releases from active service. SG : 320.2–1.
[54] Ltr, TAG to Chief of each arm or service, 19 Dec 41, sub : Officer filler and loss replacements for ground arms and services. SG : 320.2–1.
[55] Ltr, SG to TAG, 1 Jan 42, sub : Procurement objective, Medical Department officers, Army of the United States. AG : 210.1.
[56] 1st ind, TAG to SG, 24 Jan 42, to ltr cited in footnote 55.

ber of Regular Army dental officers, varying from 2 in the Fifth Corps Area to 13 in the Fourth, would be allotted to corps area activities.[57]

On 12 April 1942 The Surgeon General was instructed by Services of Supply (SOS) to establish Medical Officer Recruiting Boards to commission officers in the field. This action was intended mainly to speed the lagging procurement of medical rather than dental officers, for dentists were not to be accepted unless they were under 37 years of age or had been classified I–A by their draft boards.

By May 1942 it was evident that the Army would reach a strength much greater than had been anticipated in prewar plans. In that month the Military Personnel Division, SOS, estimated that 7,110 dentists would be needed by 1 January 1943, as follows:[58]

```
Services of Supply ------------------------------------------------- 2,699
Operations and AGF ------------------------------------------------- 2,472
Army Air Force ----------------------------------------------------- 1,755
Pools ---------------------------------------------------------------- 184
```

As of 31 March 1942 there were 3,373 dental officers on duty and it was estimated that only 587 more could be obtained from the Reserve; it would therefore be necessary to make 3,150 new appointments in the Army of the United States (AUS) during the remainder of 1942.[59] On 3 July 1942 The Surgeon General reported that the procurement objective of 500 officers, authorized on 24 January, had been filled and he requested an additional objective of 4,000 dentists.[60] This time his request was approved in full within a few days.[61]

Some difficulty was expected in obtaining 4,000 more dentists for on 9 July 1942 The Adjutant General directed the corps areas to add dental officers to all Medical Officer Recruiting Boards and granted authority, for the first time, to consider applications for original appointments from the following:[62]

    1. Dentists between the ages of 37 and 45.
    2. Dentists qualified only for limited service.
    3. Dentists whose training and experience justified an original appointment above the grade of lieutenant.

Though dentists in these categories were to be accepted only by authority of The Surgeon General, they had not previously been placed on active duty under any circumstances. At about the same time the Dental Division, SGO, was directed to call to active service all physically qualified lieutenant colonels and colonels of the Reserve, a step which had been postponed as long as possible

---

[57] Ltr, TAG to all CA comdrs, 27 Jan 42, sub: Allotment of Regular Army officers for duty with the Corps Area Service Commands. AG : 320.2.
[58] Memo, Brig Gen James E. Wharton for Pers Off, SGO, 11 May 42. SG : 320.2–1.
[59] Ibid.
[60] Ltr, Lt Col Francis M. Fitts to CG, SOS, 3 Jul 42, sub: Procurement objective, Dental Corps, Army of the United States. SG : 320.2–1.
[61] Ltr, TAG to SG, 8 Jul 42, sub: Procurement objective, Army of the United States, for duty with Dental Corps (Surgeon General). SG : 320.2–1.
[62] Ltr, TAG to CGs all CAs, 9 Jul 42, sub: Dental Corps members for certain Medical Department recruiting boards. AG : SPX 210.31.

THE PROCUREMENT OF DENTAL OFFICERS 55

due to the difficulty of assigning men in the higher grades to appropriate positions.[63] Misgivings concerning dental procurement proved unfounded at this time. On 1 September 1942 dental representatives were removed from the Medical Officer Recruiting Boards and the latter were instructed not to accept any new dental applications.[64] A few days later the Dental Division, SGO, notified its liaison officer with the ADA that the objective of 4,000 officers authorized in July 1942, had nearly been filled and that commissions would thereafter be given only to men who had been declared Class I-A by their draft boards.[65] From September through November 1942 further procurement of dental officers was actually discouraged.

On 16 November 1942 The Surgeon General reported that there were 9,706 dental officers on duty, a number slightly in excess of current requirements. However, with mobilization plans providing for many more men than had been considered necessary at the beginning of the year, it was estimated that 17,248 dentists would be needed by the end of 1943. The Surgeon General therefore asked for a new procurement objective of 7,200 dental officers in addition to the 300 officers of the unexpended portion of the old objective.[66] This request was approved on 27 November.[67] On 15 January 1943 PAS, WMC, agreed to declare 400 civilian dentists available each month through the year, for a total of 4,800 dentists; the remaining 2,700 dental officers were to be obtained from the newly established Army Specialized Training Program (ASTP) (see chapter IV), from dentists inducted as enlisted men by Selective Service, and from students holding inactive Medical Administrative Corps Reserve commissions.[68]

During the first months of 1943, the program to meet the procurement objective of 7,500 dental officers lagged somewhat, though difficulties of dental procurement were overshadowed by the much more acute shortage of medical officers. In February the Dental Division asked that PAS speed its activities as only 269 dentists had been declared available since 1 January. In April, the Medical Department was still short 1,042 dentists and 6,677 physicians, but by May, when the situation in respect to medical officers was grave, some improvement was noted in the procurement of dental officers.[69] Though Selective Service placed dentists in the "scarce" category at about this time,[70] this action was intended only to prevent the waste of dental manpower in nonprofessional activities, and on 22 May representatives of the War Department

---
[63] See footnote 21, p. 44.
[64] Rad, TAG to CG, 1st SvC, 1 Sep 42. SG: 210.31-1.
[65] Ltr, Col Robert C. Craven to Maj Kenneth R. Cofield, 4 Sep 42. [D]
[66] Ltr, SG to CG, SOS, 16 Nov 42, sub: 1943 procurement objective, Dental Corps, Army of the United States. SG: 320.2-1.
[67] Ltr, TAG to SG, 27 Nov 42, sub: Increase in procurement objective, Army of the United States, for The Surgeon General (Dental Corps). SG: 320.2-1.
[68] See footnote 52, p. 53.
[69] Ltr, SG to ACofS, G-1, 13 May 43, sub: Procurement of physicians and dentists. AG: 210.1.
[70] WD Memo W605-23-43, 15 May 43, sub: Scarce categories of specialized skills. AG: 210.1.

and PAS found that "the dental picture was not alarming." [71] By the end of June 1943, 12,046 dental officers were on duty, and half of the year's objective had been obtained.[72]

On 7 September 1943, when about 13,500 dentists were in the service, ASF placed an arbitrary ceiling of 15,200 officers on the Dental Corps. It was then estimated that in addition to graduates of the ASTP and students holding Reserve Medical Administrative Corps commissions only 1,124 more dentists would be needed from civil life. Both PAS and the Officer Procurement Service (OPS) of the ASF were notified not to accept additional applications from dentists who were over 38 years of age or who were not physically fit for unlimited military service. This action is especially significant when it is noted that at this same time The Surgeon General was seriously considering a draft of 12,000 physicians.[73] By 9 December 1943, over 14,200 dental officers were in the military service and further procurement from civilian sources, other than from students in the ASTP or the Medical Administrative Corps Reserve, was stopped.[74]

On 16 December 1943, The Surgeon General agreed, at the request of the Veterans Administration, to commission all dentists of that agency who were under 63 years of age, and about 170 dental officers in this category were ultimately accepted. These men remained in their normal duties with the Veterans Administration.[75]

Peculiarly, serious difficulties in dental procurement did not arise until the Dental Service approached its maximum strength in the spring of 1944, and then the principal problem was not to obtain replacements, but to find vacancies for graduates of the ASTP and for such dentists as might be inducted by Selective Service. At that time the Dental Corps numbered nearly 15,000 officers, many of whom had already been on active duty for 2 to 3 years. Very few of these men could be returned to civilian life under existing directives, and natural attrition had proved to be much less than expected. On the other hand, the ASTP had been established early in 1943 to provide about 825 dental officers every 9 months, and unless vacancies could be found for them they would have to be released to private practice after the Government had given them draft exemption and paid for a considerable part of their professional training.

The Dental Division and the War Department did not agree on the best solution for this problem. The Dental Division was influenced mainly by the fessional training.

---

[71] Minutes of Conf between the Directing Board, PAS, and representatives of the WD, 22 May 43. On file Natl Archives, PAS files, WMC.

[72] Annual Report . . . Surgeon General for CG, ASF, (1943). HD: 319.1–2.

[73] Draft of proposed call on Selective Service for the conscription of 12,000 physicians, submitted to The Surgeon General on 9 Oct 43 by Lt Col Durward G. Hall. [D]

[74] Ltr, Col Durward G. Hall to Exec Off, PAS, 10 Dec 43, sub: Cancellation of further procurement of dentists. [D]

[75] Annual Rpt, Procmt Br, Mil Pers Div SGO, 1943. HD: 319.1–2.

through the discharge of surplus, overage officers or by the reclassification of the inefficient. The effectiveness of this step was largely nullified, however, by the fact that the dental ASTP would graduate its last student in April 1945, in contrast to the medical ASTP which would continue to provide replacements until January 1948. No authority was given at this time to commission graduates holding Medical Administrative Corps Reserve commissions or dentists who might be inducted, though the latter could be discharged under existing regulations.[85] On 28 August 1944 The Surgeon General was further advised that some 300 senior students holding Medical Administrative Corps Reserve commissions could be placed on active duty on graduation.[86]

Peak strength of the Dental Corps was reached in November 1944, when 15,292 officers were on duty.[87] At the end of 1944 there were 15,110 dental officers in the service.[88] Only 1,418 dentists had been commissioned during the year, as follows: [89]

Graduates of the dental ASTP	997
Graduates with Reserve MAC commissions	94
Civilians (other than inductees)	324
Dentists inducted as enlisted men	3

From 1 August through 31 December, 503 officers had been discharged, mainly to create vacancies for younger men, and at the end of the year 212 still awaited separation under previous commitments.[90]

By 1945 the dental procurement picture was beginning to change. The Dental Corps remained at just a little under authorized maximum strength, but the only prospective replacements were the 218 senior ASTP students who were to graduate in April and 180 students holding Reserve Medical Administrative Corps commissions, many of whom might be rejected for physical defects. Nine hundred former ASTP students would graduate after April, but they had been unconditionally released by the Army in June 1944 and the Military Personnel Division of the SGO was very doubtful if G-1 could be "sold" on any new procurement program from civilian life.[91]

Early in February 1945 a dental officer with the Military Personnel Division, SGO, noted the possibility of a later shortage of dentists, and that office warned the Director of the Dental Division that future procurement was pre-

---

[85] AR 615-360, 25 May 44.

[86] Ltr, Maj F. E. Golembieski to SG, 28 Aug 44, sub: Appointment of inactive Medical Administrative Corps dental graduates. Quoted in semiannual report, Pers Serv, SGO, 1 Jul-31 Dec 44, Incl 10. HD: 319.1-2.

[87] Memo, Mr. Isaac Cogan for Chief, Dental Cons Div, SGO, 8 Oct 46, sub: Basic data for Dental Corps. SG: 322.0531. The figure given includes officers with the Veterans Administration, traveling, or sick. It does not include officers on terminal leave, officers enroute home for discharge, or officers sick in hospital, not expected to return to duty.

[88] Data from Resources Anal Div, SGO. [D]

[89] Annual Report, Pers Oprs Br, Pers Serv SGO, 1944. HD: 319.1-2.

[90] Memo, Maj Ernest J. Fedor for Chief, Procmt Br, Pers Serv SGO, 17 Jan 45, sub: Dental Corps active duty strength. HD: 314.

[91] Ibid.

carious and that conservation of dental officers would be necessary.[92] More revealing was a note attached to this correspondence, in which the Director of the Military Personnel Division recommended to his own personnel that "we slow down on the Release and Separation Board in the Military Personnel Division; take no more (dentists) in nor request any new procurement objective; let attrition go below the ceiling and gamble on redeployment and partial demobilization overtaking us." Apparently it was believed at this time that most procurement troubles would be over with the expected end of hostilities, and if dental officers were required for the postwar period they could be obtained through Selective Service. The possibility that demobilization might actually result in a temporary increase in the demand for dental treatment had been mentioned as early as June 1944, but it seems not to have been considered too seriously.[93]

When the war ended in Europe the Dental Corps numbered 14,700 officers, providing an overall ratio of 1.8 dentists for each 1,000 troops, or 2.6 per 1,000 in the United States and 1.3 per 1,000 overseas.[94]

Soon after V-E Day The Adjutant General suggested a review of the procurement objectives for dental officers to determine if they might not be reduced in view of changed conditions. In reply The Surgeon General noted that previous sources of replacements were rapidly drying up and he asked that: [95]

1. Present authority to commission Medical Administrative Reserve Corps graduates, applying only to those who had been enrolled in the senior class as of 1 July 1944, be extended throughout 1945.

2. Authority be granted to commission any dentist inducted as an enlisted man, rather than discharge him under current instructions.

It was not expected that these measures would suffice to maintain the existing strength of the Dental Corps, but it was believed that they would enable the Dental Service to meet the lessened demand for treatment which might accompany a decrease in the total strength of the Army. No action was taken on this request. By July 1945 The Surgeon General anticipated a shortage of 475 dental officers by the end of the year, and he recommended that the Dental Corps be maintained at 15,000 officers (exclusive of those with the Veterans Administration) until March 1946. He further advised that 805 new dental officers be obtained, as follows: [96]

Students holding MAC commissions	70
Inducted dentists	35
Former ASTP students	700

---

[92] Memo, Lt Col Durward G. Hall for Maj Gen R. H. Mills, 8 Feb 45, sub: Dental Corps officers. SG: 322.0531.
[93] See footnote 83, p. 58.
[94] See footnote 87, p. 59.
[95] Memo, SG for AG, Appointment and Induction Br, Appointment Sec, 4 Jun 45, sub: Procurement objective for appointment in the Army of the United States. AG: 210.1 (G-1).
[96] Memo, Brig Gen R. W. Bliss for ACofS, G-1, 6 Jul 45, sub: Ceiling and procurement objective for Dental Corps officers. HD: 314.

1. During the early stages of mobilization some men had been commissioned who were physically or mentally incapable of performing their duties efficiently. Their presence decreased the effectiveness of the entire Dental Service.

2. Long before the start of actual hostilities many Reserve officers had volunteered for active duty in the emergency. After 3 years of service, during which their colleagues at home had enjoyed exceptionally high incomes, these officers were anxious to return to their offices as soon as they could be spared. It was believed that if ASTP graduates were released while the older men were held in the Army the resulting drop in morale would be catastrophic.

The Dental Division therefore wished to replace older men with recent graduates who had no family ties and who might be expected to be available during the demobilization period.

The War Department, on the other hand, apparently attached more importance to the following considerations:

1. Any great turnover in dental personnel would mean wasted effort in training replacements.

2. Officers with several years of service were considered the most valuable to the Army, and it was doubted if recent graduates of the curtailed dental course would be equal in ability to men with 5 to 20 years of practical experience.

3. Line officers and enlisted men who had proved themselves in combat could be replaced only at the cost of American lives; they had to be retained until the last battle was won. To release dental officers, who generally lived a less dangerous and rigorous life, while combat personnel had to remain in the fighting, might seriously impair the morale of the latter.

For these reasons the War Department at first preferred to keep the older officers in service, even at the expense of discharging recent graduates under the Army training program. It later changed its attitude to conform more nearly to that of the Dental Division, but this did not occur until the graduating class of June 1944 had been lost and the dental ASTP had been terminated.[76]

On 11 March 1944 The Surgeon General, at the request of the Dental Division, advised the Military Personnel Division, ASF, that the authorized ceiling for dental officers had been reached; in addition, that approximately 1,294 ASTP students would graduate during the remainder of the year. At the same time he noted that many dental officers were in a "limited service" status and he recommended that the following be relieved from active duty in numbers sufficient to make room for the younger men:[77]

---

[76] Data on reasons for War Department opposition to the discharge of older dental officers in early 1944 have been difficult to obtain, and reliance has had to be placed on information given by officers on duty in the War Department at the time. Considerable material has been obtained from Maj Ernest J. Fedor, who was dental liaison officer with the Military Personnel Division, SGO, during much of the war. There is some reason to believe that the War Department saw the advantages of replacing the older officers, but that it wished to avoid a categorical statement of policy which would receive wide publicity and which might lead to criticism by line personnel who could not be included.

[77] Memo, Col Robert J. Carpenter, Exec Off SGO, for Dir Mil Pers Div, ASF, 11 Mar 44. SG: 322.0531.

1. Any dentist over 45 years of age who was classified "limited service."

2. Dentists over 38 years of age who were recommended for release by corps area commanders. This provision was expected to authorize the discharge of men who were not sufficiently incompetent to be released under existing criteria, but who were of doubtful value to the dental service.

This request was disapproved on the grounds that existing directives were adequate to assure the discharge of inefficient officers. The primary purpose of this proposal, to create vacancies, was apparently given little consideration.[78] On 1 April 1944, however, Lt. Col. Durward G. Hall, of the Military Personnel Division, SGO, reported to The Surgeon General that he had received informal, verbal authority to exceed the official ceiling for short periods of time to permit the commissioning of some ASTP graduates, and that he had also been instructed to release enough dentists over 40 years of age to maintain the required level. G-1 and ASF refused to confirm these agreements in writing, however, and Colonel Hall was doubtful concerning the advisability of putting them in effect.[79]

On 16 May 1944 the Director of the Dental Division was informed by the Military Personnel Division, SGO, that due to a lack of vacancies no graduates of the class of June 1944 would be commissioned in the Army, though some names would be referred to the Veterans Administration and the Navy.[80] About 225 dental ASTP graduates were actually commissioned at this time by the Navy.[81] Shortly thereafter the dental ASTP was terminated, except for senior students who would finish their courses by 1945.[82] While The Surgeon General advised against this step, even he apparently underestimated the difficulties which would be encountered in maintaining a Dental Service for a million or more men in the postwar period, after wartime officers had been discharged and Selective Service had been terminated. On 5 June 1944 he stated that while it "might be desirable from some points of view to grant at least some appointments to ASTP graduates," such action was "not justified in view of the present strength of the corps."[83]

A partial change of attitude on the part of the War Department General Staff was registered in July 1944 when the Commanding General, ASF, was directed to commission qualified ASTP students graduating after June 1944 if they were not desired by the Navy.[84] Necessary vacancies were to be created

---

[78] Memo, Brig Gen R. B. Reynolds, Mil Pers Div, ASF, for SG, 25 Mar 44, sub: Relief from active duty of temporary officers of Dental Corps over 40 years of age on permanent limited duty status. HD: 314.

[79] Memo, Lt Col Durward G. Hall for Dep SG, 1 Apr 44. [D]

[80] Memo, Maj Ernest J. Fedor for Maj Gen R. H. Mills, 16 May 44, sub: Disposition of dental ASTP graduates who will complete their course in dentistry during the month of June 1944. [D]

[81] Ltr, Capt W. F. Peterson to SG, 10 Oct 44, sub: ASTP dental students commissioned in the U. S. Naval Reserve. [D]

[82] See discussion of the Dental ASTP in chapter IV.

[83] Memo, Brig Gen R. W. Bliss for CG, ASF, 5 Jun 44, sub: Requirements for Dental Corps officers. SG: 322.053-1.

[84] Memo, Maj Gen M. G. White for CG, ASF, 18 Jul 44, sub: ASTP dental program. Quoted in semiannual report, Pers Serv, SGO, 1 Jul–31 Dec 44. HD: 319.1-2.

On 18 July the General Staff approved these recommendations.[97] It must be noted, however, that the Army had no hold on former ASTP students who did not choose to volunteer, and instructions to the service commands actually specified that no persuasion would be used in recruiting from that category. Nor were applications from civilian dentists, other than former ASTP students, to be accepted.[98] This limited, largely voluntary program produced very little result.

Soon after the collapse of Japan all procurement of officers was stopped by a blanket order issued by The Adjutant General.[99] By this time the Dental Corps was down to 13,600 men, and on 20 September the Deputy Surgeon General requested that the commissioning of MAC students be resumed to permit the earlier discharge of older dentists. This time no mention was made of procuring former ASTP students then in civilian status.[100] This request of the Deputy Surgeon General was approved about a month later, but it could have little effect in any event since there were only 173 MAC students remaining in the schools, and rejections for physical disability were high because a large proportion of the physically fit had given up their Reserve status to enter the ASTP.[101] By the end of the year the strength of the Dental Corps was down to 9,600 men.[102] Serious personnel difficulties were still not anticipated in this period as evidenced by General Mills' statement in October that, even though dentists were being discharged in connection with the reduction of the Army, no major procurement program was being considered.[103]

With the sudden end of the war, pressure for the release of veteran Medical Department officers mounted rapidly, to a point where a congressional investigation was threatened. In particular, the Office of The Surgeon General was flooded with letters protesting the fact that men with several years of service were being held in the Army while students who had been given deferment and whose education had been partially paid for by the Government were being released to private practice.[104] Nevertheless, it was found necessary to maintain considerable forces to meet unexpected postwar responsibilities.

Information on the total number of dentists to serve with the Army Dental Corps during the war is not completely reliable. The Strength Account-

---

[97] Ltr, TAG to SG, 18 Jul 45, sub: Ceiling and procurement objective for Dental Corps officers. AG : 210.1 (G-1).

[98] Ltr, CG, ASF, to CG, 1st SvC, 25 Jul 45, sub: Procurement of dental officers. AG : 210.1.

[99] Ltr, TAG to all agencies having procurement objectives, 2 Sep 45, sub: Cancellation of procurement objectives. AG : 210.1.

[100] Ltr, Maj Gen Geo. F. Lull to ACofS, G-1, 20 Sep 45, sub: Waiver of procurement objectives for appointment as second lieutenants MAC-AUS (students, interns) as first lieutenants, Medical and Dental Corps, AUS. AG : 210.1.

[101] Ltr, TAG to SG, 13 Oct 45, sub: Appointments of second lieutenants, MAC-AUS, as first lieutenants, Medical and/or Dental Corps, AUS. AG : 210.1.

[102] See footnote 88, p. 59.

[103] Ltr, Maj Gen R. H. Mills to Capt D. E. Cooper, 26 Oct 45, no sub. SG : 210.8.

[104] Nearly the whole of SGO file 322.0531 for the year 1946 is taken up with complaints against the release of former Dental ASTP students.

ing Branch, AGO, reported that 16,775 dentists were called to active duty from 1 January 1939 through 28 February 1946,[105] for a total of about 17,100 men, including Regular Army and Reserve personnel already serving at the start of the war. The Resources Analysis Division, SGO, however, estimated that about 18,000 dentists were on duty between October 1940 and the end of 1945.[106]

SOURCES AND METHODS OF PROCUREMENT FOR DENTAL OFFICERS, WORLD WAR II

General Considerations

On V-E Day the Army Dental Corps was made up of the following categories: [107] [108]

Component	Number of officers	Percentage of total strength
Regular Army	266	1.7
National Guard	117	0.8
Organized Reserve	3,106	20.3
AUS (ASTP graduates)	1,802	11.8
AUS (from civil life)	10,011	65.4

Regular Army

Since Regular Army dental officers were chosen in highly competitive examinations and received thorough training they were generally well qualified in the broad aspects of their profession. A few of the 250 Regular Army dental officers were unfitted for higher administrative duties by temperamental or other defects, but the majority were well trained in that field (see chapter IV) and they filled key positions with credit to themselves and the service. Prewar clinical training, however, had not encouraged the development of skilled specialists. In an era when a high proportion of posts was small, the average Army dentist had to be able to handle a case of periodontoclasia, treat a fractured mandible, construct a denture, or supervise a station laboratory, and emphasis was placed on all-round ability rather than on qualification in a single narrow field. Few dental officers had been able to limit their practices to one branch of dentistry. With the exception of certain outstanding individuals, therefore, the Dental Service had to rely heavily on Reserve officers or former civilians to provide the more complicated types of treatment.

The Regular Army Dental Corps was also unbalanced in respect to age and experience. Of the 269 officers on duty in April 1942, nearly 100 had been

---

[105] See footnote 32, p. 48.
[106] Memo, Mr. Isaac Cogan for Dir, Dental Div, 29 Aug 46, sub: Dental Corps officers, historical data. SG: 322.053-1.
[107] Ibid.
[108] The total given here, 15,302, is slightly higher than the number actually on duty on V-E Day as it includes a few officers who had been released but whose discharge had not yet been reported. For other data on race, age, and clinical qualifications see chapter IV.

in the service for 24 years or longer; another 100 had approximately 5 years or less of active duty, leaving only about 70 men with from 6 to 23 years of service. One hundred and two dental officers were in the grades of colonel or lieutenant colonel, 146 were in grades of captain or lieutenant, and only 21 officers were in the grade of major, where maximum physical vigor was combined with at least 12 years of experience.[109] This situation was unavoidable since it had originated in the rapid expansion of the Dental Service during and immediately following the First World War, and it would be corrected by natural attrition over a period of years.

At best, the Regular Army Dental Corps provided only about 1½ percent of the 17,000 to 18,000 dentists who were on duty with the land forces at some time during the war.

National Guard

The 250 dental officers in the National Guard at the start of the war provided a nucleus of personnel who had had some service with their units in the field and who were available on very short notice. New commissions in the National Guard brought the total taken on active duty from that source to 311 officers,[110] but like the Regular Army, the Guard was too small to provide a significant part of the total treatment required in a major mobilization. In general, the training and efficiency of National Guard dentists was comparable to that of Reserve officers, with the difference that they had generally had the benefit of slightly more practical experience.

The Organized Reserves

On 6 September 1938, 5,197 officers were enrolled in the Dental Reserve, a figure exceeding the authorized total by 97 officers. At that time it was expected that 5,100 Reserve dentists, plus about 500 Regular Army and National Guard officers, would be sufficient for the force of about 4 million men which might be mobilized in an emergency. So little concern was felt over dental procurement that the granting of new Reserve commissions was immediately stopped,[111] and it was not resumed for more than two years.[112] During this period the Dental Reserve lost 771 officers, and 30 June 1941 it was down to a strength of 4,428 men, distributed in the following grades:[113]

Colonel	7
Lieutenant colonel	96
Major	354
Captain	909
Lieutenant	3,062

---

[109] Army Directory for 20 April 1942.
[110] See footnote 49, p. 53.
[111] See footnote 36, p. 51.
[112] See footnote 45, p. 52.
[113] See footnote 42, p. 52.

Prior to the start of hostilities in Europe a negligible number of Dental Reserve officers had been on active duty with the Civilian Conservation Corps. A few more had been taken on duty in connection with increases in the Air Force and for reinforcement of the defenses of Panama. Thus, on 30 June 1940, 101 Reserve dentists were on voluntary active service.[114]

On 18 November 1940, maximum age limits for initial active duty with the Reserve were established as follows:[115]

1. For troop duty, not more than five years above maximum prescribed for initial appointment in the grade held.

2. For duty other than with troops:

Colonel	60 years
Lieutenant colonel	58 years
Major	54 years
Captain	50 years
Lieutenant	47 years

On 19 February 1941 it was directed that Reserve officers would be assigned on the same basis as Regular Army officers, with no restrictions on the positions they might fill.[116]

At the end of June 1941, there were 2,090 Reserve and National Guard dental officers on active duty.[117] By the end of the year the number had reached about 2,900.[118] On 7 November 1941 it was directed that, with a few exceptions, dentists taken on active duty directly from civilian life would thereafter be commissioned in the Army of the United States, which was the temporary emergency force, rather than in the permanent Reserve.[119] On 15 April 1942, when about 3,220 Reserve and National Guard dental officers had been called,[120] The Surgeon General reported that the Medical Department Reserve was nearly exhausted, so far as physically fit officers in usable grades were concerned, and that emphasis would thereafter have to be directed toward the procurement of civilians with no previous military training.

From 1 January 1939 through February 1946 a total of 3,606 Dental Reserve officers were called to active duty.[121] However, it cannot be stated what proportion of the 4,428 dental reservists listed on 30 June 1941 saw active

---

[114] Ibid.

[115] Ltr, TAG to CGs Hawaiian, Panama Canal, Philippine, and Puerto Rican Depts; each Chief of Arm and Service; and each CA Comdr, 18 Nov 40, sub: Reserve officers, resident in overseas departments, for extended active duty under Public Resolution 96, 76th Congress. AG: 210.31-1.

[116] Ltr, TAG to all Comdrs of CAs and Depts, each Chief of Arm and Service, and CGs 1st, 2d, 3d, and 4th armies, 19 Feb 41, sub: Administrative status of Reserve officers on extended active duty. AG: 210.31 ORC.

[117] See footnote 42, p. 52.

[118] See footnote 55, p. 53.

[119] Ltr, TAG to CGs of all armies, CAs, and Depts, Chiefs of Arms and Services, and chiefs of other sections of the WD Overhead, 7 Nov 41, sub: Policies relating to appointments in the Army of the United States under the provisions of PL 252, 77th Congress. AG: 210.1.

[120] Ltr, Lt Col John A. Rogers, SGO (no addressee indicated), 23 Apr 42, sub: Appointment in the Army of the United States (Medical Department). SG: 320.2-1.

[121] See footnote 49, p. 53.

duty, because additional commissions were granted between that date and 7 November 1941 when new commissions in the Reserve were discontinued. It seems probable that the figure was close to 75 percent.

Before Selective Service and PAS could be established the Reserve supplied trained dental officers when they were immediately needed. In general, these officers performed their duties creditably. Their training had not always been sufficient, however, to enable them to fill the more critical positions, and the classification of Reserve officers had not been accurate enough to permit assignment of specially qualified individuals to appropriate functions. Above all, the wartime experiences of many Reserve officers led them to doubt the advantages of belonging to that organization. Prior to the war the principal inducements for entering the Reserve, besides patriotism, had been (1) assurance that the dentist would serve in the field for which he was trained, and (2) the prospect that in time of emergency the superior training of the Reserve officer would put him in a favorable position for promotion and assignment. Events showed that there was little danger that any dentist would have to serve in enlisted status, and the Reserve dentist in the grade of captain or lieutenant seemed to have little more chance for promotion than the dentist called directly from civil life. As previous incentives for accepting Reserve commissions diminished in importance it seemed probable that postwar procurement for that organization would have to be stimulated by financial remuneration in the form of pay for the time expended or as retirement privileges.

Interviews with senior dental officers have brought out the following comments concerning the effectiveness of the Dental Reserve Corps:[122] [123]

1. The patriotism, zeal, and professional qualifications of the average Reserve dentist were above criticism.

2. The Dental Reserve supplied essential officers during the most critical period of the mobilization for war, before the Selective Service System was in effective operation. Officers were obtained in a more orderly way through the Reserve than would have been possible through Selective Service, at least until the establishment of the PAS.

3. Reserve officers in the lower grades were able to assume their military duties immediately, with little or no additional training. Some, though not all, of the senior officers successfully filled key positions when the Dental Service was filled out with former civilians with no previous experience.

4. Some senior officers of the Reserve were found to lack the experience and training required in important positions, and since routine chair work was not appropriate for their high grades their proper assignment was extremely difficult. This was not necessarily the fault of the officer himself since he had usually fulfilled the requirements for promotion to the field grades, but sporadic

---

[122] Final Report of The Surgeon General, Medical Department Personnel, included in ASF report on Logistics in World War II, 1945. HD: 319.1–2.

[123] See footnote 21, p. 44.

correspondence courses and occasional 2-week periods of active duty were simply not sufficient preparation for major administrative duties which bore little resemblance to the officer's peacetime activities. In some aggravated cases senior officers of the Reserve had actually given up the practice of their profession years before and were engaged in other occupations. When such men were called upon to instruct juniors or to operate larger installations, the Dental Service inevitably suffered.

5. Prior to the war, classification of Reserve officers was defective and little accurate information was available concerning their true qualifications. As a result, most Reserve dentists were immediately assigned to tactical commands where it was believed they could be most useful, and many clinical experts were lost to professional centers where they were badly needed. The men themselves were discouraged when their special skills were not employed.

6. In the year of the "phony" war, before Pearl Harbor had emphasized the national danger, Reserve officers were called from their homes and practices to staff the clinics of an Army assembled primarily for training purposes. Meanwhile, their competitors enjoyed the "boom." Under these conditions some Reserve officers felt that they had been called upon to make uncalled-for sacrifices for their patriotism. If they had been encouraged by the thought that they would get quicker promotion in the coming expansion, their disappointment was even more acute when some of these same competitors demanded, and received, higher grades as the price of volunteering for active duty, while the Reserve officer remained assigned to a tactical unit where promotion was stagnated. (This complaint was more frequent in the Medical Corps than in the Dental Corps, where few initial appointments were given above the grade of captain.) Also, the very fact that a Reserve officer had some training in military matters often led to his assignment to a tactical organization, where opportunities for the practice of his profession were poorest, while the man without military experience was sent to a hospital where he maintained or improved his skill and where he lived under much more pleasant conditions. Finally, when it was announced in 1944 that ASTP graduates would be released to private practice, while Reserve officers with 3 years or more of service would be kept in the Army, criticism from Dental Reserve officers reached a new peak, though the Office of The Surgeon General was in no way responsible for that decision. The experiences of some of these officers led them to advise young graduates to stay out of the Reserve and take their chances on induction, especially since there was little probability that they would have to serve as enlisted men in any event.[124]

World War II experience also indicated the need for more comprehensive training and more practical experience for Dental Reserve officers in the higher grades.

---

[124] Personal Ltr, Dr. Charles W. Freeman, Dean, Northwestern University Dental School, to Maj Maurice E. Washburn, 21 May 46. SG : 322.0531.

ASTP, Medical Administrative Corps Reserve, Enlisted Reserve

The procurement of some 1,900 dental officers through the ASTP, and of approximately 1,200 through the MAC and Enlisted Reserves, is discussed in Chapter IV. These men were generally recent graduates who entered the service in the lowest grade, directly from school. They were already obligated to render military service, and had not been engaged in essential civilian practice, so their procurement offered no special problems.

Selective Service and Dental Procurement

It has been pointed out that until the spring of 1942 the Dental Service was expanded mainly with officers from the Reserve and National Guard. The Surgeon General was able to pass on every application for these branches, to insure compliance with professional, moral, and ethical standards, and the number taken from civil practice did not constitute a serious threat to civilian dental care. As these sources approached exhaustion, however, and as prospective requirements loomed larger, emphasis was switched to the procurement of dentists engaged in private practice who lacked previous connection with the Armed Forces. By V-E Day nearly two-thirds of the Dental Corps consisted of men taken directly from civil life.[125] As it became necessary to dip deeper into the reservoir of civilian practitioners The Surgeon General had to rely on other agencies to assist in locating eligible men, determining if they could be spared from their communities, and inducing them to accept active duty.

The first official, nonmilitary agency to enter the dental procurement field was the Selective Service System. As the only authority which could order an individual into the Armed Forces, this organization had great potential importance for the Dental Service, but for some time after it was established late in 1940 its activities proved more embarrassing than helpful, for the following reasons:

1. The Selective Service law provided for the deferment of persons essential to the national health or welfare, but blanket deferment on an occupational basis was specifically prohibited. The responsibility for determining which individuals were actually indispensable rested mainly on the local draft boards. Neither the heads of the Selective Service System nor the members of local boards were at first seriously concerned over the possibility that a shortage of dental personnel might develop, and the latter did not hesitate to induct dentists who were not at the moment urgently essential in their communities. On the other hand, the ADA and The Surgeon General believed that the dental personnel situation was cause for alarm, and that serious difficulties could be avoided only if every dentist were employed according to his skills.[126]

---
[125] See footnote 106, p. 62.
[126] Memo, Brig Gen Albert G. Love for ACofS, G–1, 25 Mar 41. HD: 314.

Since there were very few vacancies in the Dental Reserve, it appeared that dentists inducted into the Army would have to serve as enlisted men in duties which could be performed equally well by less highly trained personnel. The Surgeon General warned the War Department that it would be the target of widespread criticism from the profession and from civilian communities if the services of badly needed dentists were wasted in relatively minor activities.

2. Selective Service boards were not technically qualified to pass on questions of professional qualifications or ethics, nor were they greatly concerned with such matters. They therefore tended to induct dentists who could not have been commissioned by the Army, even if vacancies had existed. In some instances, in fact, the boards apparently selected for induction those dentists who were considered least valuable to the community, and such men were likely to be of doubtful value to the services as well.[127]

The Surgeon General was powerless to prevent the induction of dentists by Selective Service, but he attempted, unsuccessfully at first, to provide for the commissioning of qualified inductees in the Dental Corps. On the same day that the Selective Service System was established The Surgeon General reminded The Adjutant General that commissions in the Medical Department Reserve had been suspended since December 1939 [128] and that professional personnel who would later be in short supply would probably be inducted as enlisted men. He recommended that commissions be offered any inducted physician, dentist, or veterinarian, and those who faced imminent induction.[129] A notation on this letter states that it was "returned informally," apparently without action. Substantially the same request was repeated on 26 October 1940,[130] and on 29 October the corps areas were authorized to resume commissioning Medical Department personnel to fill actual vacancies.[131] Dental vacancies were practically nonexistent at this time, however, so this directive had little effect so far as the Dental Corps was concerned. In November 1940 The Surgeon General asked the corps areas to save the few available dental vacancies for men who might be inducted,[132] but even this slight gain was shortlived since the granting of new commissions was again suspended on 8 December 1940.[133] Procurement to fill vacancies in the Medical Department was again resumed on 19 December [134] but The Surgeon General again reported that there

---

[127] Interv by the author with Maj Gen R. H. Mills (6 Oct 47) and Maj Ernest J. Fedor (24 Nov 47).

[128] Commissions in the Dental Reserve had actually been suspended since September 1938.

[129] Ltr, Col Larry B. McAfee to TAG, 16 Sep 40, sub: Appointment in the Medical, Dental, and Veterinary Corps Reserve. [D]

[130] See footnote 44, p. 52.

[131] See footnote 45, p. 52.

[132] The original radiogram from The Surgeon General has not been found. It is mentioned in "Preparedness and War Activities of the American Dental Association: A résumé." J. Am. Dent. A. 33 : 80, 1 Jan 46.

[133] Ltr, TAG to CA and Dept Comdrs, 8 Dec 40, sub: Suspension of Appointments in the Officers' Reserve Corps. [D]

[134] Ltr, TAG to each CA and Dept Comdr, and SG, 19 Dec 40, sub: Appointments in the Medical Department Reserve. [D]

THE PROCUREMENT OF DENTAL OFFICERS

The action of the Army in making it possible to offer commissions to inducted dentists solved only half of the problem, however. It still did not prevent the more or less indiscriminate conscription of men who were not immediately needed or wanted by the Armed Forces or who were in essential civilian positions. By the spring of 1941 Selective Service itself was beginning to show some alarm over the professional personnel situation, and on 22 April it cautioned the local boards that a shortage of dentists *might* impend.[150] This tentative warning was confirmed on 30 April.[151] Local boards were then reminded that (1) they still had full responsibility for determining if a dentist was indispensable in his own community, (2) the Army did not need dentists for the time being, and (3) if a board felt that a dentist should be inducted anyway he should be notified that he might apply for a commission as soon as he entered active duty. This directive had the effect of discouraging the draft of dentists, though it did not categorically prohibit such action.

In January 1942 Selective Service advised its boards that it was essential that all dentists be used where their services would do the most good, and it directed that the recently formed PAS, WMC, be consulted in determining essentiality.[152] This regulation was obviously not intended to confer blanket exemption on dentists, however, since the boards were notified at the same time that when dependency was the only cause for deferment it should be kept in mind that the salary of a commisioned officer was normally sufficient for the support of a family. In February 1942 the Director of the Dental Division reported that dentists were still being inducted, and he recommended that Selective Service modify its regulations to prevent the conscription of Medical Department personnel except with the advice and consent of the PAS.[153] No formal action was taken on this request, but within 2 months the ADA reported that Selective Service boards were generally deferring dentists, at least until the PAS could be placed in full operation.[154] In December 1942 Selective Service again advised the local boards to give careful consideration to the occupational deferment of dentists,[155] and the conscription of professional personnel was thereafter a very minor problem, though it did not cease entirely.

---

[150] Memo, Dir, Selective Service System, for all State Directors, No. I-62, 22 Apr 41, sub: Occupational deferment of students and other necessary men in certain specialized professional fields (III). On file Natl Hq Selective Service System.

[151] Telegram, Dir, Selective Service System, to all State Directors, 30 Apr 41. On file Natl Hq Selective Service System.

[152] Memo, Dir, Selective Service, for all State Directors (I-363), 28 Jan 42, sub: Occupational deferments of medical doctors, dentists, and doctors of veterinary medicine. *In* Memoranda to all State Directors 1940-43. Washington, Government Printing Office, 1945.

[153] See footnote 149, p. 70.

[154] The procurement and assignment service for physicians, dentists, and veterinarians. J. Am. Dent. A. 29: 653, Apr 1942.

[155] Selective Service Occupational Bulletin No. 41, 14 Dec 42, sub: Doctors, dentists, veterinarians, and osteopaths. *In* Occupational Bulletins 1-44, and Activity and Occupation Bulletin 1-35. Washington, Government Printing Office, 1944.

As noted above, during the first years of the war Selective Service was most often blamed for inducting professional personnel who were not wanted by the Armed Forces. During this period the War Department, WMC, and the professions tended to deprecate the activities of Selective Service in mobilizing physicians, dentists, and veterinarians as an indiscriminate threat to essential civilian medical care and to the economic use of scarce personnel, and late in 1941 all of these agencies approved the formation of PAS, WMC (to be discussed later in this chapter), as an organization which was expected to supplant Selective Service in this field. Though liaison between PAS and Selective Service was imperfect at first, the system was functioning by the end of 1942, at least to the extent that Selective Service boards were inducting very few physicians or dentists who had not been cleared by PAS.

Unfortunately, a serious weakness was revealed in this program early in 1943 when voluntary procurement for the Medical Department began to lag. Fifty percent of all physicians and 17 percent of all dentists declared "available" by PAS refused to accept commissions, and the Medical Corps, in particular, faced a critical and mounting shortage of personnel.[156][157] But when the War Department and PAS decided that the time had come for Selective Service to exercise its powers,[158] those powers were found to be inadequate, at least under existing policies. Among the reasons for this situation, the following were most important:

1. While Selective Service had been criticized for inducting professional personnel, it had done so only under the same policies that applied to any other category, according to a priority based mainly on age, physical condition, and absence of family responsibilities. It was a fundamental principle of Selective Service that every man should be considered for military service on the basis of such impersonal factors, and boards were now as reluctant to induct an individual merely because he happened to be a physician or dentist as they had been to exempt him for the same reason earlier in the war. But the supply of young professional men with few dependents was small. Because of the long period of training required, medical personnel tended to be older than their contemporaries in industry; because they enjoyed a good income and constituted a stable element in the community they tended to acquire families soon after entering practice. It was now found that in spite of earlier complaints the majority of physicians, dentists, and veterinarians were immune to induction under current criteria.

PAS protested that from 70 to 80 percent of all recalcitrants were not subject to induction because of age or dependency.[159] One state director reported

---

[156] See footnote 52, p. 53.

[157] Another author has declared that 26 percent of 7,259 dentists declared available by PAS refused to accept commissions. See State Officers' Conference. J. Am. Dent. A. 31: 1574–1576, 15 Nov 44.

[158] Rpt of Conference between Col Harley L. Swift, Off Dir Mil Pers, ASF, and representatives of PAS, 20 Mar 43. Off file Mil Pers Div, SGO, PAS file.

[159] Minutes of Meeting, Directing Board, PAS, 31 Jul 43. Off file Mil Pers Div, SGO, PAS file.

THE PROCUREMENT OF DENTAL OFFICERS 69

were almost no vacancies in the Dental Corps.[135] A notice in the Journal of the American Dental Association for December 1940, that any inducted dentist could apply for a commission, proved premature.[136] On 22 January 1941 the Chief of the Dental Division again recommended that physicians, dentists, and veterinarians who received low call numbers, or who were inducted, should be offered commissions,[137] but no action was taken at this time.

Meanwhile, other interests had become involved in the matter. Two days after Selective Service was inaugurated Senator James E. Murray introduced a bill providing that any licensed physician or dentist who met established mental and physical standards should be commissioned in lieu of induction.[138] This measure also provided for the deferment of medical and dental students, interns, and residents. At first it was reported that the Army was not opposed to this bill,[139] but on 16 December 1940, the War Department formally registered its disapproval, based on the following considerations:

1. It was felt that rigid regulations favorable to any one branch were not justified. If all Medical Department personnel were given commissions on induction, engineers, lawyers, and other groups would feel entitled to the same treatment.

2. It was believed that deferment of persons actually essential to the preservation of the nation's health could be accomplished without legislation and that mandatory legislation would handicap the administration of Selective Service.[140]

No final action was taken on this measure before the end of the congressional session, and substantially the same bill was reintroduced on 6 January 1941.[141] Before hearings could be held, however, an amended version was introduced which provided not only for the commissioning of inducted dentists and the deferment of students, but for the deferment of teachers in medical and dental schools.[142] Hearings were held on this bill from 18 to 20 March 1941 [143] and the Army again opposed passage, adding as another reason the fact that it did not wish to be placed in the position of having to commission any physician or dentist who might be inducted, regardless of his professional, ethical, or

---

[135] 1st ind, SG, 20 Jan 41, to ltr from Lt Col T. W. Wren to CG, 8th CA, sub: Application for appointment in the Dental Corps Reserve. [D]

[136] Fairbank, L. C.: Dentistry in mobilization. J. Am. Dent. A. 27: 1972, Dec 1940.

[137] Memo, Brig Gen Leigh C. Fairbank for Brig Gen William E. Shedd, 22 Jan 41, sub: Reserve commissions for physicians, dentists, and veterinarians subject to induction into the military service. HD: 314.

[138] S. 4396, 76th Cong., introduced 18 Sep 40.

[139] Committee on Legislation. J. Am. Dent. A. 28: 989–990, Jun 1941.

[140] Ltr, SecWar (Henry L. Stimson) to Hon Morris Sheppard, Chairman, Sen Committee on Mil Affairs, 16 Dec 40. Quoted in "Report of Hearings Before the Committee on Military Affairs, United States Senate, 77th Congress, on S. 783, 18–20 Mar 41." Washington, Government Printing Office, 1941, p. 144.

[141] S. 197, 77th Cong., introduced 6 Jan 41.

[142] S. 783, 77th Cong., introduced 6 Feb 41.

[143] Report of Hearings before the Committee on Military Affairs, United States Senate, 77th Congress, on S. 783, 18–20 Mar 41. Washington, Government Printing Office, 1941.

moral status.[144] Since both medical and dental officers testified against the measure it must be assumed that in spite of his repeated attempts to get authority to commission inducted dentists The Surgeon General was also opposed to the Murray bill, probably because it left him no chance to reject the few men who were undesirable because they had graduated from substandard schools or because they had engaged in unethical practice. The combined opposition of the War Department and of Selective Service blocked the passage of this legislation.

Meanwhile, as The Surgeon General had foreseen, the War Department was flooded with protests from congressmen, civilian communities, and the profession, at the wasteful use of physicians and dentists as enlisted soldiers. Since The Surgeon General was in agreement with these complaints, and had been prevented from taking corrective action by higher authority, he washed his hands of the whole matter and referred all protests to The Adjutant General as "pertaining to your office." In January 1941 the Chairman of the Military Preparedness Committee of the ADA discussed this question with Senator Claude Pepper, and the latter directed a letter of inquiry to the Secretary of War. When this communication was referred to The Surgeon General, he submitted an analysis of probable needs showing that the Reserve would be depleted by June 1942, and again proposed that procurement for the Dental Reserve be resumed.[145] However, when the ADA in February 1941, recommended an increase in the Dental Reserve Corps from 5,100 officers to 8,000 officers, The Surgeon General opposed such action. It was stated later that he felt that this number of men could not be used, and to enroll officers in the Reserve, beyond the number which would be called to active duty, was equivalent to granting occupational deferment, which was a prerogative of Selective Service.[146] [147] It must be kept in mind that at this time the country was still nearly a year away from active participation in the war.

As a result of the recommendations of The Surgeon General, the numerous protests received, and the threat of legislative action if existing policies were not changed, the War Department finally, on 5 May 1941, authorized the granting of a commission to any inducted dentist who was found to be qualified.[148] Senator Murray stated that his bill had forced consideration of the problem, and this was implied, if not admitted, in General Fairbank's statement that the action of 5 May had "followed participation of Army representatives in hearings on the Murray bill." [149]

---

[144] Ibid.
[145] 2d ind, SG to TAG, 18 Feb 41, on ltr, SecWar to TAG, 27 Jan 41. SG: 080 (ADA).
[146] See footnote 50, p. 53.
[147] Camalier, C. W.: Preparedness and war activities of the American Dental Association: A résumé. J. Am. Dent. A. 33:80, 1 Jan 46.
[148] See footnote 48, p. 53.
[149] Memo, Brig Gen Leigh C. Fairbank for SG, 25 Feb 42, sub: Procurement of dentists for military service. HD: 314.

that out of 130 physicians declared eligible, only a handful had been induced to apply for commissions, and he complained that the remainder were not at all impressed with the possibility that they might be inducted as enlisted men.[160] Even if he were drafted, the professional man had little to fear since he would in all probability be offered a commission without delay, and he often preferred to take the slight risk involved when he refused to comply with PAS recommendations. When it was suggested that Selective Service take over PAS' functions even The Surgeon General was doubtful that the situation would be improved by such action as long as such a large proportion of professional men were deferable for age or dependency.[161]

2. Selective Service regulations were generally drawn up on the assumption that an inductee would serve as an enlisted man, with an enlisted man's pay and allowances. In determining eligibility for induction these regulations did not recognize that the professional man would immediately be commissioned and enjoy an income adequate to support a family in moderate circumstances.

3. During the first part of the war the Armed Forces, the WMC, and public officials had repeatedly warned the Selective Service System that it was taking professional personnel from communities where they would later be needed urgently, and that such personnel should not be inducted without strong reason. Now it was becoming clear even to laymen that these warnings had been well founded, and the growing shortage of physicians and dentists in his own area made the member of a Selective Service Board extremely reluctant to approve the induction of additional men in these categories, even at the request of PAS.[162]

The only solution to this problem was for Selective Service to place a call on its local boards for the required number of physicians and dentists on an occupational basis. As noted above, however, this action would have been a radical departure from established policies, and as such it was extremely distasteful to the Selective Service System. Prior to this time no man had been inducted merely because he happened to be a cook or truck driver who was critically needed by the Armed Forces, and any modification of this principle was regarded with apprehension by that agency. But the situation in respect to professional personnel was not entirely comparable to that of cooks and truck drivers; unlike the latter, physicians and dentists could not be trained in a few weeks or months in an emergency, and they could be obtained in large numbers only from civilian life. If the normal operation of Selective Service failed to produce the number required, more drastic steps were necessary. In October 1943 the War Department reluctantly made a formal call on Selective Service for the conscription of 12,000 physicians.

---

[160] Ltr, Dr. Creighton Barker to Lt Col Durward G. Hall, 27 Dec 43. [D]
[161] See footnote 69, p. 55.
[162] Interv between the author and Maj Ernest J. Fedor, Dental Liaison Off, Mil Pers Div, SGO, 25 Nov 47.

The dental personnel situation, which had always been less critical than the medical, was much improved by the summer of 1943, and dentists were not included in the proposed draft of physicians. In fact, other developments eventually prevented even the proposed induction of physicians, but not until an important precedent had been established; it was finally recognized by the Armed Forces, PAS, and Selective Service that the latter might have to undertake the priority induction of specific groups whose special skills were essential to the national defense if sufficient personnel could not be procured voluntarily.[163]

From the end of 1942 until May 1946 Selective Service played a small part in the procurement of dental officers and very few dentists were inducted as enlisted men. Sixty-one applications for commissions were received from conscripted dentists during 1943, of whom 46 were accepted.[164] Only seven officers were commissioned from the ranks from 1 January 1944 through August 1945. Thirty-five applications were rejected in the same period but this figure means little because men who were refused commissions could, and did, make new applications at frequent intervals; it is probable that most of the applications received in 1944 and 1945 came from men who had been rejected for good reasons a year or more before.[165]

With the end of hostilities the dental personnel picture began to deteriorate and Selective Service again became a factor in procurement. ASTP had graduated its last dental student in the spring of 1945. The shortage of civilian dentists was acute, and even recent graduates could count on incomes of as much as $10,000 yearly in private practice. Above all, effective pressure to volunteer for military service for patriotic reasons was almost eliminated. Yet the Army still had several million men scattered all over the world who had to be furnished dental care. Under these circumstances the military had no alternative but to ask for a draft of dentists.[166] This draft shattered all precedents for it was the first and only time during and immediately following the war that Selective Service asked its boards to induct men from a specific occupational group.[167] (Very few dentists were actually drafted in 1946 since the Army took every precaution to insure that men threatened with induction would be offered commissions with the least possible delay.) [168]

Information on the number of dentists who actually served any considerable time as enlisted men during the war is indefinite. Selective Service re-

---
[163] This principle was later made the basis for the draft of dentists in 1946.
[164] History of the Army Dental Corps, Personnel, 1940–43, p. 41. HD: 314.7-2 (Dental).
[165] Info compiled by the author from annual procurement summaries received from the Mil Pers Div, SGO.
[166] Memo, Maj Gen Norman T. Kirk for ACofS, G-1, 17 May 46, sub: Procurement objective for Dental Corps officers. SG: 322.0531.
[167] Info given the author by Dr. Matheus Smith, Natl Hq, Selective Service System, 24 Nov 47.
[168] Col (later Brig Gen) James M. Epperly, Dental Div, SGO, estimated that only about 4 dentists were inducted by their boards before they could be granted commissions. Personal interv with author, 10 Nov 47.

ports that 558 dentists were inducted and that 49 enlisted during the life of that agency.[169] Army records, on the other hand, indicate that only 263 inducted dentists and 14 who enlisted voluntarily were commissioned between 1 January 1941 and 30 June 1945.[170] A few additional were commissioned after 30 June 1945, but the total number of enlisted dentists commissioned by the Army probably did not exceed 300 officers. Since the Navy did not accept any inducted dentists [171] these figures, if correct, would indicate that some 300 dental graduates actually continued to serve in enlisted status.

This conclusion is open to question, however, on the following grounds:

1. A few dentists who were inducted against the advice of the Army after the middle of 1944 were immediately discharged. In AGO records these men would be shown to have been discharged as enlisted men, though their period of service was extremely short.

2. It is probable that a certain number of laboratory technicians, dental assistants, or even dental students, were mistakenly listed as "dentists" in Selective Service forms. These men would of course not be eligible for commissions in the Army.

Col. Louis H. Renfrow, of the Selective Service System, has said that "all but a very few" of the inducted dentists were commissioned.[172] Similarly, Maj. Gen. Robert H. Mills stated that only a handful of inducted dentists were not commissioned.[173] On the other hand, Maj. Ernest Fedor, formerly of the Military Personnel Division, SGO, reported that that office received some 100 to 125 applications for commissions which were rejected for various reasons, including the following:

1. A few unfortunates were unable to convince a board of line officers that they possessed the superior intelligence, or met the generally higher standards, demanded of an officer.

2. Some applicants were refugee dentists of doubtful background and ability who had volunteered for military service as an aid to establishing citizenship.

3. Some dentists held no state licenses, or had not practiced since graduation from dental college. Others had abandoned the practice of their profession for many years. The Army refused to commission such personnel.

4. Some dentists had been engaged in grossly unethical practice or had been convicted of felonies.

5. A few dentists actually refused commissions because they were in locations near home which they feared to lose, because they preferred their current

---

[169] Personal ltr, Col Louis H. Renfrow, Selective Service Natl Hq, to the author, 10 Sep 47. HD: 314.

[170] Info given the author by Mr. Kirkman J. Rhodes, Strength Accounting Br, AGO, 8 Sep 47.

[171] Info given the author by Comdr J. V. Westerman, Bu Med and Surg, USN, 25 Nov 47.

[172] Renfrow, L. H.: Dentistry in the Selective Service System. The Mil. Surgeon 101: 423, Nov 1947.

[173] See footnote 127, p. 68.

duties, or because they felt their opportunities for an early discharge were better as enlisted men than as officers.

The Army could not use the above categories in its clinics, and it is doubtful if any useful purpose would have been served by releasing most of them to return to civilian life.

It seems probable that a little over 100 men technically classified as dentists served as enlisted men in the Army during the war. On the other hand, there is every indication that most dentists whose qualifications were not open to serious question were either offered commissions or discharged. This opinion has been confirmed by the Selective Service System,[174] the Dental Division,[175] and organized dentistry.[176]

The Procurement and Assignment Service, War Manpower Commission

The background and activities of the Procurement and Assignment Service are covered in detail in Lt. Col. Alfred Mordecai's "History of the Procurement and Assignment Service for Physicians, Dentists, Veterinarians, Sanitary Engineers, and Nurses, War Manpower Commission." [177]

Briefly, PAS was formed in October 1941 as a Division of the Office of Defense Health and Welfare Services. Its mission was to insure that scarce medical personnel would be used to the best advantage of all concerned, so that the needs of the Armed Forces and of critical defense areas could be met with minimum hardship for the civilian population. In April 1942 PAS was transferred to the War Manpower Commission and functioned under that bureau for the remainder of the war. From the beginning, PAS was operated in close cooperation with the Armed Forces, USPHS, the civilian professions, and the Selective Service System. At the time of its organization PAS consisted of the following:

1. A central policy board of 5 members (later increased to 8), including Dr. C. Willard Camalier as a representative of the dental profession.

2. Nine advisory subcommittees (later increased to 15) which were concerned with the various medical branches. At first a single committee on dentistry was included, but later a separate committee on dental education was added.

3. Nine corps area subcommittees, each consisting of 2 physicians, 1 dentist, 1 medical educator, 1 dental educator, 1 veterinarian, and 1 hospital representative. These corps area subcommittees were at first expected to be the principal operating units, but they proved unwieldly and the state subcommittees eventually assumed most administrative functions.

---

[174] See footnote 172, p. 75.
[175] See footnote 127, p. 68.
[176] See footnote 147, p. 70.
[177] See footnote 52, p. 53.

could determine how many dentists should be retained to meet the reasonable needs of the civilian population.

In June 1942 the directing board of PAS decided to undertake a nationwide survey of dental resources as a basis for establishing state allocations.[183] The Committee on Dentistry carried out this survey with the assistance of USPHS and the results were reported on 20 February 1943.[184] The findings of this committee have already been discussed in this chapter under "Limitations on the Number of Dentists Available from Civilian Practice."

When it had been determined how many dentists were in practice in any area, and how many were required for civilian care, state chairmen were assigned quotas based on current military needs. When procurement reached its fastest tempo in the first months of 1943 PAS was obligated to declare 400 dentists available each month.[185]

The first procedure adopted by PAS and The Surgeon General for the procurement of medical personnel involved the folowing steps:[186]

1. The Surgeon General notified the central office, PAS, of his requirements for officers.

2. The central office, PAS, made up lists of names from its files and forwarded them to the SGO liaison officer with the appropriate professional organization for ethical and educational clearance.

3. The SGO liaison officer sent the lists to the state PAS chairmen concerned. The latter eliminated all men considered essential and returned the lists to the central office, PAS.

4. The central office, PAS, mailed individual application forms and authorizations for a physical examination at an Army installation.

5. Physical examination reports were mailed, by the surgeons completing them, directly to The Surgeon General. Completed applications were returned by the individual to the central office, PAS, where they were checked for accuracy by an SGO liaison officer, and if correct they were sent to The Surgeon General.

6. If the applicant was acceptable to The Surgeon General all papers in the case were forwarded to The Adjutant General, who offered the man a commission. The Surgeon General notified any applicant whose request for a commission was rejected.

This system proved to be very cumbersome in operation and it was simplified considerably in the spring of 1942 when the Medical Officer Recruiting Boards were established by The Surgeon General. These boards were organized in each state, with authority to contact prospects, pass on their professional qualifications and ethical standing, and offer commissions in the grades of

---
[183] See footnote 18, p. 41.
[184] See footnote 19, p. 42.
[185] See footnote 52, p. 53.
[186] Ibid.

lieutenant or captain on the spot. The boards often set up their offices in the same quarters occupied by the state PAS, and cooperation was close and informal. PAS retained the sole right to declare any man available, however, and the boards were instructed to process no physician or dentist who was not cleared by the state PAS chairman.[187][188][189]

When the functions of the Medical Officer Recruiting Boards were taken over by OPS, ASF, at the end of 1942, The Surgeon General again had to pass on the acceptability of applicants and the procurement process again became more complicated. The field offices of OPS then contacted prospects in cooperation with local PAS representatives, completed applications, and forwarded them to The Surgeon General. If the prospective officer appeared to be acceptable his application was sent to the central office, PAS, which forwarded it to the state chairman for clearance as to availability. The latter sent the application to the SGO liaison officer with the appropriate professional society for ethical and professional clearance, and it was then returned to The Surgeon General for final action. The clearance of the state PAS chairman was an essential part of the application.

When professional personnel who had been declared available by PAS refused to apply for commissions the case was turned over to Selective Service for appropriate action.

Opinions concerning the effectiveness of PAS, in respect to the procurement of dentists, varied. Certainly some agency was needed to determine availability and advise Selective Service and The Surgeon General on matters affecting medical manpower. This function PAS seems to have performed with reasonable satisfaction. But its name suggested that PAS was expected to go further and actually present to the Armed Forces the names of qualified men who would accept commissions if they were physically fit, and in this activity it was less successful. Half of the physicians declared available, and a smaller proportion of the dentists, refused to volunteer for military service. In the critical days of early 1943 both the Army and Navy expressed considerable dissatisfaction concerning PAS' inability to provide replacements. The agency was accused of "pussyfooting" and it was stated that PAS chairmen should "get tough," that younger men were needed as state chairmen, or even that Selective Service should take over PAS functions. The shortage of dental officers was less acute than that of medical personnel, but a representative of the Dental Division also expressed some concern over the lagging procurement of dentists during the first 2 months of 1943. Much of this criticism seems to have stemmed from a misunderstanding of the limited powers of PAS and of its proper function. If the PAS had had effective backing from Selective Service any man declared available would have hurried to apply for a com-

---

[187] Ltr, TAG to CG, 1st CA, 28 Apr 42, sub: Medical Officer Recruiting Boards. AG: 210.31.
[188] Memo, SG for Medical Officer Recruiting Boards, 27 May 42, sub: Memorandum to Medical Officer Recruiting Boards. Natl Archives, PAS files, WMC.
[189] Ltr, SG to Medical Officer Recruiting Boards, 20 Jun 42: Instructions. [D].

4. Thirty-nine state subcommittees (some covered more than one state; one state had two committees) consisting of a chairman and subordinate committees on medicine, dentistry, veterinary medicine, and, eventually, sanitary engineering and nursing. The chairman of the state dental committee was nominated by the state dental society and he, in turn, nominated the members of his committee.

5. County or district subcommittees for each profession, as required. Chairman of these committees were nominated by the district or county dental societies, and in turn they nominated their own assistants. These committees were advisory only, and no one but the state chairman could declare a dentist available, but as a matter of custom the recommendations of the local chairmen were accepted in the absence of compelling reasons to the contrary.

6. The Professional and Technical Employment and Training Division of the War Manpower Commission. Though a separate agency, this unit assisted PAS by maintaining rosters of medical personnel, with data on special qualifications, if any.

When PAS began to function, early in 1942, it met a definite need in the procurement picture. As long as most physicians and dentists were obtained from the Reserve, with very few commissions granted to men with no military experience or training, The Surgeon General was able to contact prospective officers, pass on their professional qualifications, and place them on active duty. Even when larger numbers of dentists had to be procured he was able to decentralize this function to corps area Medical Officer Recruiting Boards with fair success. But when it became necessary for the Army and Navy to take nearly 30 percent of all the dentists in the United States it was essential to insure not only that the Armed Forces got the officers they required, but that the reasonable needs of the civilian population, especially in critical defense areas, were considered. Selective Service was familiar with local conditions but it lacked the technical information for such a project, and its efforts to procure medical personnel before the inauguration of PAS generally resulted only in increased confusion. Very early in the war the professional societies had attempted to list all professional personnel and record essential data on specialties, and at first they made some effort to induce younger men to volunteer for military service, but many dentists failed to return questionnaires,[178] and the men who were "selected" for Army duty by their colleagues were resentful and inclined to question the justice of the method followed. No matter how impersonal the proceedings, when a society tried to decide which of its own members were most eligible, the resulting protests and charges of favoritism generally made it glad to turn the whole problem over to an impartial, semi-official agency with no axe to grind.

The PAS agreed to produce the required officers for the Army, advise Selective Service concerning the availability of medical personnel, and assure

---

[178] Committee on Dental Preparedness, Résumé of activities. J. Am. Dent. A. 27 : 1970, Dec 1940.

the dental profession and the nation that dental manpower would not be wasted and that the needs of local communities would be considered. To carry out these aims it inaugurated two projects: (1) It made a strong effort to list every dentist in the country with supplementary data on special abilities, educational background, age, dependents, et cetera. (2) It set up the mechanism for determining how many men could be spared from any given area, selecting those who were most eligible and declaring them available to the military.

The ADA had originally sent out a questionnaire to all dentists for whom it could obtain addresses in October 1940,[179] but lists were incomplete and the response was not too good; over a year later only 75 percent of the questionnaires had been returned, and in some states only about half of the dentists replied.[180] The questionnaires received by the ADA were eventually turned over to PAS and they provided useful information in the first stages of that agency's operations, but PAS found it necessary to cooperate with the National Roster of Scientific and Specialized Personnel in sending out new questionnaires in February 1942.[181] Data so obtained were available to the Central Board, State Chairmen, or the military.

The question of the availability of dentists for military duty involved several factors, including the following:

1. How many dentists were in practice in the United States?

2. How many dentists would be required to meet the minimum needs of the civilian population?

3. Which areas could best spare the dentists needed by the Armed Forces? An overall survey of medical personnel had been made very early in the operation of PAS, but at first local chairmen were relied upon to determine the availability of dentists.[182] This policy did not prove satisfactory, however, for the following reasons:

1. Dental manpower was distributed very unevenly over the nation. Some cities had more than one dentist for every 1,000 persons, while some rural areas had less than one dentist for 5,000 individuals. PAS representatives in the latter districts felt called upon to deliver at least a few dentists, though they could not, in fact, be spared. The representative in a big city might declare a large number of men available and still obtain only a small proportion of the dentists which could have been taken without endangering civilian practice.

2. The southern states, which generally had the lowest proportion of dentists to total population, had already supplied the most dentists on a volunteer basis during 1940 and 1941.

3. No uniform yardstick had been established by which local chairmen

---

[179] Committee on Dental Preparedness. J. Am. Dent. A. 27: 1658, Oct 1940.
[180] Procurement and assignment agency for professional personnel in the Army. J. Am. Dent. A. 28: 2026–2030, Dec 1941.
[181] See footnote 52, p. 53.
[182] See footnote 19, p. 42.

mission to prevent his induction as an enlisted man, but it was apparent from the start that professional personnel were not much worried over the possibility of being drafted.[190] The Assistant Executive Officer of Selective Service himself admitted that his organization had had great difficulty in supporting the OPS in its efforts to obtain medical officers and that local boards often refused to take the advice of PAS.[191] PAS was an advisory body only; it had no authority to apply official pressure to recalcitrants. It could supply technical knowledge which Selective Service did not possess, but Selective Service had to exercise any compulsion required. It would therefore appear that the first consideration, if an agency similar to PAS is to be established in the future, should be a definite arrangement for effective cooperation between that body and Selective Service.[192]

PAS was also criticized by a representative of the Dental Division for failing to pass on the ethical qualifications of dentists. It was stated that local PAS personnel were afraid to commit themselves in doubtful cases, merely declaring the man available and leaving it up to The Surgeon General to refuse or accept him.[193] This, again, would appear to have been the proper function of The Surgeon General's liaison officers with the professional societies, rather than of PAS.

It was also inevitable, with so much at stake, that personalities and professional jealousy should sometimes enter the picture. PAS necessarily had to give the directors of schools and hospitals a certain amount of freedom to determine which members of the staff were essential and which could be spared. One hospital director was categorically accused of using his influence in this respect to force younger physicians to play his political games under threat of induction into the Army.[194] It was also felt that methods used by local personnel were not always wisely chosen. It was reported, for instance, that in some large cities, where individuals could not be known personally, the local chairmen contacted the supply houses to see who ran up the largest bills, and declared these men essential on the grounds that they were obviously doing the most work![195] Such abuses were apparently infrequent, however, and there seems to be no reason to believe that PAS was not as impersonal in its actions as any human agency could be. Certainly PAS personnel gave unselfishly of their time and energy in a thankless job.

---

[190] See footnote 160, p. 73.

[191] Ltr, Richard H. Eanes, Asst Exec Off, Selective Service System, to Maj Gen Geo F. Lull, 21 Mar 44, sub: State Director advice No 206. [D]

[192] It must be admitted, however, that local PAS representatives were sometimes suspected of declaring medical personnel available under pressure from higher authority, and then informing Selective Service Board members that they did not actually believe these individuals could be spared. Information from Maj Ernest Fedor, given the author 25 Nov 47.

[193] See footnote 21, p. 44.

[194] The confidential letter carrying this accusation has been seen by the author, but no useful purpose would be served by divulging the names of individuals and institutions concerned.

[195] See footnote 162, p. 73.

At the end of the war the Director of the Dental Division stated that PAS had proved "workable." [196]

After giving PAS credit for preventing the induction of dentists as enlisted men, to which it was not entitled, the American Dental Association noted that: [197]

> The Procurement and Assignment Service, through its State and local committees, brought the selection of dentists for service down to a level where local factors could play an important part. Admittedly, it did not work perfectly, and inequalities can be found without too much research. But the fact remains that the Procurement and Assignment Service did a better job than any previous similar agency. Dentists should see to it that, in any future crisis, it is given sufficient authority to make its program more effective.

PAS took a very minor part in dental procurement for the Army after 9 December 1943.

Medical Officer Recruiting Boards

As it became necessary to procure large numbers of medical personnel directly from civil life in 1942 The Surgeon General was authorized to establish decentralized boards which could locate prospective officers, pass on their professional and ethical standing, and offer them immediate commissions in one of the two lower grades without reference to the SGO. The corps areas were instructed to form these boards in April 1942 [198] but they were of minor importance to dental procurement for several months since there were very few vacancies in the Dental Corps at that time. When The Surgeon General was authorized a new procurement objective of 4,000 dentists in July 1942, it was directed that a dental officer would be added to each of the 30 boards which were then operating in 25 States.[199] The Surgeon General's objective was reached very rapidly, and dentists were removed from the remaining boards on 1 September 1942.[200] At the same time the boards were instructed to process no more dental applications except for men classified I-A by Selective Service. Initial quotas for physicians were also being met, and the first board had already been closed for this reason on 26 June 1942. By 21 October 1942 most boards had suspended operations because there was no longer a need for their services. The OPS, ASF, came into operation in November 1942, and the Medical Officer Recruiting Boards did not have an opportunity to demonstrate their effectiveness in the personnel crisis of 1943.

The Medical Officer Recruiting Boards were more important to the Medical Corps than to the Dental Service and they are discussed at length in other sections of the Medical History. In general, Medical Department officers,

---

[196] See footnote 122, p. 65.
[197] The right to gripe: The fifth freedom. J. Am. Dent. A. 33 : 118–122, 1 Jan 46.
[198] Ltr, TAG to CG, 1st CA, 28 Apr 42, sub: Medical officer recruiting boards. AG : 210.31.
[199] See footnote 62, p. 54.
[200] See footnote 64, p. 55.

working closely with PAS, were able to approach individuals and professional societies more effectively than laymen, and the activities of the Medical Officer Recruiting Boards were compared favorably with those of the nonprofessional Officer Procurement Service Boards which succeeded them. The fact that nearly 4,000 dentists were commissioned in less than 2 months showed that boards operating under The Surgeon General could play an important part in dental procurement if the need arose and they had the opportunity.

Officer Procurement Service, ASF

On 7 November 1942 the War Department directed that all direct commissions from civil life would thenceforth be handled through an Officer Procurement Service operating under ASF.[201] For most branches of the Army, officer replacements were being obtained largely from officer candidate schools at the end of 1942, and very few men without previous military experience were being considered. Instructions given OPS indicate that no small part of its mission was to keep a tight rein on direct commissions from civil life, to keep them to a minimum, and this negative attitude seems to have colored its early operations. But the Medical Department was faced with a different problem; it needed officers and it needed them in a hurry, and they could be obtained only from civil practice. The Surgeon General made no secret of the fact that in his opinion OPS hindered rather than helped procurement, and that it was a poor substitute for his own Medical Officer Recruiting Boards.

Soon after OPS started to function in February 1943, The Surgeon General expressed great dissatisfaction with the results attained and recommended that if no improvement were noted by the end of March, the Medical Officer Recruiting Boards be reestablished. On the same day the Dental Division complained of the slow procurement of dental officers since the first of the year, and the delay was blamed on OPS since PAS reported that the needed dentists were available. By May 1943 the dental personnel situation was less disturbing, but the shortage of medical officers remained so acute that the SGO began to consider a special conscription by Selective Service.[202] The procurement of medical officers continued to lag until ASTP graduates became available, but whether the difficulties encountered were due to deficiencies of OPS, or to the fact that civilian medical resources were approaching exhaustion, is a matter of opinion. Since the procurement of dental officers under OPS offered no problems not common to all Medical Department procurement, detailed discussion of that agency will be left for the general medical administrative history.

American Dental Association

The American Dental Association was of course deeply interested in the procurement of dental officers. Soon after the start of hostilities in Europe

---
[201] WD Cir 367, 7 Nov 42.
[202] See footnote 69, p. 55.

in the fall of 1939, the Director of the Dental Division asked the ADA to establish a committee to consult and cooperate with the military.[203] At the time no action was taken, but when the request was repeated in December a "Committee on National Defense" (later called the "Committee on National Preparedness") was appointed without further delay.[204] Corresponding committees were formed in each state.

It appears that The Surgeon General initially expected the ADA to play a major role in the procurement of dental officers, and in July 1940, he specifically requested the Association to undertake the following program:[205]

1. The Association to conduct a survey of the dental profession through its state and local societies.

2. The local societies to canvass their members to determine which of these would be willing to serve, which could be spared for military service, and which should remain at home because of age, physical disability, or essentiality in civilian capacity.

3. The local societies to list those who were selected for possible military duty according to their professional qualifications, listing as oral surgeons, prosthetists, etc., only those of outstanding ability. Also, to select qualified men to serve on examination boards.

4. The state societies to maintain a roster of all available members.

5. The American Dental Association to maintain a numerical roster of available men, by states.

6. The Medical Department of the Army to have one or more selected officers on duty with the American Dental Association when and if necessary.

7. The War Department, corps areas, or regional officers to call upon the American Dental Association for dentists by specialties, as and when required.

8. The American Dental Association to call upon the states according to their quotas for the dentists required; the states, in turn, to call upon the local societies for their quotas.

The plan discussed above would have placed almost the entire burden of procurement on the ADA; the Army was merely to request a certain number of dentists with the desired qualifications and the ADA was to deliver them. The Association would have assumed the duties later assigned to PAS in that it would have had to determine local needs, specify the dentists which could be spared, and maintain a roster according to individual qualifications. In addition it would have accepted much of the responsibility of Selective Service in determining individual eligibility for military duty and, presumably, in exerting the pressure necessary to induce dentists to accept commissions in the Army.

The ADA was apparently favorably inclined toward the plan because it would give some assurance that dentists would not be taken indiscriminately,

---

[203] President's Page. J. Am. Dent. A. 28: 982, Jun 1941.
[204] See footnote 154, p. 71.
[205] Ltr, Maj Gen James C. Magee to Dr. Arthur H. Merritt, Pres ADA, 6 Jul 40. SG: 080 (ADA) T.

without regard to the needs of their communities, and because it would give the organization an opportunity to perform a valuable service.

A program for an immediate survey and classification of all civilian dental personnel was submitted to the Board of Trustees of the ADA in September 1940.[206] It was approved without delay and $20,000 appropriated for the purpose, in addition to $5,000 for expenses of the Preparedness Committee. Questionnaires were mailed in October of the same year.

Unfortunately, serious defects soon developed in the scheme to use the ADA as the principal dental procurement agency. The Association lacked official status, and about 25 percent of the questionnaires sent to individual dentists were ignored. Also, the local ADA officers were too close to their membership to have the objective attitude and impersonal status required of any official who is to determine which men will be taken from the community for military service. There is no evidence that the endeavors of the ADA in this respect were anything but disinterested, but some dentists objected strongly to being picked for the Armed Forces by their competitors, and charges that political influence was being exerted were inevitable under the circumstances. Antagonism resulted among local members, and the whole task soon proved very distasteful to those who had to carry it out. Further, when a dentist refused to accept a commission after being recommended by the ADA the latter had no authority to enforce its decision.

The ADA was happy to relinquish its thankless task to PAS in 1942. It played an important part in the inauguration of that organization, and it maintained close liaison with it throughout the war.[207] It turned over to PAS the data it had obtained through its survey of civilian dentists, providing that body with much valuable information on which to proceed while plans were being made for PAS' own survey of June 1942. The ADA also cooperated closely with the Dental Advisory Committee of the Selective Service System.[208]

The ADA rendered an important service to The Surgeon General by assuming responsibility for determining the professional and ethical status of prospective dental officers. In May 1942[209] a representative of the SGO was placed on duty with the national headquarters of the ADA and the Association furnished him the information on which to decide whether or not a man's standing in the profession made him acceptable for the Army Dental Corps. Membership in the ADA was not required, but dentists who did not meet recognized ethical standards, who were graduates of substandard schools (mainly foreign), who did not possess valid licenses to practice, or who had been convicted of serious offenses, were rejected for military service in the Dental Corps.

---

[206] See footnote 203, p. 84.
[207] Committee on Dental Preparedness: A procurement and assignment agency. J. Am. Dent. A. 28: 2057–2060, Dec 1941.
[208] See footnote 147, p. 70.
[209] WD SO 131, 19 May 42.

The part played by the ADA in the rehabilitation programs for Selective Service registrants is discussed in chapter VI.

The ADA consistently objected to the induction of dentists and dental students as enlisted men. It backed the Murray bills to commission inducted dentists and defer dental students and instructors, and it made vigorous efforts to have the Dental Reserve increased in 1940 and 1941 to permit the commissioning of inducted dentists.[210] It also sponsored a plan to provide care for the patients of dentists in the Armed Forces and to keep the latters' practices intact until their return.[211]

ATTRITION IN THE ARMY DENTAL CORPS

In the period from 7 December 1941 through 31 December 1946, 2,107 dental officers were lost to the Army, as follows: [212] [213]

Cause	Total	Cause	Total
Killed in action	20	Over 38, no suitable assignment	448
Died of wounds	5	Key man in industry or Government	3
Declared dead	0	Hardship	8
Missing in action (subsequently returned to duty)	1	Honorable discharge	4
Captured	38	Resignation	64
Deaths from accident, aircraft	8	Reclassification, honorable and other than honorable	28
Deaths from accident, not aircraft	15	Dishonorable discharge	6
Died of disease	56	Conditions other than honorable	29
Suicide	2	Other	12
Other nonbattle deaths	10	Unsatisfactory service	2
Retirement	15	Necessary to national health	1
Physically disqualified	1,328		
Overage	4		

(See chapter IX for losses due to demobilization.)

From 7 December 1941 to 30 June 1945, an average of about 50 dental officers were lost each month, for all causes. This was a rate of about 5.2 percent a year of the average of 11,400 dental officers on duty during this period. This rate was far from uniform, however, and was artificially stimulated in 1944 to permit replacement of some veterans by younger ASTP graduates.

In general, combat losses, or discharges for disabilities resulting from wounds, were almost negligible so far as the overall manpower problem was concerned. Only 20 dentists were returned to the Zone of Interior for serious injuries during the period 7 December 1941 through 31 December 1946, and not all of these officers were lost to the Service. Thus, losses from battle action

---

[210] See footnote 147, p. 70.
[211] Ibid.
[212] Casualty data are for the period 7 December 1941 through 31 December 1946. Army Battle Casualties and Nonbattle Deaths in World War II, Final Report, 7 Dec 41–31 Dec 46. Strength and Acctg Br, AGO.
[213] Statistics for the remaining causes are for the period 7 December 1941 through 30 June 1945. Compiled from data on file in the Personnel Stat Unit, Administrative Services Div, AGO.

(killed, died of wounds, captured, or missing) amounted to 1.5 percent of the mean Dental Corps strength overseas during the 4 war years, or about 0.38 percent per year. (See also chapter IV, p. 117, for casualty data, 7 Dec 41–31 Dec 46.)

Administrative discharges accounted for 624 separations, or 30 percent of the total. Of these, 448 were men over 38 years of age who were released to create vacancies for younger ASTP graduates, and to the extent that these separations were optional they need not be considered in the personnel problem.

By far the largest proportion of all losses, 63 percent, were due to physical disqualification. The 1,328 dentists discharged for this reason in the period reported amounted to 12 percent of the average of 11,400 officers on duty, or about 3.5 percent each year. It has already been pointed out that few physical discharges resulted from battle injuries; most represented normal attrition under the stresses of wartime conditions. These losses were understandably higher than in peacetime when retirements for physical disability had amounted to about one-half of 1 percent a year.

About 45 dentists, or 0.4 percent of the average strength for the period, were released under conditions "other than honorable." This was only 0.25 percent of about 18,000 dentists on duty at some time during the emergency.

During the first 2 years of the war the Dental Corps was primarily concerned with obtaining enough officers to staff its expanding installations and some dentists were accepted who, for physical or other reasons, had a less than average work capacity. By 1943, however, the Army was approaching relative stability and it was possible to place greater emphasis on physical fitness and efficiency. Also, the ASTP was expected to supply a large number of graduates who had been given deferment from military service and had received at least a part of their training at Government expense. It was highly desirable that these men be taken into the Dental Corps rather than released to return to civilian practice. Finally, a certain amount of "turnover" in the Dental Service was necessary to provide a balanced force from the standpoint of age and total service. Efforts to improve the efficiency of the Dental Corps and to create vacancies for young replacements took two main directions: (1) to relieve from active duty those officers whose physical condition limited their assignment or prevented them from working normal hours, and (2) to eliminate those few officers whose efficiency was below accepted standards.

Release of Limited Service Officers. As early as July 1943 the War Department had directed that line officers qualified only for limited service might be released, but physicians, dentists, and chaplains had been specifically excepted.[214] A similar order of 1 November 1943 applied to dentists,[215] but

---

[214] Radiogram, Maj Gen M. G. White, ACofS G-1, 10 Jul 43, quoted verbatim in History of the Army Dental Corps, 21 Feb–1 Apr 44, Bi-weekly Dental Service Reports. HD : 024.

[215] Ltr, TAG to CGs AAF, AGF, ASF, 1 Nov 43, sub: Instructions relative to retention of officers on active duty for limited service. AG : 210.85.

was again modified in January 1944 to exclude physicians, dentists, and chaplains.[216] In February 1944 the Director of the Dental Division recommended that dental officers once more be included in the category which could be separated when found eligible only for limited service, but at the time no action was taken. In March 1944, with the urgent need for creating vacancies for prospective ASTP graduates (see discussion this chapter, pp. 56–59), this recommendation was resubmitted, and on 18 April 1944 The Adjutant General published a directive providing that dental officers were to be released if: (1) they had been commissioned for general service and were later found to be qualified only for limited service, or (2) if they had originally been accepted for limited service but had suffered deterioration of their physical condition while in military service.

Some difficulty was encountered in persuading all concerned to give effective support to the policy of April 1944. In August 1944 ASF complained that even retiring boards were returning limited service dentists to active duty with the recommendation that they be used in administrative functions when they could not work at the chair.[217] ASF pointed out the lack of administrative positions in the Dental Service and advised that since plenty of physically qualified young dentists were available from ASTP the retention of limited service officers was not desired. About 2 months later, however, the policy of ASF was modified by the War Department to permit major commands to retain limited service dental officers if it could be certified that their services were required and could be used efficiently.[218]

Except for a few senior students the dental ASTP had been terminated by the end of 1944 and replacements were more difficult to find. The Surgeon General therefore abandoned the attempt to have all limited service dentists released,[219] and on 23 December 1944 [220] the ASF directive which made the separation of such officers mandatory was rescinded. It cannot be determined how many dental officers were released under this program since they were included in the larger category separated for physical disabilities. Also, many officers classified for limited service only were separated under other provisions, especially those pertaining to the discharge of personnel for whom no suitable assignment could be found. At any rate the number of limited service dental officers released as such was unimportant in the overall personnel picture.

Release of Officers for Whom no Suitable Assignment Existed. The first general attempt to separate the less efficient officers, other than those in the limited service category, was made in December 1943 when The Adjutant

---

[216] Ltr, TAG to CGs, AAF, AGF, ASF, 13 Jan 44, sub: Instructions relative to retention of officers on active duty for limited service. AG: 210.85.

[217] ASF Cir 272, 24 Aug 44; ASF Cir 274, 25 Aug 44.

[218] WD Cir 403, 14 Oct 44.

[219] Memo, Maj Ernest J. Fedor for Dir Mil Pers Div, 28 Nov 44, sub: Relief from active duty of Dental Corps officers. HD: 314.

[220] ASF Cir 420, 23 Dec 44.

THE PROCUREMENT OF DENTAL OFFICERS

General authorized major commands to release officers over 45 years of age "for whom no suitable assignment could be found." [221] In January 1944 the age limit for such separations was reduced to 38 years.[222] It was pointed out that a number of officers in all branches had rendered valuable service during mobilization, but that due to physical defects or other circumstances over which they had no control they could not be placed in appropriate positions now that the Army was entering a new phase of the war. Such of these men as were surplus in their commands, who did not come under other regulations permitting their discharge, and whose service had justified separation under honorable conditions, were to be released without prejudice.

The separation of dental officers under this directive proceeded very slowly and eventually more specific action was initiated. In May 1944 the War Department noted that recommendations for the release of dentists had been based primarily on personal desires rather than the good of the service, and ordered a general survey of all dental officers with a view toward selecting for discharge those who were least effective.[223] The Surgeon General ordered replacement pools, where dental officers awaited assignment, to refer to a general hospital for disposition any dentist unable to do a full day's work. Other officers in these pools, who were over 38 years of age and could not be assigned to appropriate positions, were to be interviewed to determine if they would accept voluntary separation. By the end of 1944, 121 dentists were released on the basis of such individual recommendations, but that number was far short of the figure required to permit the commissioning of available ASTP graduates.[224]

In order to reduce the dental replacement pools which then numbered 811 officers, and to permit the commissioning of an anticipated 900 ASTP graduates, ASF directed The Surgeon General, on 10 August 1944, to recommend specific quotas to be separated by the various major commands.[225] Order of priority for discharge, without regard to age, was to be:

1. Officers who were not physically capable of doing a full day's duty operating at a dental chair.

2. Officers marked "limited service" who required special consideration as to climate, diet, type of work, or who were qualified for assignment within the United States only.

3. Officers in the lower efficiency rating brackets.

4. Officers in a limited service status, other than those in "2" above.

5. Officers in other categories whose relief from active duty could be accomplished under current War Department directives.

---

[221] Ltr, TAG to Divs of WDGS, 8 Dec 43, sub: Relief from active duty of officers for whom no suitable assignment exists. SG: 210.8.

[222] Ltr, TAG to Divs of WDGS, 12 Jan 44, sub: Relief from active duty of officers for whom no suitable assignment exists. SG: 210.8.

[223] WD Memo W605-44, 25 May 44.

[224] Semiannual Rpt Procmt Br Mil Pers Div SGO, 1 Jul to 31 Dec 44, pars. 1 o, p. q. HD.

[225] Memo, Brig Gen Russel B. Reynolds, Dir Mil Pers Div ASF, for SG, 10 Aug 44, sub: Relief from active duty of Dental Corps officers. Filed as incl 11 to rpt cited in footnote 224.

The authority to release officers in the categories listed, regardless of age, was an exception to War Department policy and at the time was applied only to the Dental Corps.

In order to protect officers eligible for separation under this policy but who had rendered faithful and valuable service, the aforementioned directive was, at the suggestion of the Assistant Chief of Staff G-1, later modified to eliminate any reference to inefficiency. As finally published it provided for the release of:[226]

> 1. Officers who were not physically capable of doing a full day's duty operating at a dental chair.
> 2. Officers marked "Limited Service" who required special consideration as to climate, diet, type of work, or who were qualified for assignment within the United States only.
> 3. Officers whose relief from active duty could be accomplished under current War Department policies.
> 4. Officers selected by The Surgeon General who could be released with least detriment to the service. This category was to be used after exhausting categories "1" through "3" above. . . .

In compliance with the 29 August 1944 directive, The Surgeon General recommended on 2 September 1944 that 1,209 dental officers be separated in the United States as follows:[227]

Service Commands (10 to 15 percent in each area)	516
Surgeon General (to be released from pools)	376
Army Air Forces	200
Army Ground Forces	75
Office, Chief of Transportation	35
Military District of Washington	7

A second list covering officers overseas was submitted on 28 September.[228] It recommended the release of 5 percent of the dentists in each theater, for a total of 212 officers. The Adjutant General approved in toto the overseas request but in the United States a preliminary quota of only 250 dentists was authorized for separation.[229] This was subsequently increased to 290 [230] and it was expected that new allotments would be announced between January and May 1945. By the end of 1944, 239 dental officers had been released under this program in the Zone of Interior [231] and the overseas quota of 212 officers was being processed,

---

[226] Memo, Brig Gen Russel B. Reynolds for SG, 29 Aug 44, sub: Relief from active duty of Dental Corps officers. Filed as incl 11 to rpt cited in footnote 224.
[227] Memo, Col J. R. Hudnall for CG ASF, 2 Sep 44, sub: Relief from active duty of Dental Corps officers. Filed as incl 11 to rpt cited in footnote 224.
[228] Incl 12 to footnote 224, Memo, Maj Gen R. H. Mills for CG ASF, 28 Sep 44, sub: Relief from active duty of Dental Corps officers. HD.
[229] See footnote 224, p. 89.
[230] 1st ind, TAG to CofT, 4 Nov 44, on Ltr, Lt Col A. Kojassar, OCT, to TAG, 12 Oct 44, sub: Relief from active duty of Dental Corps officers. SG: 210.8.
[231] See footnote 224, p. 89.

but by that time the personnel situation had changed considerably and no further "mass" quotas were announced. On 29 December 1944 a new War Department circular summarized and liberalized earlier provisions for the relief of officers for whom no assignment could be found, who were essential to national health and interest in a civilian capacity, or who suffered unusual hardships because of their military service, and future releases for causes other than physical disability were generally carried out under that circular.[232] No further pressure was applied to speed the separation of older or less efficient men. (See pp. 87–88).

Release of Dentists Needed in their Local Communities. For some time before the end of 1944 the Procurement and Assignment Service had tried to have released from active duty Army physicians who were urgently needed in their communities. Results had been insignificant, however, both because The Surgeon General could spare very few officers and because PAS at first showed little critical judgment in drawing up its recommendations.[233] As a result of a conference early in January 1945, PAS notified its state chairmen for physicians that the Army would consider separating a few medical officers though no men would be released who were under 39 years of age, who were qualified for general service, or who were practicing a specialty in the Medical Department. Great care was recommended in selecting only the most worthy cases.[234] Dental officers were not mentioned in the instructions to PAS state chairmen, but before the end of demobilization some 18 officers were actually separated as essential to national health or interest.[235]

Release of Dental Officers for Hardship. Release of dental officers for hardship, also authorized by War Department Circular 485, 29 December 1944, took place slowly prior to the end of the war. By the end of June 1945 only eight dentists had been separated for this cause. In August 1945, however, the War Department directed that increased consideration be given this factor as a cause for release from active duty before eligibility was established under normal separation criteria.[236]

Slowed "Turnover" Immediately Prior to V-E Day. At the end of 1944, the dental ASTP was approaching its termination and it appeared that in the future very few replacements would be available from this source. On 17 January 1945, a representative of the Military Personnel Division, SGO, warned that unless conservation of dental officers was practiced the procurement of dentists from civil life would have to be resumed by the end of June.[237] Alerted

---
[232] WD Cir 485, 29 Dec 44.

[233] A note accompanying a report of a conference between Army and PAS representatives in January 1945 states that "They (PAS) threw everything at us before; lists were meaningless." On file with Ltr, PAS to state chairmen for physicians, 27 Jan 45, sub: Release of physicians from the Army Medical Corps to return to practice. SG: 210.8.

[234] Basic communication referred to in footnote 233.

[235] Data given to the author by the Strength Accounting Br AGO, 13 Feb 48.

[236] By the end of August 1947 a total of 45 dental officers had been discharged for hardships. See also footnote 235, above.

[237] See footnote 90, p. 59.

by this warning, it was announced on 8 February 1945 that dental officer personnel then on duty would be considered as being within a critical and scarce category.[238] Further, that separations for causes other than those authorized by the provisions of War Department Circular 485 (see p. 91) would be limited insofar as practicable.[239] While the application of this rigid conservation policy enabled the Dental Corps to maintain its strength at the level required, it also slowed down the "turnover" of its officer personnel. This created a personnel situation which was far from favorable, and which at the end of the war (see chapter IX, Demobilization), was subject to a great deal of criticism.

STANDARDS FOR COMMISSION IN THE ARMY DENTAL CORPS

Physical Standards

With minor exceptions (e. g., dental standards for Medical Department officers and chaplains early in the war) physical standards for commissioning in the Dental Corps were the same as for all other branches.[240] Approximately one-third of all applicants were rejected for physical defects.[241]

The Dental Division was very reluctant to commission dentists who could not work a full day, who could not serve in unfavorable climates, or who were otherwise unavailable for general assignment. The first deviation from this policy came in July 1942 when Medical Officer Recruiting Boards were directed to accept dentists in the limited service category, apparently anticipating that sufficient officers could not otherwise be obtained.[242] By September 1942, procurement objectives were being filled without difficulty and The Surgeon General directed that only men threatened by induction would be commissioned, automatically eliminating limited service applicants.[243] With the granting of a new procurement objective for 7,200 dental officers in November 1942, restrictions on the commissioning of dentists were temporarily lifted and those in limited service categories again accepted, though The Surgeon General passed on all applications and it is probable that the number approved was kept as low as possible. On 8 September 1943 the PAS was asked not to declare available any dentists who were classified for "limited service" only. No additional dentists were accepted in that category during the remainder of the war, and with the first of 1944, efforts were concentrated on eliminating such officers already in the Dental Corps (see discussion this chapter, pp. 87–88).

---

[238] See footnote 92, p. 60.
[239] Ibid.
[240] See AR 40–105 for physical standards for military service at different periods of the war. Also, MR 1–9, 31 Aug 40. HD.
[241] Ltr, Col Robert C. Craven to Dr. John W. Leggett, 1 Sep 42. [D]
[242] See footnote 62, p. 54.
[243] See footnote 65, p. 55.

THE PROCUREMENT OF DENTAL OFFICERS 93

Age restrictions for dental officers varied considerably from time to time. In November 1940 it was directed that Reserve dentists would be called to active duty only when they were under the following maximum ages: [244]

First lieutenant	47 years
Captain	50 years
Major	54 years
Lieutenant colonel	58 years
Colonel	60 years

In August 1941 these provisions were modified to require that dentists on duty with troops be not over 56 years old, or 58 years if they were on Army staffs. Age-in-grade requirements were simultaneously removed.[245]

But while trained Reserve officers were generally accepted for active duty as long as they were not over the prescribed maximum age, the principal need was for young, vigorous men who could be assigned to combat units or to overseas areas with unfavorable climates. Most of this group were taken directly from civil life, without previous experience, and commissioned in the lowest grade. For these reasons the Dental Division desired to limit, as far as possible, procurement outside the reserve to men under 37 years of age who were eligible for general military duty and for whom the grade of lieutenant or captain would be appropriate. But the Dental Corps also wanted to be able to offer a commission to any dentist who might be threatened with early induction, so the maximum age limit went to 39 years during the periods when the Selective Service age limit was set at that figure. For brief periods when procurement threatened to lag, the upper age limit was raised to 44 or even 45 years.

When The Surgeon General established his Medical Officer Recruiting Boards in April 1942 he was instructed to accept older physicians to the extent necessary to permit him to obtain men with the necessary professional qualifications, but applicants for the Dental Corps were still to be accepted only if they were under 37 years of age.[246] The following month this directive was modified to allow the commissioning of dentists over 37 who were classified I-A by their Selective Service Boards,[247] and in June 1942 The Surgeon General informed The Adjutant General that a few men between the ages of 37 and 50 would be commissioned, but only with the express approval of The Surgeon General in each case.[248] It was implied that such exceptions to general policy would be made only to permit the commissioning of outstanding individuals, and the records support that inference. As a matter of fact, routine instruc-

---

[244] See footnote 116, p. 64.

[245] Ltr, TAG to CGs of all Armies, Army Corps, Divs, CAs, Depts, Def and Base Comds, COs of Exempted Stas, Chiefs of Arms and Servs, Chief of Armored Force, Chief AAF, CG, AF Combat Comd, and Chief of Staff, GHQ, 23 Aug 41, sub: Extension of tours of active duty, reserve officers. SG: 210.31-1.

[246] See footnote 198, p. 82.

[247] Ltr, Lt Col J. R. Hudnall to Lt Col A. R. Nichols, 16 May 42, sub: Medical officer recruiting board, letters of appointment and related forms. [D]

[248] Ltr, Lt Col Francis M. Fitts to Off Procmt Div, AGO, 24 Jun 42, sub: Officer procurement for the Army of the United States. SG: 320.2-1.

tions to the Medical Officer Recruiting Boards a week later again directed that dental officers were to be appointed only if they were under 37 years of age.[249] With the authorization of a new procurement objective of 4,000 dentists on 8 July 1942, the boards were temporarily instructed to accept applications from dentists up to 45 years of age, though applications from men over 37 still had to be approved by The Surgeon General.[250]

In January 1943 The Surgeon General directed that only dentists under 38 years of age would be considered, but on 19 May the Secretary of War was notified that dentists would be accepted up to age 42, or age 44 if classified I–A. In June 1943 the service commands were authorized to accept dentists between the ages of 38 and 44 if they had been declared available by the PAS, had refused commissions, and had been recommended for induction by Selective Service, but it is believed that this procedure was followed in very few cases.[251] In September 1943 the PAS was requested not to declare available any dentists who had reached the age of 38. By the end of 1943 The Adjutant General had authorized the release of dentists over 45 years of age for whom no suitable assignment could be found,[252] and this age limit was subsequently lowered to 38.[253] In March 1944 the Dental Division recommended that all dentists over 40 years of age be released, but this request was denied by ASF.[254] [255]

On V-E Day the age distribution of the Dental Corps was as follows:[256]

Age	Number of officers	Percentage of all officers
Under 30	3,902	25.5
30–34	4,086	26.7
35–39	4,958	32.4
40–44	1,423	9.3
45–49	581	3.8
50 or over	352	2.3

Professional and Ethical Standards

Educational requirements for dental officers were relatively simple; the applicant had to be a graduate of a standard school acceptable to The Surgeon General. All American schools were approved, including those limited to Negro students. The question of foreign schools was troublesome to the Medical

---

[249] Telegram, TAG to Medical Officers' Recruiting Board, 9th CA, 2 Jul 42. AG: 210.31.
[250] See footnote 62, p. 54.
[251] Ltr, TAG to CG, 5th SvC, 8 Jun 43, sub: Induction of physicians and dentists 38 years of age and over. SG: PAS files, Mil Pers Div.
[252] Ltr, TAG to Divs of WD Gen Staff, CGs AGF, AAF, ASF, Def Comds, Overseas Theaters and Depts, 8 Dec 43, sub: Relief from active duty of officers for whom no suitable assignment exists. SG: 210.8.
[253] Ltr, TAG to Divs of WD Gen Staff, CGs AGF, AAF, ASF, Def Comds, Overseas Theaters and Depts, 12 Jan 44, sub: Relief from active duty of officers for whom no suitable assignment exists. AG: 210.85.
[254] Memo, Exec Off, SGO, to Dir Mil Pers Div, ASF, 11 Mar 44. HD: 314.
[255] The original of the communication rejecting The Surgeon General's request of 11 March 1944 has not been found. This letter, dated 25 March 1944, is quoted verbatim, however, in a report of the Dental Division for the period 21 Feb–1 Apr 44, on file in Bi-weekly Reports file. HD: 024.
[256] See footnote 106, p. 62.

Corps, but the number of graduates of foreign schools applying for dental commissions was negligible.

During the first year of the war an applicant for the Dental Corps was required to have a valid license to practice in a state or territory, but in January 1943 this requisite was dropped, as far as recent graduates were concerned, to make it possible to accept the latter immediately, without waiting for them to take a board.

The enforcement of ethical standards involved some knotty problems. It was of course directed that only dentists in good standing in the profession would be commissioned, but the definition of ethical practice, and its application in specific cases, was not always easy. In the absence of evidence to the contrary, membership in the ADA was a prima facie indication of acceptability, but approximately one-third of the dentists in the United States were not members of the ADA and these men had to be considered on their own merits. In some cases it was charged that actual membership had been required locally. In New York City, for instance, the Allied Dental Council complained that its members had been asked if they belonged to the 2d District Dental Society (ADA) when they applied for commissions at the city recruiting board.[257] It was not specifically stated that they would otherwise be rejected, but rightly or wrongly that inference was drawn. The Surgeon General immediately replied that membership in any society was not a requisite for a commission in the Army.[258] But the ADA was allowed to set the ethical standard for acceptance by the Dental Corps, and to pass on the standing of individuals through the SGO liaison office at ADA national headquarters, resulting in occasional protests from groups having less rigid requirements. In May 1943, for instance, a number of members of a New York society met with representatives of the Dental Division to protest refusal of the 2d District Dental Society to certify them to the Army, mainly on the grounds that they were "advertisers." They were informed that "dentists in New York City . . . must conform to the code of ethics laid down by the 2d District Dental Society."[259] A few days later the protesting dentists were called to a joint meeting with representatives of the 2d District Society and they were informed that if they met the requirements of that organization (i. e., removed the offending signs) they would be certified. Many dentists followed this advice and were accepted.

The practice of allowing the ADA to pass on the ethical status of nonmembers may be questioned, but it is difficult to see how the problem could have been solved in any other way. The ordinary citizen is assumed to be honest if he is not convicted of a crime, and the merchant who gains an advantage in

---

[257] Ltr, Dr. M. J. Futterman, Chairman, National Victory Committee, Allied Dental Council, New York, to SG, 24 Jun 42. [D]

[258] Ltr, Maj Gen R. H. Mills to Dr. M. J. Futterman, 30 Jun 42. [D]

[259] Statement, Col Robert C. Craven to Co-chairman of Mil Affairs Committee, 2d District Dental Society, 17 May 43. [D]

a business deal is considered to be a smart operator, but the ethics of the commercial world are not applicable to dental practice; if the merchant delivers goods other than those specified the fact is readily apparent and redress can easily be made, but the quality of the dentist's work can be determined only after many years have elapsed, and after irreparable damage may have been done. The dentist is therefore in a unique position of trust in that he must consider not only his own interests but those of his patients as well. To protect its patients, and its own good name, the dental profession has found it necessary to set for itself standards which are materially higher than those prescribed by law, which are generally drawn up to meet commercial requirements. This has been accomplished through the only organization representing any large proportion of American dentists, the ADA.

Not all of the criteria established by the ADA have been accepted by nonmembers of that body. Advertising, for instance, tends to substitute the press agent's skill for a laboriously acquired professional reputation, but in itself it may not indicate gross moral deficiency. It was therefore held in some quarters that the fact that a dentist had advertised for patients was not an adequate reason for barring him from the Army Dental Corps. As a matter of past experience, however, advertising had so often been associated with other, more objectionable practices that it was certainly a danger signal to be given considerable weight in determining whether or not a dentist was of the type wanted for Army installations. In general the ADA standards had been found satisfactory in operation, and their acceptance by the Dental Corps would appear to have been justified. Moreover, The Surgeon General had neither the information nor the organization with which to undertake the evaluation of thousands of dentists, and the ADA was the only body which had both. It has been suggested that the PAS should have assumed responsibility for determining ethical and professional standing, but if it had been given that task it would almost certainly have had to go to the ADA for the information on which to act.

COMMISSIONS ABOVE THE GRADE OF FIRST LIEUTENANT

During the war the Dental Division generally disapproved of granting initial commissions above the lowest grade, and even when an allotment of higher grades was authorized it was seldom filled. This policy was voluntarily adopted without pressure from higher authority in either the SGO or the War Department. The first major procurement objective of the war, granted in January 1942, provided for the procurement of 5 majors, 20 captains, and 475 lieutenants, but it was filled almost entirely in the grade of lieutenant.[260] When the Medical Officer Recruiting Boards were established in April 1942 The Surgeon General was permitted to offer sufficient commissions above the

---

[260] See footnote 56, p. 53.

lowest grade to attract qualified applicants, but a few weeks later the boards were specifically directed that dentists would be commissioned in the grade of first lieutenant only, except in special cases, and with the approval of The Surgeon General.[261] In June 1942 The Surgeon General notified The Adjutant General that a few dentists above the age of 37 would be given commissions as captains or majors with the approval of the Chief of the Dental Division, but implied that such cases would be very rare.[262] In September 1942 an officer of the Dental Division stated that captaincies would be given only to men over 40, with special qualifications. A few appointments above the lowest grade were made in 1943, but by 1 January 1944 only 2 dentists had been commissioned as majors and 163 as captains.[263] At least one of the above majors was commissioned for the Veterans Administration, and most subsequent commissions above the grade of captain were for that organization.

The policy of the Dental Division in respect to granting higher original commissions was criticized by PAS, which felt that its task would have been easier if it could have offered captaincies or majorities to hesitant applicants. Some dental societies also felt that qualified specialists or older men with families should be given grades above that of first lieutenant. The position of the Dental Division was that for each dentist appointed as a captain or major some officer who had volunteered a year or more before would be deprived of promotion. It was felt that men already in the service generally had as much to offer as the dentists who were holding out for advanced grades, and there could be no question but that the former were better qualified from the military point of view. Only in exceptional cases did clinical proficiency justify giving a dentist without military background a commission in a higher grade than had been offered the man who volunteered immediately after Pearl Harbor. The situation was also complicated by the absence of definite standards for determining clinical qualifications; as long as there were no recognized boards to say whether or not a dentist should be classed as a specialist, claims to special ability were made very freely, and to have granted dentists advanced grades on the basis of their own statements would in many cases have resulted in an injustice to the Government and to the officers already commissioned. There can be no doubt, however, that qualified oral surgeons or prosthetic specialists were not attracted by the grades they were offered in the Dental Service, and this fact was noted in personnel summaries submitted at the end of the war.[264] If the policy of assigning dental officers to units in the grade of *either* captain or lieutenant is followed in the future it will be possible to offer captaincies to the more experienced dentists without jeopardizing the

---

[261] Ltr, SG, no distribution indicated, but apparently directed to Medical Officer Recruiting Boards, 23 Apr 42, sub: Appointment in the Army of the United States (Medical Department). SG: 320.2-1.
[262] See footnote 247, p. 93.
[263] Brown, P. W.: Procurement of dental officers from civil life, p. 32. HD: 314.7-2 (Dentistry—Army Dental Corps).
[264] See footnote 122, p. 65.

rights of earlier volunteers. The establishment of recognized specialty boards will also make it possible to commission qualified dentists as captains or majors on an equitable basis, with a minimum of protest from nonboard members. But only a limited number of vacancies exist in the higher grades, and if they are used carelessly, to lure reluctant dentists when procurement becomes more difficult, the earlier volunteers will suffer, and morale may be expected to drop.

THE DEFERMENT OF INSTRUCTORS IN DENTAL SCHOOLS

(See Chapter on "Personnel and Training.")

THE NONPROFESSIONAL USE OF DENTAL OFFICERS

The number of dentists in the United States has never exceeded the bare minimum required to meet the most urgent requirements. When the Armed Forces took nearly a third of all civilian dentists the remainder were able to care for the nonmilitary population only with the greatest difficulty. No more men could be spared without endangering the health of war workers, school children, and the general public. It was therefore imperative that the available supply of dental officers be used with the utmost economy.

Under some circumstances a military dentist had to be prepared to assume nonprofessional duties. A dental officer with a small task force attacking a Pacific island, for instance, could not hope to accomplish much dental work during the assault phase, and he could generally render the most valuable service by acting as assistant to a medical officer. Also, during the first part of the war, medical organizations, and even tactical units, were sometimes so short of trained personnel that any officers with military experience had to fill key positions until replacements could be trained. In these situations dental officers were used as executives or even as detachment commanders. Regulations provided that dentists could not command any unit, but these directives were often ignored.[265] When the Dental Division recommended in 1942 that an order be published prohibiting the use of dentists for other than their proper clinical or administrative duties, the Military Personnel Division of the SGO flatly refused approval on the grounds that dental officers were at that time indispensable in many auxiliary positions.[266]

There was less justification for the tendency to use dental officers in minor duties which could have been performed by administrative personnel with a few months of training. In the case of tactical commands this abuse often resulted from the circumstances surrounding the formation of new units in the Zone of Interior. As new organizations were assembled there was usually an interim period during which most dental care was furnished by the permanent station

---
[265] See footnote 21, p. 44.
[266] Ibid.

dental clinic. At this time assigned dental officers often lacked their equipment, and the full complement of enlisted personnel had not yet arrived. A field hospital, for instance, had little clinical work to perform until it went overseas, yet it had a full quota of administrative positions to be filled by inexperienced officers. Under these conditions it was almost routine practice to assign the three dental officers to nonprofessional tasks since they had free time and the other officers were busy coping with unfamiliar jobs.

But when such a unit arrived overseas the situation changed completely. The dentists were immediately overwhelmed with demands for treatment, but the assignment to outside duties often continued. The dental surgeon of the Middle East theater found that two dentists in one hospital were together acting as mess officer, supply officer, transportation officer, finance officer, censor officer, and sanitary officer.[267] The dental surgeon of the China-Burma-India theater reported that "We really have plenty of dental officers en route to and in the theater if they could be properly placed and put on their proper duty, but we still have plenty with supply units, messing with minor staff jobs, censoring mail, running messes, etc." [268]

The improper utilization of dental officers during the first years of World War II also derived in part from the prewar doctrine that the dentist's normal duty in combat was to assist the surgeon. This conception had in turn resulted from the admitted circumstance that under the World War I organization the Dental Service could not function too effectively in a forward area and some other duty had to be found for the dental officer of a unit in action. The period of actual combat in World War I was too short to reveal the danger of this policy, but as the Second World War progressed it was found that evacuations for dental emergencies soon reached important proportions when routine treatment was neglected over any considerable period of time; the dental officer could render the most important service to his command by giving all his time to his proper professional duties. The dental surgeon of the European theater reported that "the dental officers were used purely as auxiliary medical officers in most instances . . . until the medical officers realized that men were getting into the chain of evacuation for dental reasons only, showing that the best utilization of dental officers was not being made." [269] A conference of senior dental surgeons, called by The Surgeon General in February 1945, recommended that: [270]

> The utilization of dental officers as auxiliary medical officers, as a routine procedure, is condemned. . . . the dental needs of a division require the full and most efficient utilization of its dental personnel in dental activities at all times.

---

[267] Jeffcott, G. F.: Dental problems in the Middle East Theater of Operations. Mil. Surgeon 96: 54–58, Jan 1945.
[268] Personal ltr, Col Dell S. Gray to Col Rex McK. McDowell, 1 Jul 44. [D]
[269] Ltr, Col Thomas L. Smith, Dental Surg, ETO, to SG, 6 Feb 45, sub: History of the Dental Division, Headquarters, ETOUSA, from 1 Sep through 31 Dec 44. HD: 730 (Dentistry) ETO.
[270] Memo, Maj Gen R. H. Mills to Brig Gen F. A. Blesse, 8 Feb 45. [D]

It was ultimately clear that if dental officers could not render regular dental care under the existing organization, that organization would have to be changed. (See discussion of the division Dental Service in chapter VIII.)

Until the middle of 1942, dental officers' services were also misused to some extent in permanent installations of the Zone of Interior. (See chapter I, page 14.) This practice was prohibited in the Zone of Interior by a War Department directive of 31 July 1942 which provided that in the future dentists would be used only in the operation or supervision of the Dental Service, and that dentists currently performing other functions would be replaced as soon as substitutes could be trained.[271] The Air Force issued a similar directive on 7 September 1942.[272]

World War II experience supported the following conclusions in respect to the proper use of dental officers:

1. The number of dentists available in an emergency will normally be strictly limited. It will be sufficient only if they are used with the greatest economy.

2. If the dentists assigned to combat units are used for other than professional duties, except for very short periods of time, evacuations for dental emergencies may be expected to result in an excessive loss of manpower when it is most urgently needed.

3. It is essential that the Dental Service be organized to permit dental officers to function with a minimum of interruption due to tactical operations. If dental officers cannot treat the soldiers of their commands during combat they should be removed and used for the care of units in reserve.

4. Some line officers who do not appreciate the need for regular dental care in their commands will probably continue to use dentists in nonessential activities until prevented by a specific official directive or by a reorganization of dental facilities.

Early steps to prevent the misuse of dentists were reasonably effective in the Zone of Interior, but they had no direct application outside the United States. Changes in the organization of dental facilities in tactical units and the development of the mobile operating and prosthetic units improved the situation overseas to some extent, but the nonprofessional use of dentists was not altogether eliminated before the end of hostilities. Finally, in October 1945, the War Department directed all commands, Zone of Interior and overseas, that no medical, dental, or Army Nurse Corps officers would be used in positions which could be filled by officers of other corps of the Medical Department.[273]

---

[271] Ltr, TAG to CGs all Svcs, 31 Jul 42, sub: Utilization of dental officers for professional duties. AG: 210.312 (Dental Corps).

[272] AAF Reg 25-4, 7 Sep 42, sub: Utilization of dental officers with the AAF. On file in the Office of the Air Surgeon, USAF.

[273] WD Cir 307, 6 Oct 45.

THE RELOCATION OF CIVILIAN DENTISTS

The program to relocate civilian dentists who were excess to the needs of their communities, so that they could provide dental treatment in areas where they were more critically required, was of course not a responsibility of the Armed Forces. It did affect the overall utilization of dental manpower, however, and the Army was even more directly concerned when it had to furnish dental care at such locations as the Oak Ridge atomic bomb plant. Actually, the relocation program seems to have received very little attention during the war, either because it was considered unnecessary or because it was considered impractical by those who would have had to enforce it.

Early in 1944 Congress appropriated $200,000 to be used to encourage dentists and physicians to move to districts where health care was precarious. Volunteers were to be paid $250 a month for 3 months to enable them to get a start in the new location, and all moving expenses were to be paid. Local communities were to carry one-quarter of the total expense in each case.[274] The small amount of money appropriated indicates that the effort was experimental, and practical results of the voluntary relocation program were actually negligible. Only 7 applications were received, and 3 dentists were moved; 1 other moved with Federal assistance but with no expenditure of funds. The project was abandoned in June 1944.[275]

In theory PAS could have brought about the relocation of dentists by declaring them nonessential in their own areas, making them subject to conscription if they did not move to critical districts. But such action depended upon effective support from Selective Service, and it has already been seen that such support was lacking. Moreover, PAS itself showed little interest in the matter. Dr. C. Willard Camalier, who was Chairman of the War Service Committee of the ADA, and also a member of the Directing Board, PAS, had reported that:[276]

> . . . while we have no figures on the matter, I am inclined to feel that very little, if any, of this (relocation) was done.
>
> As a member of the Procurement and Assignment Directing Board, I was quite well aware of the fact that the Armed Services were taking so many dentists from civil practice that those left were kept so busy that it would not have been profitable for them to locate in other sections of the United States. They would have all they could possibly look after in their own areas. In several instances, such as Michigan, near the war plants, and a few points down South, officers of the U. S. Public Health Service were detailed to care for the needs of the population. Dentists under the auspices of the Army were utilized at Oak Ridge, Tennessee.

Whether or not the relocation program was necessary, or whether it would have produced more tangible results if a more sustained effort had been made

---

[274] Congress provides fund for relocation of civilian dentists. J. Am. Dent. A. 31 : 166, Jan 1944.
[275] Relocation program for dentists halted June 30. J. Am. Dent. A. 31 : 1021, Jul 1944.
[276] Personal ltr, Dr. C. Willard Camalier to the author, 16 Oct 47. [D]

by all concerned, is not a matter for consideration here. It seems clear, though, that dentists who are very busy in their home communities will not voluntarily move to other locations; if such redistribution becomes unavoidable in a future emergency some compulsion or extra remuneration must be provided.

UTILIZATION OF FEMALE DENTISTS

Three bills to authorize the commissioning of female dentists were introduced in Congress between June 1943 and March 1945.[277][278][279] The Dental Division and the Army opposed enactment of all of these bills on the grounds that there was no shortage of male dentists in the Armed Forces and that to commission females would raise special problems of housing and assignment.[280] After 1944 it was also noted that the Army was already being criticized because it could not accept all ASTP graduates. Another consideration, which was implied but not stated in these protests, was that the factor which limited the number of dentists available to the Armed Forces was not a numerical shortage of male dentists but the necessity for leaving sufficient personnel to meet the minimum needs of the civilian population. It would have served no useful purpose to commission women and then leave a corresponding number of ablebodied males to care for their patients. Probably as a result of Army disapproval, none of the bills to commission female dentists was passed by Congress.

POSTWAR PROCUREMENT FOR THE DENTAL CORPS

On 10 August 1945 the War Department announced that it was considering a plan for increasing the Regular Army Dental Corps by offering commissions to dental officers who had demonstrated their capabilities during the emergency period.[281] The necessary legislation was passed by Congress on 28 December 1945,[282] and the procedure to be followed was published by the War Department on the following day.[283] The integration program was designed to bring the total number of officers in the Regular Army to 50,000, an increase of a little under 34,000 officers. The Dental Corps was authorized an additional 476 officers, to bring its total strength to 743 dentists.[284]

[277] H. R. 2892, 78th Cong., introduced by Representative John J. Sparkman, on 7 Jun 43.
[278] H. R. 1704, 79th Cong., introduced by Representative John J. Sparkman, on 23 Jan 45.
[279] S. 731, 79th Cong., introduced by Senator Claude Pepper, on 13 Mar 45.
[280] For criticism of the bills to commission female dentists see: (1) Ltr, SecWar to Hon Andrew J. May, 22 Jul 43. (2) Ltr, SecWar to Hon Elbert D. Thomas, 8 May 45. (3) Memo, Maj Gen R. H. Mills for Mil Pers Div SGO, 27 Mar 45. All in HD: 314.
[281] WD Cir 243, 10 Aug 45.
[282] Public Law 281, 79th Cong., 28 Dec 45.
[283] WD Cir 392, 29 Dec 45.
[284] Data given the author by Col James M. Epperly of the Dental Div SGO, on 15 Jan 48.

SUMMARY, DENTAL OFFICER PROCUREMENT PROGRAM

The dental officer procurement program of World War II was successful in that more than 15,000 qualified dentists were obtained for the Army under very difficult conditions. The principal defects revealed were: [285]

1. During the early part of the war applicants were accepted without regard to their true availability, endangering civilian dental practice in some areas.

2. The policy of commissioning almost all applicants in the lowest grade protected earlier volunteers but it lost the services of some expert clinicians who might profitably have been accepted as captains or majors in spite of their lack of military experience. Deviation from World War II policy, in a limited number of selected cases, will probably prove advisable in any future mobilization.

3. The classification of officers according to special skills was not accurate enough, especially during the first years of the war, to permit the most efficient assignment and utilization of personnel. Clinical specialists were sometimes assigned to small tactical units rather than to hospitals or other large installations where their services could best be used.

4. Experience at the end of hostilities, when dental officers had to be held in the service after other officers were released, and when conscription was necessary to procure even a part of the replacements needed, clearly demonstrated the need for a slow but constant turnover of dental personnel during a long war. Older men with families and with established practices will be willing to serve in the Army during the early stages of an emergency, but they will bring strong and effective pressure to bear if, after they have served for 2 or 3 years, they see recent graduates of the dental schools returning to civilian life to take over their practices. The situation of a dental officer in this respect is different from that of a line officer. No able-bodied young man who is eligible for service in the infantry, for instance, will be allowed to evade military duty after he graduates from high school or college; he will be taken into the Army without delay, and his status will generally be inferior to that of the man who came on duty at an earlier date. But the shortage of dentists in the United States is such that recent dental graduates will not ordinarily be taken into the Armed Forces for nondental duty. If they cannot be used as dental officers because of a lack of vacancies they will be allowed to set up offices in civilian communities to provide badly needed dental care. It is easy to understand the older dentists' position that the younger men should be given their share of military service, releasing officers who have already had several years of active duty. When Dr. X, who had served 3 years in the Army, with 2 years overseas, received a letter from his wife saying that young Dr. Y, who had graduated the year before, had now taken over most of Dr. X's practice

---
[285] See footnote 122, p. 65.

his morale took a severe dip. When Dr. X was later held in the Army after other officers with similar service were being released, his general distaste for all things military was converted to an active resentment which would color his future actions as a member of the dental profession and as a citizen.

If the Army Dental Corps consists almost entirely of officers with several years of service when hostilities end, these men will have to be released without delay; at about the same time compulsory procurement may be terminated, resulting in a critical personnel crisis. By the very nature of their business, dentists cannot afford to give up the practices which they have taken years to build to accept temporary, voluntary, military service in the postwar period. If the older men are gradually replaced by recent graduates during the war a more balanced Dental Corps will result, demobilization at the end of hostilities will be more orderly, and personnel difficulties will be minimized during the difficult period of transition from war to peace.

5. The procurement program was characterized by frequent changes of policy which confused and irritated cooperating agencies and the dentists themselves. The ADA complained of this situation as follows:[286]

> When war came, the Army opened and closed commissions in the Dental Corps with such eccentric rapidity that dentists and state Procurement and Assignment chairmen were in a perpetual quandary. On one day a large procurement objective would be set and on another the Dental Corps would be closed and dentists in the process of getting commissions, having closed their offices would be sent back to civilian life. The Army Specialized Training Program was initiated with the proper flourish of military trumpets as the answer to the problem of providing the Army with a continuing supply of dental personnel. This program was barely in full motion when one entire class of dental graduates was sent into civilian life because "procurement objectives" allegedly had been reached. . . . Under this mistaken knowledge of its own needs the Army eventually shut down the entire dental ASTP and permitted many potential dental officers to return to civil life instead of completing their training as replacements for veteran officers. So certain was the Army that the matter of dental personnel was well in hand that, at about this time, the Dental Corps was again closed.

This criticism was of course extreme, and not fully justified. So far as is known, dentists in the process of being commissioned were always accepted for service if they met physical requirements. The frequent changes in policy complained of generally paralleled War Department changes in estimates of the forces needed to meet new developments, and the extent to which the flow of dentists into the Armed Forces could have been smoothed out is a matter of opinion. Procurement objectives were admittedly changed on short notice, however, and a more consistent program would certainly be desirable, to the extent it could be achieved under emergency conditions.

---

[286] Dental officers pay again. J. Am. Dent. A. 33 : 755–757, 1 Jun 46.

CHAPTER IV

Personnel and Training

COMPOSITION OF THE DENTAL CORPS

Important items in a discussion of officers of the wartime Dental Corps are background, age, and previous military preparation. Information is not available concerning all of the 18,000 dental officers who served in the Army between 1 October 1940 and 31 December 1945,[1] but a cross-sectional view of the 15,302 officers who were either on duty 31 May 1945 or had been released shortly before that date [2] reveals the following:[3]

Distribution by Age

Age	Number	Percent	Approximate years of practice before entering the Army*
Under 30	3,902	25.5	0–2
30–34	4,086	26.7	3–7
35–39	4,958	32.4	8–12
40–44	1,423	9.3	13–17
45–49	581	3.8	18–22
50–over	352	2.3	23–over

*Years of practice based on average age at graduation of 25–26 [4] and assumption that men on duty in 1945 averaged 2 years of military service.

Distribution by Race

Race	Number	Percent
White	15,131	98.89
Negro	132	0.86
Chinese	25	0.16
Japanese	8	0.05
Others	6	0.04

Distribution by Component

Component	Number	Percent
Regular Army	266	1.7
National Guard	117	0.8
Organized Reserve Corps	3,106	20.3
AUS (obtained through ASTP)	1,802	11.8
AUS (obtained from civilian life)	10,011	65.4

---

[1] Memo, Mr. Isaac Cogan for Dir, Dent Cons Div, SGO, 29 Aug 46, sub: Dental Corps officers—historical data. SG: 322.053-1.

[2] The number of dental officers actually on duty on V-E Day was about 14,700. When the data given here were calculated in June 1945 reports of separations during the preceding month were incomplete.

[3] See footnote 1 above.

[4] Strusser, H.: Dental problems in postwar planning. J. Am. Dent. A. 32: 991–1003, 1 Aug 45.

Distribution by Specialty

Specialty	Number	Percent
Oral Surgeon (MOS 3171)	65	0.4
Exodontist (MOS 3172)	325	2.1
Periodontist (MOS 3174)	20	0.1
Prosthodontist (MOS 3175)	255	1.7
Staff Dentist (MOS 3178)	170	1.1
No specialty (MOS 3170)	14,467	94.6

The "average" dentist was about 33 when he entered the Army (assuming 2 years of service in 1945) and had been in private practice nearly 8 years. Though well-qualified as an operative dentist, he was not likely to have had extensive training as a specialist. Only 4 per 1,000 were oral surgeons and only 1 per 1,000 was a periodontist. Nearly two-thirds had entered the Army with no previous experience in the Armed Forces, and though professionally competent, almost all of this group needed more or less additional military training before they were fitted to fill responsible positions. This was the "raw material" from which the Army Dental Service was assembled.

ASSIGNMENT OF DENTAL OFFICERS

The proportion of dentists in service command installations in the United States, in the Air Forces, and in tactical organizations in the United States and overseas fluctuated with the progress of mobilization and with changes in the course of the war. The greatest number of dentists on duty at any time was 15,292 in November 1944.[5] Subsequent strength reductions were not significant until after V-E Day. The maximum figure in the United States was reached a year earlier, in November 1943, with a total of 11,544 men (Air Forces, service commands, and tactical units).[6] The largest number on duty with the Air Forces (United States and overseas) was about 3,739 in May 1945. The number of Army dentists overseas increased from about 1,000 (10 percent) in December 1942 to 3,221 (22.5 percent) in December 1943 and 6,017 (39.8 percent) in December 1944. The maximum number abroad was reached in March 1945 when 7,111 dental officers, or 48.1 percent of all Army dentists, were on foreign service, but the highest ratio was not reached until May 1945 when the 7,103 dentists overseas were 48.3 percent of the total on duty. At the end of 1945 only 2,886 (30.0 percent) of all dentists were overseas. The maximum number of Air Forces dentists overseas was 1,103 (29.5 percent) in May 1945.[7]

---

[5] Memo, Mr. Isaac Cogan for Chief, Dent Cons Div, SGO, 8 Oct 46, sub: Basic data for Dental Corps. SG: 322.0531.

[6] Unpublished data from the Resources Analysis Division, SGO, given to author in Oct 1946.

[7] Unpublished data from the Personnel Division, Office of the Air Surgeon, given to author on 1 Oct 46.

PERSONNEL AND TRAINING

The approximate authorized percentages of dentists in different types of assignments on 31 March 1944 were as follows:[8]

	Percent
Tables of organization units (U. S. and overseas)	36.9
Army Service Forces, U. S. (Exclusive of T/O Units)	32.3
Army Air Forces, U. S. (Exclusive of T/O Units)	21.1
Theater overhead (Exclusive of T/O Units)	.7
Replacement pools	6.8
Other	2.2

This ratio was of course subject to constant change as emphasis was transferred from training activities in the United States to combat operations overseas. During the early part of the war a majority of dentists were required for work on new men in Army Service Forces and Air Forces installations in the United States. Later they were needed in the units actually engaged in operations (T/O units overseas and in the United States).

PROFESSIONAL CLASSIFICATION OF DENTAL OFFICERS

At the start of mobilization there was no effective plan for the classification of dental officers according to special qualifications. Some attempt was made locally to assign dentists to appropriate work but these efforts were hampered by the absence of any standardized system by which the specialized abilities of an officer could be determined at a glance. Too much reliance had to be placed on the dentist's own estimate of his qualifications, so that men with not much more than a desire to do a certain type of work were designated as specialists, while other trained officers were placed in routine jobs.[9]

On 21 October 1943 The Adjutant General directed that dental officers would be evaluated in respect to professional qualifications on the basis of questionnaires to be sent to The Surgeon General.[10] At about the same time a War Department Technical Manual (TM 12–406) described six classifications for dentists, as follows:[11]

MOS 3170 (Dental officer) general practitioner.
MOS 3171 (Oral surgeon, dental) fully qualified oral surgeon. Should have extensive experience in oral surgery and have been a member of a hospital staff. Internship, residency, or fellowship desirable.
MOS 3172 (Exodontist) qualified as extraction specialist. Extensive training in exodontia, and internship or residency desirable.
MOS 3174 (Periodontist) qualified to treat investing tissues of teeth. Extensive training or experience very desirable.

---
[8] Memo, Chief, Oprs Br, SGO, for CG, ASF, 5 Jun 44, sub: Requirements for Dental Corps officers. SG: 322.0531–1.
[9] Final Rpt for ASF, Logistics in World War II. HD: 319.1–2 (Dental Division).
[10] Ltr SPX 220.01 (6 Oct 1943) OC–E–SPGAP–MB–A, 21 Oct 43, sub: Correct classification and assignment of Army Service Forces officers and enlisted men. AG: 220.01 (19 Sep 43) (1).
[11] TM 12–406, Officer classification, commissioned and warrant, 30 Oct 43.

MOS 3175 (Prosthodontist) qualified to construct bridges and dentures. Extensive training or experience essential.

MOS 3178 (Dental officer, staff) qualified to advise surgeons of major units on the operation of the dental service. Must have previous military experience.

(All dentists were required to be graduates of accepted schools, licensed to practice dentistry, and actually engaged in ethical practice at the time of entry into the Army.)

Early in 1944, TM 12–406 was amended to authorize the use of modifying letter symbols in connection with the MOS numbers, of medical officers only, to indicate relative ability within a specific field. Thus a surgeon of moderate skill might be designed "MOS D 3150," while a surgeon with outstanding background and experience would be listed as "MOS A 3150."[12] This refinement, however, was not applied to other Medical Department officers, possibly because there were then in existence no recognized civilian standards for dental and veterinary specialists.

Original classifications of medical, dental, and veterinary officers were made from information contained in the "Classification Questionnaire of Medical Department Officers."[13] Later adjustments in classification were made from reports of "Reevaluation Data for Medical Department Officers."[14] In the case of dental officers, the assignment of an MOS number was carried out in the Dental Division, SGO.

The Director of the Dental Division, SGO, found that these measures aided in the appropriate assignment of dentists, but that they were not a complete solution of the problem. He stated after the war that:[15]

> . . . the system is very weak because there is no "measuring rod" and no "official" check or follow-up to determine an officer's true classification . . . There are too many officers classified as oral surgeons and as prosthodontists who in reality have had no formal training in those specialties and whose experience in these fields has been very limited. . . . The fact that a man's MOS states that he is an oral surgeon does not really mean that he is a qualified oral surgeon. . . . Although the present mechanics set up for the classification of dental officers is a definite advancement over that used at the beginning of the war, it definitely is not an effective instrument in the assignment and utilization of manpower.

The solution recommended was a "clearer definition of the meaning and intent of the several classifications as well as the setting up of additional criteria for selection; a dental classification section in Personnel Service, SGO, with sufficient personnel, which can currently follow up on all changes of classification, and which can check effectively on qualifications as well as on assignments of Dental Corps personnel."[16]

---
[12] TM 12–406, C 1, 10 May 44.
[13] WD AGO Form 178–2, 1 Jan 45.
[14] WD AGO Form 178–3, 1 Aug 45.
[35] See footnote 9, p. 107.
[16] Ibid.

PROMOTION

In time of peace, promotion in the Dental Corps of the Regular Army was based on the same regulations which governed promotion in the Medical Corps, providing for original appointment in the grade of first lieutenant, with periodic advancement thereafter on the basis of total service.[17] Total service required for promotion to the various grades above that of lieutenant was as follows:

Captain	3 years
Major	12 years
Lieutenant colonel	20 years
Colonel	26 years

For reasons which are not clear, Reserve officers could be promoted even more rapidly, after the following periods of total service:[18]

Captain	4 years
Major	9 years
Lieutenant colonel	15 years
Colonel	22 years

Regular Army dental officers were required to pass examinations on both professional and military subjects, except that candidates for advancement to the two highest grades were examined only on military problems.[19] Reserve officers had to pass examinations in military subjects or complete specified correspondence courses appropriate to the higher grade.[20] In addition, they had to attend at least one summer camp of 2 weeks duration prior to each promotion.

Original commissions in the grade of first lieutenant helped to equalize the status of the professional officer, who generally entered the service at an older age, with that of the line officer who started his career several years earlier and who generally obtained his education at Government expense. Promotion solely on the basis of time-in-grade was criticized because it did not reward the outstanding officer nor provide an incentive to special efforts. It did, however, eliminate political influence as a factor in advancement and left the officer more opportunity to exercise his own judgment without fear of reprisal as long as his performance and behavior met accepted standards.

With mobilization, key positions in a rapidly expanding Army had to be filled quickly by procedures which could be applied to Regular, Reserve, and temporary officers. On 1 January 1942 most of the peacetime promotion regulations were suspended, and advancement was thereafter based on the following factors:[21]

---

[17] AR 605-50, 30 Jul 36.
[18] AR 140-5, 16 Jun 36.
[19] AR 605-55, 11 Oct 35.
[20] See footnote 18, above.
[21] WD Cir 1, 1 Jan 42.

1. Completion of a minimum specified time-in-grade.
2. Recommendations from superiors, attesting to the officers' qualifications.
3. Existence of a vacancy in the desired grade. Under these provisions dental officers enjoyed the same promotion status as members of other branches, at least in theory. In practice, unfortunately, stagnation of promotion in the Dental Corps soon became so serious that it was the cause for frequent criticism during the latter part of the war.[22]

A minor reason for the lack of opportunity for advancement in the Dental Service was of course the relatively low rate of attrition among dental officers.[23]

Another factor was the difficulty encountered, under emergency conditions, in determining which officers were best qualified for promotion. Little effort was made to transfer eligible officers from posts where no vacancies existed to installations where opportunities were better. At the worst, an officer's efficiency might actually reduce his chances for advancement since he was more likely to be held at the old, established installation, while the less desirable officer might be transferred to a new facility where more vacancies could be expected. A considerable element of chance was thus introduced into the promotion program, and men who were lucky enough to be in the right place at the right time advanced rapidly while equally competent men held the same grade for the duration of the war.

By far the most important reason for slow promotion in the Dental Corps, however, was the lack of positions in the Dental Service calling for grades above that of captain.

In the Zone of Interior, where the size and mission of installations varied widely, local commanders were given considerable freedom to determine what grades would be allotted to individual activities, as long as prescribed totals were not exceeded. The commanding general of a service command, for instance, received a total authorization of grades for his entire area, and he could distribute them among the respective corps pretty much as he pleased, according to their relative strength, his own estimate of responsibilities involved, or any other factors which seemed important. Similarly, the commander of a post or hospital might or might not allocate to the Dental Service enough of the field grades at his disposal to make reasonable promotion possible. Only in the case of very gross and obvious discrimination was the local commander likely to be called upon to justify his actions in this respect. The advantage of this policy was that promotion was placed in the hands of officials who were familiar with duties and responsibilities in the installation concerned; the disadvantage was that personal factors might play a considerable part in determining who should be advanced. Also, under regulations then in effect the dental officer could not personally support his recommendations concerning the grades needed by his activity, and he had to rely on the good will and aggressiveness of the surgeon, who alone served on the commander's staff.

---

[22] See chapter I.
[23] See chapter III, p. 56.

Under such circumstances it was perhaps inevitable that opportunities for promotion in the Dental Service varied greatly in different commands and installations in the Zone of Interior, and that serious inequities were possible. The normal allotment of dentists for a 25-chair clinic, for example, was considered to be 1 lieutenant colonel, 5 majors, and 19 captains or lieutenants,[24] but this ratio was seldom attained. One general hospital was reported to have no dental officer in field grade in spite of the fact that it had 15 majors in other branches.[25] Since the senior dentist was always a subordinate of the senior medical officer the former's grade tended to be set below that of the surgeon, and this lower grade of the dental surgeon was in turn reflected in lower grades for his subordinates throughout the Dental Service. At the end of 1943 only 1.6 percent of all service command dentists were colonels, 3.3 percent were lieutenant colonels, and 11.6 percent were majors; the proportion of medical officers in these top grades was approximately twice as great.[26]

The composition of tactical commands was not left to the discretion of commanders, but was prescribed by rigid "tables of organization." An infantry regiment could have two dentists in the grade of captain or lieutenant, and no deviation in number or grade was permitted. A captain in such a regiment could be promoted only if he could be transferred to another organization where a vacancy existed. Some limitation on promotion was obviously required to prevent a top-heavy accumulation of officers in grades not justified by their duties and responsibilities. As constituted during World War II, however, tables of organization provided few field grade vacancies in tactical commands.

In an infantry division, only 1 of the 12 dental officers was a major. Even a field army, with from 300 to more than 600 dentists, provided relatively few positions for field grade officers. In a "type" army of three corps and supporting troops, there were only 9 majors and 1 full colonel (the army dental surgeon) among about 244 dental officers in troop units. Among the 70 dentists with army hospitals the situation was better since this group included 16 majors and 3 lieutenant colonels, but of the total of about 314 dentists in this "type" army only 1 (0.3 percent) was a colonel, 3 (1.0 percent) were lieutenant colonels, and 25 (8.0 percent) were majors.

Hospitals in the overseas areas generally fared better than combat commands. Field hospitals, evacuation hospitals, and the smaller station hospitals (under 250 beds) provided no field grades for dentists in the first part of the war, but a 250-bed station hospital had a major, and all station hospitals with over 500 beds included both a lieutenant colonel and a major among their 4 or 5 dental officers.[27] A 1,000-bed general hospital had a lieutenant colonel, and a 1,500-bed or 2,000-bed general hospital had a full colonel, a lieutenant colonel,

---

[24] ASF Cir 389, 16 Oct 45.
[25] The Surgeon General's Conference with Service Command Surgeons, 10 December 1943. HD: 337.
[26] Info from Strength Accounting Br, AGO, given to author on 6 May 46.
[27] Data extracted from the T/O's for combat and medical units.

and a major on its staff of dentists. The larger number of these medical installations in the communications zone raised the proportion of field grade dental officers in that area, but not to a sufficient degree to assure reasonable promotion in overseas areas as a whole.

Because the Air Force had very few hospitals the limitations imposed by tables of organization worked an especial hardship on its overseas dental personnel, and the ratio of Air Force dentists in the two top field grades (United States and overseas, combined) was only about half the meager ratio allotted to the Dental Service as a whole.[28]

The fact that dental officers had less opportunity to reach the grades above that of captain is shown in the following tabulation which lists the percentage of all officers of the Dental Corps, Medical Corps, and total Army in each grade as of 30 April 1945:[29]

Grade	Dental Corps	Medical Corps	Total Army*
General	------	------	0.18 (-----)
Colonel	0.83	2.35	1.24 (1.69)
Lieutenant colonel	2.71	7.34	3.36 (4.56)
Major	10.38	21.61	8.24 (11.20)
Captain	67.25	56.50	23.33 (31.70)
First lieutenant	18.83	12.20	37.42 (50.85)
Second lieutenant	------	------	26.23 (-----)

*Figures in parentheses provide a distribution of the total Army officers excluding generals and second lieutenants. The percentages for the total Army (not in parentheses) are based on total commissioned officers including generals as well as second lieutenants.

In August 1945 the Medical Corps had 9 major generals and 46 brigadier generals, while the Dental Corps had 1 major general and 1 brigadier general.

Comparisons between the proportions of medical and dental officers in the grades of lieutenant and captain slightly favor the latter, but cannot be considered significant since any lieutenant could be promoted captain as soon as he had spent the required time in grade. It is more difficult to explain the wide discrepancy in the general grades, but this situation probably had little effect on morale as very few dentists could hope to become general officers under any circumstances. It is in the range of the field grades that the dental officer was at the greatest disadvantage, and inability to reach those grades was the greatest cause for dissatisfaction with promotion policies. The ratio of colonels and lieutenant colonels in the Dental Service was about one-third that in the Medical Corps, and about one-half that in the Army as a whole if generals and second lieutenants are not considered. The ratio of majors in the Dental Corps was about half that in the Medical Corps, and less than the ratio for the Army as a whole if generals and second lieutenants are not considered, in spite of the fact that most dental officers started one grade higher than most officers of branches outside the Medical Department.

---
[28] See footnote 7, p. 106.
[29] Strength of the Army, 1 May 45.

The unfortunate results of slow promotion in the Dental Corps were described as follows by the dental surgeon of the Middle East theater: [30]

> A condition which had a very adverse effect on the morale of dental officers . . . was relative discrimination in the grades to which dentists could hope to attain. This is a familiar complaint, but it was well founded. When twenty-five percent of medical officers were in field grade, for instance, only seven and one-half percent of dental officers could reach field grade. The inevitable result . . . was that dental officers found themselves passed at regular intervals by men of other branches with less experience and ability. I do not wish to imply that the discrimination existed only between the Medical and Dental Corps, nor can the blame be placed on medical officers commanding in this theater. . . . I merely draw attention to the condition as it undoubtedly existed. Dental officers, like the rest of the Army, recognized that in time of national emergency individuals must be prepared to sacrifice their own personal welfare for the successful prosecution of the war. They had given up their practices and their homes because they felt they could make an important contribution toward winning that war, and as long as they had this conviction they were glad to give their best efforts, with or without promotion. But when a dental officer was passed again and again by men of other branches who were less experienced, no more intelligent, and certainly no harder working, he inevitably arrived at the conclusion that his own work was not considered important. I need not elaborate on the danger of such an attitude.

The Director of the Dental Division, SGO, stated in 1945 that: [31]

> There is no doubt that proportionately there are more position vacancies for brigadier generals, colonels, and lieutenant colonels in the Medical Corps by virtue of the fact that the medical officer commands the hospitals. . . (but) it is believed generally in the Dental Corps that the ratio of Medical Corps officers to Dental Corps officers, in accordance with strength figures, is not equitable. It was extremely difficult for officers of the Dental Corps to understand such a vast difference in all field grades, and there was only one general result—lowered morale.

During the war a number of efforts were made to improve the status of dental officers in respect to promotion. In 1943 the American Dental Association claimed that failure to insure equal promotion for dentists violated the act of 6 October 1917 (40 Stat. 397) which provided that officers of the Dental Corps would have the same grades, proportionately distributed, as officers of the Medical Corps.[32] These charges were based on the contention that Section 10 of the National Defense Act, as amended by Section 10, act of 4 June 1920 (41 Stat. 766), which prescribed promotion by length of service, had merely amplified the principle established in the act of 1917, but The Judge Advocate General ruled that the law providing for promotion by length of service had rescinded the earlier legislation, and that there was no legal requirement that

---

[30] Address by Col George F. Jeffcott before the Association of Military Surgeons in New York on 2 Nov 44. This paragraph was omitted from the version of that talk which was published in The Military Surgeon, Jan 1945.

[31] See footnote 9, p. 107.

[32] Ltr, Dr. J. Ben Robinson, Pres ADA, to Maj Gen James C. Magee, 5 Feb 43, no sub. SG: 080 (American Dental Association).

the Medical and Dental Corps should have the same proportion of officers in each grade.[33]

In January 1943 the Director of the Dental Division, SGO, initiated important steps to speed the promotion of lieutenants. Prior to this time tables of organization or tables of allotment had prescribed specific numbers of lieutenants for the Dental Service of units or installations, and in many cases the result was complete stagnation of promotion, regardless of length of service. The situation was particularly serious in the smaller tactical commands, where the lieutenant of an infantry regiment was practically "frozen" in grade since changes in personnel were infrequent after the unit was once organized. The Director of the Dental Division requested that tables of organization which included dental lieutenants be amended to read "lieutenants or captains," thus making it possible to advance dentists out of the lowest grade when they met other requirements for promotion, regardless of the existence of a position vacancy. This recommendation was adopted for both medical and dental officers of table-of-organization units in May 1943.[34] It was extended to include Zone of Interior installations in July of the same year.[35] The effect in tactical units was immediate, but some difficulty was encountered in Zone of Interior installations since service commands were operating under maximum ceilings in each grade, and they hesitated to advance Medical Department officers when such action would use up position vacancies previously earmarked for other activities.[36] By January 1944, however, the proportion of captains in the Dental Corps had risen from about 25 percent to over 48 percent, and by V-E Day 68 percent of all dental officers were captains and only 19 percent were lieutenants.[37]

Partially successful efforts were also made to increase the grades held by dentists in hospitals, which provided almost the only opportunity for promotion to field grade. In 1942, for instance, a 300-bed station hospital was authorized only a captain and a lieutenant, but by 1944 the allotment was a major and a captain. Similarly, the major, captain, and lieutenant of a 750-bed evacuation hospital were each authorized the next higher grade. A major was added to the tables of organization of the 1,000-bed general hospital. In general, an effort was made to have the senior dental officer of any hospital given the same grade held by the chiefs of the medical or surgical services.[38]

The Deputy Surgeon General [39] stated in October 1943 that brigadier generals would be appointed in the Dental Corps to act as dental surgeons of the three principal theaters, but no such action was taken until February 1945,

---

[33] 1st ind, Chief Mil Affairs Div, JAGD, 2 Nov 43, on ltr, Chief of Legal Div, SGO, to JAG, 28 Oct 43, sub: Rank of dental officers. SG: 322.0531-1.
[34] WD Cir 122, 18 May 43.
[35] WD Cir 169, 24 Jul 43.
[36] See footnote 25, p. 111.
[37] See footnote 29, p. 112.
[38] See footnote 9, p. 107.
[39] Memo, Brig Gen George F. Lull, for Pers Div, G-1, 26 Oct 43. SG: 322.053-1.

when Col. Rex McDowell, of the Dental Division, SGO, was promoted. In 1945 the Director of the Dental Division, SGO, asked for legislation to authorize 1 major general and 4 brigadier generals for the Dental Service, with 1 each of the latter to be assigned to the Air Forces, the Ground Forces, and the Service Forces, but no action was taken on this request.[40]

Efforts to increase the authorization of field grades for dentists in tactical commands, outside of hospitals, were generally unsuccessful. A single dental officer in a battalion was unlikely to be granted a grade higher than that held by a company commander who was responsible for over 200 men. It is probable that some improvement would have been possible if the Dental Service of the larger elements, such as the division, could have been organized into larger detachments, in which higher grades for those officers having increased professional or administrative responsibility would have been justified. Such an organization had more important advantages than the possibility of increasing the allotment of field grades (see chapter VIII), but it was attempted only on an experimental basis during World War II.

In general, the opportunities for promotion in the Dental Corps were increased during the war, especially in respect to the company grades, but the Director of the Dental Division, SGO, stated at the end of hostilities that the measures taken had not been adequate, and that "there was no real solution reached with reference to field grades."[41]

MORALE

Official wartime reports seldom mentioned morale problems among dental officers, suggesting that deficiencies were not considered serious. From the practical point of view, dentists certainly rendered loyal and effective service during the period of hostilities. Unfortunately, there is good evidence that many dental officers left the Armed Forces, including the Army, with the feeling that they had not received fair treatment, and relations between the Dental Corps and the civilian profession left much to be desired as the Medical Department faced the postwar era.[42] The ADA, in particular, was called upon to defend itself from the bitter criticisms of members who felt that their interests had not been adequately guarded,[43] and these criticisms were passed on to the Dental Services of the Armed Forces with interest.

Many complaints could of course be ascribed to the age-old military privilege of "griping." Also, it would be too much to expect that wartime

---

[40] Memo, Maj Gen R. H. Mills for Col B. C. T. Fenton, 21 Sep 45. This memorandum has been seen by the writer, but it was not placed in permanent files of SGO.

[41] See footnote 9, p. 107.

[42] Series of editorials in Oral Hygiene from July to October 1943. See also (1) The Army Dental Corps. J. Am. Dent. A. 32: 487–488, 1 Apr 45. (2) Sauce for the goose. J. Am. Dent. A. 32: 888–889, 1 Jul 45. (3) New regulations for the Army Dental Corps. J. Am. Dent. A. 32: 1290, 1 Oct 45. (4) Theory and fact in dental legislation. J. Am. Dent. A. 32: 1301–1308, 1 Oct 45. (5) The right to gripe: The fifth freedom. J. Am. Dent. A. 33: 118, 1 Jan 45.

[43] Ibid. (4).

service should be pleasant, and in the haste of mobilizing the nation's defense resources it was probably inevitable that some men should get more favorable assignments than others, that promotion should not always be equitable, and that misassignments should be made. Such injustices will probably continue to exist under emergency conditions in spite of all efforts to end them. On the other hand, some criticisms were undoubtedly justified, and even those which appear to have been exaggerated deserve consideration since imagined deficiencies were often as detrimental to morale as those which were real.

Among the more important causes of dissatisfaction were the following:

1. Unfavorable promotion status. (See discussion, this chapter.)

2. A fairly widespread opinion that the Dental Service was unnecessarily dominated by medical officers. (See discussion under "Medicodental Relations" in chapter I, pp. 7–15.)

3. Unfavorable assignments and lack of opportunity for promotion for members of the Reserve called to active duty early in the war. Reserve officers were among the first to be brought into the service, before other dentists were being taken from civilian life in large numbers. Because they had had some military training they were often placed in tactical units where dental practice was limited to routine, minor operations, and where promotion was notoriously slow. The inexperienced man, on the other hand, was more likely to be placed under supervision in a large clinic or hospital where military knowledge was less important. Here his opportunities for improving his professional skill were better, probability of advancement was increased, and the chance of being shipped overseas to a combat theater reduced. The Reserve officer tended to feel that he had been "sold down the river" because he had taken sufficient interest to prepare himself for military service before war broke out. This matter is discussed in greater detail in chapter III.

4. The establishment, especially during the early part of the war, of "amalgam mills" where long hours were spent at the chair doing routine operative work which offered little stimulation to professional interest. The situation was sometimes complicated further by the prescription of daily "quotas" which each officer had to meet. Insofar as "production line" procedures contributed to efficiency and assured that the best qualified men would render specialized treatment, they were probably unavoidable. At best, approximately 90 percent of all dental care required by recruits consisted of routine restorative work, and the understandable desire of dentists to widen the scope of their experience could be gratified only to a limited extent in wartime. (See the discussion of quota dentistry in chapter VI, pp. 223–225.)

5. The handling of the dental ASTP, and related demobilization policies. First protests in this field came in June 1944 when ASTP graduates who had received part of their training at Government expense were discharged to enter private practice. (See discussions in chapters III, pp. 56–59 and IX, pp. 340–342.)

The serious drop in the morale of dental officers during the war, as expressed in postwar personnel difficulties and criticism in the professional press, was of course regrettable. At the same time it served a constructive purpose in that it emphasized defects which urgently needed attention.[44]

COMBAT ACTIVITIES, AWARDS

Dental officers shared the risks and hardships of the units to which they were assigned. They participated in Pacific landings, in assaults on Europe's fortified lines, and in airborne attacks in the Mediterranean. One dentist served as commanding officer of an infantry regiment,[45] and another was dropped by parachute into Greece late in 1943, aiding the Greek guerillas and organizing a medical service for them until that country was liberated in 1945. After liberation of Greece this officer was instrumental in obtaining the release of British officers held as hostages by leftist Greek forces. For his efforts he received the Order of the British Empire as well as Greek and American awards.[46] Recognized and unrecognized instances of heroism and exceptional devotion to duty were too numerous to be discussed in detail. In addition to those receiving the Purple Heart for wounds received in action, 384 dental officers received other awards as follows: Legion of Merit, 24; Silver Star for gallantry in action, 10; Soldier's Medal, 2; Bronze Star, 347.[47] In October 1945 Maj. Gen. Robert H. Mills, who had been Director of the Dental Division, SGO, during more than 3 years of war, was awarded the Distinguished Service Medal, the highest award for outstanding administrative duties.

From 7 December 1941 through 31 December 1946,[48] 116 dental officers died from all causes. In this period, 20 dental officers were killed in action; 60 dentists were wounded, 5 of whom died; 38 were made prisoners of war, of which number 12 died (including 2 shown among the 20 killed in action), and 1 reported missing in action who subsequently returned to duty. (There were a total of 91 nonbattle deaths, 10 of which occurred while in a prisoner of war status.) Capt. Howard A. McCurdy, Dental Reserve, who lost his life in

---

[44] By the end of 1948 the Dental Corps had been given new administrative status, temporary promotion policies were being revised, and the military were showing an increased willingness to take the representatives of the civilian professions into their confidence when problems concerning members of those professions were encountered. "Quota" dentistry was dead, probably for good, and the more knotty question of giving individual dentists greater freedom in military practice without reducing efficiency was being considered. These changes would probably not eliminate all complaints in any future mobilization, but they promised much for long-term improvement in the efficiency and morale of the Dental Service.—Ed.

[45] Colonel Roy A. Green to return to private practice. J. Am. Dent. A. 33 : 379, 1 Mar 46.

[46] Iowa dental officer receives honor from Britain. J. Am. Dent. A. 32 : 1350, 15 Nov 45.

[47] HTM–14, 1 Aug 46, Decorations and awards awarded by the War Department and overseas theater commanders, for period 7 December 1941 thru 31 May 1946. In Decorations and Awards Br, AGO.

[48] Army Battle Casualties and Nonbattle Deaths in World War II, Final Report, 7 Dec 41–31 Dec 46. Strength and Acctg Br, AGO.

the Philippines in January 1942, was the first dental officer killed by enemy action in World War II.[49]

TRAINING OF DENTAL OFFICERS

World War I

During the First World War, over 4,000 inexperienced dental officers were called to duty in a relatively short period of time. Initially, no provision had been made for training these men, but fortunately, many had been members of the Preparedness League of American Dentists and had received some instruction in both military dentistry and military administration. The Preparedness League was formed in March 1916 to provide free dental service for men wishing to enlist in the Army and, later, to prepare potential draftees to meet induction requirements.[50] [51] It had also extended its activities to sponsor study clubs for dentists who expected to enter the Reserve, a program which was started even before the United States entered the war. A standard course of study was drawn up by the League and approved by The Surgeon General. This included instruction in anatomy, dental and oral surgery, pathology, x-ray, fractures, anesthesia, prosthetic restoration, bone grafting, first aid, military law, and military administration.[52] The Association of Deans of Dental Schools approved the plan and after June 1917 most schools made their facilities available without cost to the Government or individuals. Colonel Logan, head of the Dental Service, stated that the majority of schools cooperated in the program and that from 4,000 to 5,000 dentists completed the training.[53]

The first effort by the Army to train dentists came with the establishment of the section on Surgery of the Head in the SGO. This office sponsored classes in maxillofacial surgery for selected officers at Washington University, St. Louis; Northwestern University, Chicago; and the University of Pennsylvania, Philadelphia (Thomas W. Evan Institute). From October 1917 to March 1918 these courses provided instruction along the same lines as that given in the Preparedness League program.[54]

In March 1918, a field service school was established at Camp Greenleaf, Fort Oglethorpe, Georgia, for the instruction of dental officers and their enlisted assistants.[55] The course at Camp Greenleaf included a month of in-

---

[49] Dental officer killed in action. Army Dent. Bull. 13 : 149, Apr 1942.

[50] Beach, J. W.: Preparedness League of American Dentists. J. Nat. Dent. A. 4 : 176, Feb 1917.

[51] Beach, J. W.: Preparedness League of American Dentists—Our first birthday. J. Nat. Dent. A. 4 : 363–370, Apr 1917.

[52] Synopsis of study club course in war dental surgery for the sectional units of the Preparedness League of American Dentists. J. Nat. Dent. A. 4 : 795–797, Jul 1917.

[53] Logan, W. H. G.: Development of the dental service during the present war. J. Nat. Dent. A. 5 : 993–1004, Oct 1918.

[54] Ibid.

[55] Ibid.

struction in basic military subjects, followed by a month of study in anatomy, oral surgery, the effects of focal infection, and the fixation of fractures. Every effort was made to have new officers sent to this school, and 1,200 had been enrolled when the war ended in November 1918.

Training for Regular Army Dental Corps Officers Prior to World War II

Candidates for the Regular Army Dental Corps in the period between World Wars I and II were required to be graduates of accepted civilian dental schools and to have at least 2 years of experience in the practice of dentistry. Many were without previous military experience, however, and required both basic military training and additional professional instructions before they were qualified to assume complete responsibility for the Dental Service of a camp or post. As they reached the higher grades, dental officers also required additional training to fit them for positions of greater responsibility. The Army was therefore called upon to provide graduate instruction of all types from the most elementary to the most advanced, both military and professional.

Basic Graduate Course, Army Dental School. The first step in the preparation of a new dental officer was to supplement his previous education in oral surgery, operative dentistry, and prosthetics; subjects in which he would need to be especially proficient if called upon to take over the operation of the Dental Service at an isolated post. In a 4-month basic course at the Army Dental School in Washington (postgraduate only) the new officer received training in these specialties as well as refresher instruction in those subjects which he might have forgotten since graduation from dental school. Unfortunately, a chronic shortage of officers made it impossible to schedule these courses regularly and the last class was given in 1935. An average of seven officers took this course annually between 1930 and 1935.[56]

Officers' Basic Course, Medical Field Service School. After the professional education of the new dental officer had been brought up to date at the Army Dental School, he was sent to the Medical Field Service School (MFSS) at Carlisle Barracks for an additional 5 months of basic military instruction. With other officers of the Medical, Veterinary, and Medical Administrative Corps he studied the organization of military units, the organization and function of medical field units, preventive medicine, first aid, the evacuation of wounded, records and returns, supply procedures, and military law. He learned about Army regulations and customs of the service and he practiced close-order drill in the ranks. During 2 weeks of field maneuvers he put into practice the fundamentals he had studied in the classroom and served as part of the staff of a battalion aid station, a collecting station, and a medical regi-

---

[56] Annual Reports of Technical Activities, Army Medical Center, for the years 1930–35. HD: 319.1–2.

ment. In separate classes for dentists the new officer became familiar with dental field equipment and the administration of a dental clinic. One hundred and forty-one dental officers graduated from this course from the founding of the school in 1921 through 1939.[57]

Advanced Graduate Course, Army Dental School. As the Army dental officer approached field grade he might be sent to the advanced graduate course of the Army Dental School where he received 4 months of instruction in oral surgery, x-ray technique, prosthetics, operative dentistry, preventive dentistry, and periodontal diseases. This course was not expected to qualify the dentist as a specialist but it gave him the general background he needed to act as chief of the Dental Service at a larger post or hospital. Outstanding civilians were brought in to lecture on special subjects and all the facilities of the Army Medical School, Walter Reed General Hospital, the Dental Research Laboratory, the Army Institute of Pathology, and the Central Dental Laboratory were utilized to make this training the most effective possible. The potential value of the course was limited, however, by the small number of officers able to attend, and only 27 men graduated in the 11 years from 1930 through 1940.[58]

In 1936 the Army Dental School provided a course for professional specialists which was attended by four officers,[59] but with this single exception it did not attempt to furnish extensive instruction leading to qualification in a dental specialty.

Advanced Officers' Course, Medical Field Service School. After attaining field grade, usually before examination for promotion to lieutenant colonel, dental officers might be sent to the 3-month advanced course of the MFSS. This course was designed to fit the officer for staff duties and the administration of the Dental Services of large units. A relatively small proportion of eligible officers were able to take the course, however, and from 1923 to 1939 there were but 21 graduates.[60] A larger proportion of senior officers took the special extension course of the MFSS which covered essentially the same material and exempted the candidate from solution of a field problem in his examination for promotion to the grade of lieutenant colonel.

Instruction in Civilian Institutions. A limited number of dental officers were authorized to receive instruction in civilian institutions for periods of from a few weeks to a year. In the 11 years from 1930 to 1940 (inclusive) 32 received such training, though from 1937 to 1940 only 3 courses were authorized.[61]

Nonmedical Service Schools. Dental officers were theoretically eligible for courses of instruction at such advanced Army schools as the Command and

---

[57] Special Rpt, undated, from Col Neal Harper, DC, received in 1945. HD: 314.1-2.
[58] Annual Reports of Technical Activities, Army Medical Center, for the years 1930-40. HD: 319.1-2.
[59] Annual Reports of Technical Activities, Army Medical Center, for the year 1936. HD: 319.1-2.
[60] Annual Reports, Medical Field Service School, 1923-39. HD: 319.1-2.
[61] Annual Reports of The Surgeon General, U. S. Army, 1930-1940, Washington, Government Printing Office, 1930-1940 (cited hereafter as Annual Report . . . Surgeon General).

PERSONNEL AND TRAINING 121

General Staff School and the War College. In practice they were not ordered to these schools until after the start of hostilities in World War II, and then in almost negligible numbers.

Extension Courses. At any time in his career the dental officer was eligible to take correspondence courses published by the MFSS. These were primarily designed for Reserve officers, however, and the number of regulars enrolled was small. Command and General Staff extension courses were also open to dental officers with appropriate background, but enrollment was limited and few dentists in the peacetime establishment were able to get advanced training in general staff procedures.

Dental Internships. Dental internships were first authorized in February 1939.[62] Eight graduates of the class of June 1939 were selected and trained for 1 year in 1 of 6 major hospitals. (Walter Reed General Hospital, Letterman General Hospital, Fitzsimons General Hospital, Army-Navy General Hospital, William Beaumont General Hospital, and the Station Hospital, Fort Sam Houston.) Interns were regarded as potential candidates for the Regular Army Dental Corps and were selected on the basis of scholarship, physical fitness, and adaptability for military service. They were eligible for appointment in the Dental Corps without the 2 years of private practice required of other applicants and without competitive professional examination.[63] They received $60 monthly plus quarters and subsistence. Only about one-fifth of all applicants were accepted and the qualifications of successful candidates were high. A total of 27 interns were taken into the Dental Corps out of 28 receiving this training between 1940 and 1942. The last class of nine interns graduated in June 1943, but none of this group were taken into the permanent establishment due to the suspension of all Regular Army procurement during the war. An earnest effort was made by the Dental Division, SGO, to have these men commissioned at the end of hostilities, but the request was rejected by higher authority. Tentative plans for resumption of the dental intern program after the war called for the granting of reserve commissions to accepted candidates, who would then be called to active duty for the required period of training, with the pay and allowances of their grade.

Summary. The prewar training of the Regular Army dental officer was generally effective, but the fact that the permanent Dental Corps numbered only about 260 officers at the start of World War II meant that this source could supply only key personnel, a negligible proportion of the 15,000 officers needed to staff the Dental Service.

Training for Reserve Officers Prior to World War II

On 30 June 1941 the Dental Reserve Corps numbered 4,428 officers in the following grades: 7 colonels, 96 lieutenant colonels, 354 majors, 909 captains,

---
[62] SG Ltr 6, 14 Feb 39.
[63] AR 605-20, 19 Aug 42.

and 3,062 lieutenants.[64] From 1 January 1939 through 28 February 1946, 3,606 Reserve dentists were called to active duty,[65] including a few who were given commissions after 30 June and before 7 November 1941, when procurement for the Reserve was terminated.

Immediately following World War I the Reserve was made up largely of officers who had had some active military experience. In the period between the two World Wars, however, the Dental Reserve was maintained and augmented with men who either had had no military training whatever, or who had received limited training in connection with their professional education. These new officers required additional instruction and practical experience to fit them for the duties they would perform on mobilization.

Reserve Officers' Training Corps. For 10 years, until 1932, eight dental schools cooperated with the Army to offer courses which would qualify students for commissions in the Dental Reserve on graduation. Regular Army personnel were loaned as instructors, and students attended 30 hours of class yearly. (Credit for 60 additional hours was given for courses such as maxillofacial surgery, taken by the undergraduate as part of his regular professional training.) The course was divided into basic and advanced sections of 2 years each. Enrollment in the basic class was usually obligatory and entitled the student to no pay. A smaller number of selected students took the senior course on a voluntary basis and received a "ration allowance" of about $9 a month. Advanced students were required to attend one 6-week summer camp during which they received the pay of an enlisted man of the lowest grade ($21 monthly). Instruction was given on the organization of the Army and the Medical Department, dental reports and records, the care of maxillofacial injuries, and the operation of dental field facilities. In the summer camp the candidate drilled, set up field installations, and observed military organizations in actual operation. Of 6,854 officers commissioned in the Dental Reserve from 1922 to 1935, 2,274 or 33.2 percent were graduates of the ROTC senior course.[66] Unfortunately, the dental ROTC program was drastically curtailed as an economy measure in 1932 and the last class graduated in 1935.

Extension Courses for Reserve Officers. Before the war, the Army sponsored a series of graduated correspondence courses designed to meet the needs of Reserve officers of all degrees of experience and in all grades. Extension courses began with such basic military subjects as map reading, military law, customs of the service, and organization of the Army. They advanced to specialized instruction in sanitation, evacuation of wounded, medical reports, and the tactics of medical organizations in the field. Completion of the appropriate courses was practically a prerequisite for promotion, and the Reserve officer

---

[64] Annual Report . . . Surgeon General, 1941 (1941) p. 143–147.
[65] Officers appointed in the Dental Corps from 1 January 1939 through February 1946. Strength Acctg Br, AGO, 8 Jul 46. HD : 320.2.
[66] Annual Reports of the Secretary of War, 1922–1940, Washington, Government Printing Office, 1922–1940 (cited hereafter as Annual Report . . . Secretary of War).

was able to develop his knowledge as his responsibilities increased with each higher grade. From 1935 to 1938 an average of 8,000 Medical Department Reserve officers, or a little over one-third of the total strength, were continually enrolled in extension courses.

Summer Camps for Reserve Officers. The Medical Field Service School routinely devoted the summer period to training programs for Reserve officers. A 2-week camp was scheduled for the instruction of junior Reserve officers, another was held for those assigned to units. A 6-week camp, designed to train key personnel for larger medical units, was held for senior captains and field grade officers. Reserve dentists all over the United States were also given occasional 2-week tours of active duty at nearby posts where they received "on-the-job" training. In the 12 years before 30 June 1940, 6,034 dental officers received some type of summer camp training, though there is considerable duplication in this figure since it includes those who attended more than one camp during the period.[67] In addition, between 200 and 300 National Guard Dental officers annually attended camps conducted by that component.

Following the war, senior dental officers stated that, in general, prewar Reserve training had been adequate for the company grades, but that it had not always been extensive enough to prepare men in the higher grades to hold key positions in the Dental Service. In particular, Reserve training was found to have placed greater stress on didactic instruction rather than on practical experience. The completion of correspondence courses, plus 2 weeks of active duty every few years, was often insufficient preparation for a former small town dentist who might be called upon to operate a camp dental service for 25,000 men. These comments on the deficiencies of prewar Reserve training should not be construed as blanket criticism of the Reserve program; thousands of dentists were able to step into routine military duties without delay because they had received some preliminary training as civilians, and some Reserve officers administered major dental services with distinction. But the utilization of field grade dentists who, through no fault of their own, were inadequately trained for the duties appropriate to their grades, was a problem for the Dental Service and for the officers concerned.[68]

Training for Dental Officers During World War II

At the start of World War II the Regular Army Dental Corps and auxiliary components could together provide less than one-third of the 15,000 dental officers needed for the expanding military establishment. The remainder had to be obtained directly from civil life. Most of these new officers needed intensive professional and administrative training before they were qualified to assume unfamiliar duties in a military organization. This necessi-

---

[67] See footnote 66, p. 122.
[68] Pers interv by the author with Maj Gen Robert H. Mills, 6 Oct 47. Also pers ltr to the author from Brig Gen Leigh C. Fairbank, 9 Oct 47.

tated a large-scale expansion of all prewar programs and the initiation of extensive new facilities.

Basic Training, Medical Field Service School. The Medical Field Service School at Carlisle, Pa., assumed an important role in the training of dental officers mobilized for the emergency. Though the courses varied somewhat to meet changing conditions, the school continued throughout the war to instruct new officers in military organization and administration, the functions of field units, and the operation of the Dental Service. Before 1942 special dental lectures had been given as an incidental duty by the senior officer of the post, but in June of that year the dental representative received full faculty status.[69] At the height of the training program in 1944 the dental representative had five assistants. In the 6-week course which was in effect during most of the war, dental officers received 22 hours of special dental instruction in addition to 250 hours on general military subjects with officers of the Medical, Veterinary, and Medical Administrative Corps. The dental course covered the organization, functions, and administration of the Dental Corps, the duties of dental officers in fixed and mobile installations, dental property, the training of assistants, dental surveys, first aid to and evacuation of jaw casualties, approved splinting methods, and the relations of dental officers to other arms and services.[70]

The first change to a wartime schedule at the MFSS came late in 1939 when the normal 5-month basic course was reduced to 3 months so that an extra class could be started in the spring of 1940. In December 1940 the course was cut to 4 weeks and called the "Refresher Course." Up to this time the basic course had been intended for new Regular Army officers, but by the end of 1940 Reserve officers with some military experience were being called to active duty and it was felt that 1 month of training would be sufficient to supplement their previous preparation. Summer classes for Reserve and National Guard officers were dropped in 1940 since all officers were then being prepared for extended active duty. Extension courses were carried on until the summer of 1941. By September 1941 the pool of Reserve officers was becoming exhausted and dentists without any previous training were being called to active duty, leading to the decision to lengthen the course to 8 weeks. A critical shortage of officers in July 1942 caused the basic course to be temporarily reduced to 4 weeks but as soon as possible (December 1942) it was restored to 6 weeks and remained at that figure for most of the remainder of the war. In February 1945 the course was further extended to 8 weeks.[71] In February 1946 activities of the MFSS were transferred to Brooke Army Medical Center, Fort Sam Houston, Texas.

---

[69] History of the Army Dental Corps, 1941–43, p. 82 of Personnel Section. HD: 314.7–2 (Dental).

[70] The training of dental officers. Bulletin of the U. S. Army Medical Department, 80: 14, Sep 1944 (cited hereafter as Army Medical Bulletin).

[71] History of training, World War II, vol X, Chart 3. HD: 314.7–2.

From 1 January 1941 to 30 June 1945, 4,473 dental officers completed the basic training courses at the Medical Field Service School, as follows: [72] [73]

1941	421
1942	440
1943	1,508
1944	1,574
1945 (January to June, incl.)	530

A little over 25 percent of all dental officers on duty during the war received Medical Field Service School training.[74] It was not until May 1945 that the War Department was able to direct that all dental officers would thereafter complete field training before being assigned to a unit.[75]

Basic Training, Medical Department Replacement Pools. About the middle of 1942, training programs were instituted for officers in replacement pools at the MFSS, 4 officer replacement centers, 14 named general hospitals, several medical supply depots, and at the Gulf Coast Air Corps Training Center.[76] These pools had an authorized capacity of 200 dental officers. While officers were available for varying lengths of time, the courses were planned on a 1-month basis and were mainly "on-the-job" training in medical facilities of the installation. Since these courses were informal in nature, and since the flow of officers through the pool determined the instruction each man received, it is impossible to state how many dental officers completed this training.

Professional Training, Army Dental School. In the year ending 30 June 1940 the Army Dental School gave no professional courses for officers. In the year ending 30 June 1941 the basic graduate class, which until 1935 had been given as a 4-month course, was revived as a 3-month "Special Graduate Course" and given to two classes totaling 40 Regular Army officers. In addition, refresher courses of from 1 to 4 weeks were commenced in February 1941.[77] These were designed to train dentists in oral surgery, prosthetics, or operative dentistry in preparation for assignment as chiefs of such services in dental clinics. Refresher courses were continued until June 1942, when they were dropped after a total of 166 officers had completed the training. Four other general hospitals and the station hospital, Fort Sam Houston, also gave refresher courses during this period but the total number of officers attending these classes cannot be determined.

After 31 August 1941 the Army Dental School cooperated with the Army Medical School and Walter Reed General Hospital in giving maxillofacial

---

[72] Summary of Dental Corps officers graduated from the MFSS, 9 September 1940 to 3 August 1946. HD: 353 (1946).

[73] In addition to the figures given here, a few dental officers may have graduated in a special class of 802 Medical Department officers which passed through Camp Barkley in 1944. Reports do not break down the composition of this class by corps, but since it was scheduled to meet the needs of a large number of medical interns it is probable that few dentists were included.

[74] See footnote 9, p. 107.

[75] WD Cir 144, 16 May 45.

[76] SG Ltr 48, 23 May 42.

[77] SG Ltr 32, 5 Apr 41.

plastic courses to train teams qualified to care for these difficult injuries. Until the end of 1942 these courses were of 4 weeks' duration. They were then lengthened to 6 weeks. The last course ended in September 1943 [78] after a total of 139 dental officers had been qualified.

After 1943 no courses for officers were given at the Army Dental School.

Maxillofacial and Plastic Training, Civilian Institutions. In September 1942 maxillofacial training at the Army Medical Center was supplemented by courses given at selected civilian schools. Twelve-week courses were given at Columbia University and 6-week courses at Harvard, University of Pennsylvania, Washington University (St. Louis), Mayo Foundation (Minn.), and Tulane University (New Orleans). The last class ended in August 1944, after 287 officers had been trained, including about 148 dental officers. The number of classes given at each school varied from two to seven. During the war a total of 287 dental officers received maxillofacial training at military and civilian installations.[79]

Maxillofacial Training in Hospitals. In February 1942 it was directed that all general hospitals except Darnall General Hospital would institute training programs for maxillofacial plastic teams.[80] It was expected that these would mainly provide experience in teamwork for previously qualified individuals, but if trained personnel were not already available, authority for instruction in civilian institutions was granted.

Refresher Courses, Army Hospitals. In May 1945 refresher courses in Army general hospitals were authorized for a limited number of dental officers who had been on extended administrative duty during the war.[81] Instruction was to be for a period of 12 weeks in the clinics of the selected hospitals under the guidance of permanently assigned personnel. Since the program was still under way at the end of the war it is not known how many dental officers may have benefited from this training, but the initial response was not so large as was expected since most dentists preferred to return to their practices without delay.

Unit Training. Dental officers assigned to tactical units took part in the training programs of their organizations, learning by actual field operations the duties which they would be called upon to perform in combat. In order to provide the time for this unit training the bulk of the dental work for tactical organizations in the United States was performed by station dental clinics operating under the service commands. However, unit dentists were also assigned to these permanent station clinics for part-time duty, both to help with the rehabilitation of their personnel and for professional training. In January 1941 it was directed that: (1) unit dental officers would receive train-

---

[78] Annual Reports of Technical Activities, Army Medical Center, for the years 1942–44. HD 319.1—2.
[79] Unpublished data obtained from the files of the Training Division, SGO, by the author.
[80] AGO ltr, 27 Feb 42, sub: Training in auxiliary surgical groups. AG: 353 Med (2–19–42).
[81] AGO ltr, 1 May 45, sub: Refresher professional training for Dental Corps officers. SG: 353.

ing in medical tactics as auxiliary medical officers and in emergency treatment of jaw casualties within their respective organizations, and (2) they would receive professional training in camp or hospital dental clinics under direction of the camp or station surgeon.[82] After frequent disputes over how much time should be spent in each type of activity it was finally directed that about half of the unit dentists' time would be devoted to field training and the remainder to clinic training and duty.[83] Clinic dentists also took part in local training schedules which provided instruction in military courtesy and customs, conduct of the clinic, property, and reports and returns.[84]

Dental Consultants. In September 1944 the Dental Division was authorized to contract for the services of qualified civilian consultants to assist in training and to advise less experienced men in oral surgery and prosthetics. Fourteen dentists were made available at various times, including 10 prosthodontists and 4 oral surgeons. These men visited dental installations, advised local dental officers on procedures and the treatment of cases, and made recommendations to the Dental Division, SGO, concerning general conditions noted. Dental consultants were required to demonstrate the utmost common sense and tact, in addition to high professional qualifications, in the performance of their duties. Until they convinced local dental officers of their sincere desire to be of assistance, the latter tended to regard the consultants as "snoopers" or inspectors, rather than as educators. A few consultants also tended to recommend lengthy procedures which were admittedly superior to accepted practices, but which were not consistent with the necessary policy of "the greatest good for the greatest number." In spite of these difficulties the dental consultants showed an understanding of the problems of the Army and of the local dental officers, and their constructive advice helped materially to raise the standards of the Army Dental Service.

Film Strips and Moving Pictures. Libraries of film strips and moving pictures were maintained at each service command headquarters, in some sublibraries at large posts, and in threater headquarters. These training aids were available on call from any installation. Moving pictures of importance to dentists were "Endotracheal Anesthesia for Dental Operations," "Harelip and Cleft Palates" (three films), "Ankylosis of the Mandible" (arthroplasty), "Retruded Chin" (cartilage graft), and "Dental Extraction under Pentothalsodium." [85] A film on "Dental Health," for the general instruction of military personnel, was completed early in 1945. The basic outline for the film was developed by the Dental Division in cooperation with the Bureau of Public Relations of the ADA. The scenario was written by Signal Corps specialists,

---

[82] AGO ltr, 14 Jan 41, sub: Organization, training, and administration of medical units. AG: 320.2.

[83] AGO ltr, 31 Jul 42, sub: Utilization of dental officers for professional duties. AG: 210.312 (Dental Corps) (7–12–42) QD–A–PSM.

[84] Training. Dental Bulletin, supp. to Army Medical Bulletin 11: 175–177, Oct 1940.

[85] TB MED 4, 14 Jan 44.

and filming was completed in Hollywood under Signal Corps supervision. In 25 minutes the film described, in nontechnical language, the need for oral hygiene, the proper care of the teeth and gums, provention of caries, and the use and care of dentures.[86] Film strips were supplied on first aid for wounds of the face and jaws, bandaging, control of hemorrhage, traction appliances, clearing of the airway, and the construction of splints.[87] [88] At the end of the war a new series of film strips was being prepared covering diseases of the mouth, dental anomalies, dental caries, periodontal diseases, cysts, and tumors. These strips were to be accompanied by descriptive booklets elaborating on the conditions depicted.[89]

Publications. Three technical manuals pertaining to the Dental Service were published during the war. A handbook for dental assistants and technicians was printed in 1941 [90] and revised in 1942.[91] This manual contained chapters on the anatomy of the teeth and mouth, prosthetic procedures, dental x-ray technique, oral hygiene, duties of the dental assistant, and the keeping of dental records. Another publication on the repair and maintenance of handpieces was issued in September 1944.[92] A third manual on the dental x-ray machine was printed in January 1945.[93]

A symposium on the treatment of maxillofacial wounds was prepared by the Army Dental School in 1941, and published under the auspices of the Preparedness Committee of the American Dental Association.[94] This booklet, entitled "Lectures in Military Dentistry," was purchased by the Surgeon General's Office for general distribution among dental officers, and it was also made available to interested civilian dentists through the ADA.

Until July 1943 the Dental Corps sponsored publication of the quarterly "Dental Bulletin, Supplement to the Medical Bulletin," containing instructions and information on matters of interest to the Dental Service. After October 1943 such material was carried in the monthly Medical Bulletin and publication of the separate Dental Bulletin was discontinued. The Army took an active part in publication of the "Atlas of Dental and Oral Pathology," a volume containing descriptions of all of the more important dental lesions, with microphotographs and case histories. It had originally been prepared at the Army Institute of Pathology and published under auspices of the ADA before the war. A revised edition was published in 1942.[95]

---

[86] New training films and film bulletin available. Army Medical Bulletin 88 : 44, May 1945.
[87] Film strips approved for release. Army Dent. Bull. 13 : 57, Jan 1942.
[88] Training aids. Army Dent. Bull. 13 : 138, Apr. 1942.
[89] Dental film strips. Army Medical Bulletin 88 : 56, May 1945.
[90] Handbook for the dental assistant and mechanic. Washington, The Surgeon General, 1941.
[91] TM 8-225, Dental Technicians. Washington, Government Printing Office, 1942.
[92] TM 8-638, Engine, Handpiece, Straight; Engine, Handpiece, Angle. Washington, Government Printing Office, 1944.
[93] TM 8-634, Dental X-ray Machine. Washington, Government Printing Office, 1945.
[94] Lectures on military dentistry. Chicago, Preparedness Committee of the American Dental Association, 1942.
[95] Committee on dental museum. J. Am. Dent. A. 29 : 2260, Dec 1942.

THE WAR AND UNDERGRADUATE DENTAL EDUCATION

In time of peace the Army has customarily relied upon established civilian institutions for the undergraduate education of professional officers for the Medical Department. In both World Wars, however, the Army and Navy have felt it necessary to initiate special programs to insure the continued operation of the professional schools and to provide readily available replacements of officer personnel.

In World War II the Army and the Navy became deeply involved in the field of professional training, and for a period of approximately 1 year the majority of the nation's dental students were in military status, studying under military contracts with the dental schools. Conflicting needs of the Armed Forces for young manpower on one hand, and for a steady supply of professional replacements on the other, indicate that the Army, Navy, and Air Force must be prepared at least to advise on the deferment of students in the health sciences in any future emergency, whether or not they plan to take a more direct part in medical education.

Selective Service and Dental Education

In drawing up legislation for compulsory military service Congress consistently refused to provide for blanket exemption of any group on the basis of occupation. During discussions preceding passage of the Selective Service Act of World War II strong pleas for the deferment of professional students were made by representatives of schools and professions, but the only concession made was to permit all university students to complete the current academic year, with no general deferment authorized beyond 1 July 1941.[96] (ROTC students were permitted to finish the last 2 years of their courses.) Within 2 days after the Selective Service Act became law, Senator James E. Murray introduced a bill specifically deferring medical and dental students,[97] but it failed to receive favorable attention. The Army itself opposed the measure because it was considered contrary to the spirit of the Selective Service Act, which contemplated deferment only on the basis of individual essentiality to the war effort.[98] Between January and May 1941, similar student deferment legislation was introduced [99] [100] [101] [102] but all such bills were defeated.[103] The unfavorable response to these measures indicated that failure to grant blanket deferment to professional students was not an oversight, and that the Selective Service Act

---

[96] Selective Service in Wartime. Washington, Government Printing Office, 1943, p. 232.
[97] S. 4396, 76th Cong., introduced 18 Sep 40.
[98] Ltr, SecWar (Henry L. Stimson) to Hon Morris Sheppard, Chm Senate Committee on Mil Affairs, 16 Dec 40. Quoted in Reports of Hearings before the Committee on Military Affairs, U. S. Senate, 77th Congress, on S. 783, 18–20 March 1941. Washington, Government Printing Office, 1941.
[99] S. 197, 77th Cong., introduced 6 Jan 41.
[100] S. 783, 77th Cong., introduced 6 Feb 41.
[101] H. R. 4184, 77th Cong., introduced 26 Mar 41.
[102] S. 1504, 77th Cong., introduced 13 May 41.
[103] Selective Service in Peacetime. Washington, Government Printing Office, 1942, p. 172.

correctly interpreted Congress' determination to avoid legislation which could be construed as favorable to any special group.

On the other hand, educational facilities for the vital health professions had long been barely adequate to meet minimum needs in normal times, and it appeared that the long-range interests of the nation required the maintenance of the medical, dental, and veterinary schools, not only to meet the expanded immediate needs of the Armed Forces, but to insure adequate health care of the civilian population following the end of hostilities. Also, the schools of arts and sciences could keep in operation with student bodies made up largely of women and physically rejected men, while professional schools with their predominantly male student bodies faced probable closure if all men eligible for military service were removed. Once these complex organizations were broken up their reconstitution would be a difficult and time-consuming task. Efforts to comply with the letter of the Selective Service law and at the same time to safeguard essential professional training led to some confusion and uncertainty during the early stages of mobilization.

Early Selective Service directives concerning deferment for essentiality did not specifically mention professional students, and determination of their eligibility was left to the discretion of local boards. In February 1941, however, those boards were reminded that automatic deferment for university students would end in July, and they were directed to consider the cases of men in training for critical occupations before that time.[104] On 7 March 1941 boards were again reminded that certain students were eligible for deferment under existing regulations, and were directed to consider each applicant on the basis of the importance of the occupation, the length of time already spent in training, and the probability that the student would actually engage in the activity after his education had been completed.[105] The ADA promptly advised the deans of all dental schools to seek delay in the induction of dental students on the basis of these instructions.[106] So far as dental students were concerned, however, the effectiveness of both of these early directives was lessened by the fact that dentistry had not been declared a critical occupation. On 22 April 1941 Selective Service notified its local boards that the Office of Production Management (OPM) had warned that a shortage of dentists *might* be imminent,[107] and the position of dental students was materially improved when this tentative information was confirmed a week later.[108] On 1 May 1941 the official Selective Service news magazine emphasized in very

---

[104] Unnumbered memorandum for State Directors of Selective Service, 13 Feb 41, sub: Classification of students. *In* Memoranda to All State Directors 1940–43. Washington, Government Printing Office, 1945.

[105] See footnote 96, p. 129.

[106] Ltr, C. Willard Camalier to deans of all dental schools, 26 Apr 41. SG: 327.22–1.

[107] Memo, Dir Selective Service, for all State Directors (I–62), 22 Apr 41, sub: Occupational deferment of students and other necessary men in certain specialized professional fields (III). Washington, Government Printing Office, 1945.

[108] Telegram, Dir, Selective Service System, to all State Directors, 30 Apr 41. On file Natl Hq, Selective Service System.

strong terms the need for deferring dental students,[109] and a directive of 12 May 1941 stated: "It is of paramount importance that the supply [of dentists] be not only maintained but encouraged to grow, and that no student who gives reasonable promise of becoming a qualified dentist be called to military service before attaining that status." [110]

Under these policies a considerable number of medical, dental, engineering, and physical science students were deferred from military duty after the end of automatic deferment in July 1941. A survey made late in 1941 showed that 81 percent of all dental students 21 years of age or over were continuing their education under occupational deferment, a higher proportion than in any other group.[111] Deferment for other students ranged from 80 percent in the medical schools to 46 percent in courses in biology. In February 1942 the ADA reported that an affidavit of the dean of a dental school that an individual was a bonafide student was generally being accepted by local boards as sufficient reason for delaying induction.[112]

In March 1942 Selective Service outlined requirements for the deferment of persons in training as follows: [113]

> The applicant for deferment must be in training for a critical occupation essential to the war effort.
>
> A shortage of persons engaged in that occupation must exist.
>
> There must not be sufficient persons already engaged in training for the occupation to meet future requirements.
>
> The trainee must have advanced sufficiently in his course to give promise of successful completion.

Since it was ruled that no student could be held to "give promise of successful completion" of a university course with less than 2 years of previous instruction, deferment for professional students was automatically limited to those who had completed preprofessional training. In December 1942 Selective Service again emphasized the need for allowing dental students to continue their education, and authorized deferment after completion of the first preprofessional year.[114] On advice of the War Manpower Commission, Selective Service provisions covering the deferment of preprofessional students were further liberalized on 1 March 1943 to permit delaying the induction of any individual who would be qualified to enter a professional school by 1 July 1945 and who held a firm acceptance for admission to such school.[115]

---

[109] Deferment of students in specialized fields sanctioned to meet national defense needs. Selective Service, vol I, No. 5, 1 May 1941.

[110] Memo, Dir Selective Service, for all State Directors (I–99), 12 May 41.

[111] See footnote 103, p. 129.

[112] Dental students and instructors. J. Am. Dent. A. 29: 291, Feb 1942.

[113] Memo, Dir, Selective Service System, for all State Directors, No. I–405, 16 Mar 42, sub: Occupational classification. On file Natl Hq, Selective Service System.

[114] Selective Service Occupational Bulletin No. 41, 14 Dec 42, sub: Doctors, dentists, veterinarians, and osteopaths. In Occupational Bulletins 1–44, and Activity and Occupation Bulletins 1–35. Washington, Government Printing Office, 1944.

[115] Selective Service Occupational Bulletin No. 11, as amended 1 March 1943, sub: Student deferment. In Occupational Bulletins 1 to 44 and Activity and Occupation Bulletins 1 to 35. Washington, Government Printing Office, 1944.

The deferment of actual dental students remained fairly certain during the remainder of the war, and it will be noted later that total enrollment in dental schools materially exceeded peacetime registration. In April 1944, however, deferment of predental students was restricted to those who would be able to enter a dental school by 1 July 1944.[116] The ADA vigorously protested this action,[117] and the Director, WMC, asked the Director, Selective Service, to reconsider the order, but the request was refused. The Director, WMC, then asked the Armed Forces to give military status to enough preprofessional students to assure continued full operation of the schools, but the latter replied that the immediate need for manpower should not yield to the possible use of such students as doctors in 1949 or later, and they stated further that the current Selective Service policy had the full approval of the Army and Navy. Attempts of PAS, WMC, to have the Director of War Mobilization intervene in the matter brought the reply that the problem was clearly the responsibility of Selective Service. The PAS estimated at this time that there would be 1,446 civilian vacancies in the dental classes starting in 1945 (the Armed Forces programs, discussed later in this chapter, were expected to fill 38 percent of the available openings), and stated that if predental education were confined to veterans, women, and physically disqualified males only a small proportion of those vacancies would be filled.[118] On 23 June 1944 Representative Louis E. Miller of Missouri introduced a bill to commission 6,000 medical and premedical students, and 4,000 dental and predental students, but this legislation failed to pass.[119]

The fears of PAS were later proved to be well founded, and as a result of the discontinuance of predental education only 1,197 freshmen were enrolled in dental schools in October 1945, compared with 2,496 a year earlier.[120] It is clear that if the war had continued indefinitely very few students would have been left in the dental schools under deferment policies in effect in 1944 and 1945.

Deferment of Dental Students Through the Granting of Reserve Commissions

While Selective Service policies actually permitted a large proportion of all dental students to remain in school, the Office of Defense Health and Welfare Services, PAS, ADA, and to some extent the Armed Forces, appear not to have been satisfied that deferment was sufficiently certain under Selective Service regulations. As late as April 1942 the ADA reported continuing difficulty in insuring student deferment.[121] Also, during much of this period

---

[116] Selective Service as the Tide of War Turns. Washington, Government Printing Office, 1945, pp. 79–80.
[117] Selective Service restricts deferment of predental students. J. Am. Dent. A. 31 : 735, May 15, 1944.
[118] Procurement Service issues statement on dental students. J. Am. Dent. A. 31 : 878–880, June 15, 1944.
[119] H. R. 5128, 78th Cong., introduced 23 Jun 44.
[120] The supply of dental students. J. Am. Dent. A. 32 : 1454–1455, Nov-Dec 1945.
[121] President's Page. J. Am. Dent. A. 29 : 653, Apr 1942.

predental students had uncertain protection, and unless a steady flow of replacements into the entering classes could be maintained, a deferment for actual dental students would eventually become meaningless. These considerations, and a desire to insure the availability of young dentists on graduation, ultimately led to involvement of the Armed Forces in the field of dental education.

Even before passage of the Selective Service Act in August 1940, The Surgeon General was given authority to transfer to the Medical Administrative Corps (MAC) Reserve any medical, dental, or veterinary student who held a Reserve commission in another branch and who would therefore be subject to call to active duty.[122] These MAC Reserve officers were retained in inactive status until their professional education was completed, when they were called on active duty in the appropriate corps of the Medical Department. The number of such students was of course small, and it seems probable that this action was taken mainly to provide later replacements in scarce categories rather than because the Army then felt any responsibility for the continuation of medical education to meet postwar civilian needs. In Feburary 1941 The Surgeon General requested additional authority to grant MAC commissions to any junior or senior students in the medical, dental, or veterinary schools, basing his plea on probable future needs for the Army.[123] He pointed out that the Navy had already authorized the commissioning of medical students and that the Army would soon find itself at a disadvantage in procuring replacements unless it acted promptly. The Adjutant General disapproved this request, stating that exemption from the draft could be justified only when it was clear that students would be required in key positions in industries essential to national defense.[124]

In April 1941 pressure for military action to insure the deferment of professional students came from a new source outside the Armed Forces, and this time the need for safeguarding medical education for long-term civilian needs, as well as for the more immediate needs of the Army and Navy, was plainly advanced as an important consideration. On the advice of the Health and Medical Committee of the Office of Defense Health and Welfare Services the Administrator of the Federal Security Agency reported to the Secretary of War that he felt increasing concern over the problem of "how to insure for our military and civilian needs the requisite number of doctors and dentists, both now and in the future."[125] He noted that the Navy was granting Reserve commissions to junior and senior students, but he stated that it was also necessary to safeguard the two lower classes, and he endorsed a resolution of the Health and Medical Committee calling for first and second year students to be given the status of "cadets" and for third and fourth year students to

---
[122] See footnote 64, p. 122.
[123] Ltr, Maj Gen James C. Magee to TAG, 18 Feb 41, sub: Commissioning of junior and senior students in the Medical Department Reserve Corps. AG: 210.1.
[124] 1st ind, by TAG, 18 Mar 41, to ltr cited in footnote 123.
[125] Ltr, Paul V. McNutt to SecWar, 28 Apr 41. AG: 210.1 Med-Res (4–28–41).

be commissioned in the MAC Reserve. He stated further that even if deferment could be arranged through Selective Service a continuing supply of medical personnel should not depend upon the understanding of 6,000 local boards, thus giving a clue to the rather surprising decision to approach the problem through the military rather than through Selective Service.

The Federal Security Administrator's letter influenced the Under Secretary of War to send a memorandum to General Marshall stating that he was keenly interested in the problems of the "supply of physicians for the Medical Reserve" and that he hoped the program suggested by the Health and Medical Committee could be put in action.[126] It will be noted that through oversight or intent the reference to dentists, which had been included in the original recommendations of the Health and Medical Committee and in the Federal Security Administrator's communication, was omitted from the letter of the Under Secretary of War. The question of whether or not the Armed Forces should properly assume any responsibility for medical education to meet purely civilian needs was also avoided. The Surgeon General added his recommendation for the granting of commissions to all medical students, but he failed to mention dental students in spite of the fact that he had requested the same privilege for them less than 2 months before. Since The Surgeon General had been a member of the Health and Medical Committee which had drafted the original petition he was certainly familiar with the situation, and, presumably, favorably inclined toward including dental students in the program, and their omission may have been unintentional, in the thought that "medical students" would include dental and veterinary students as well.[127] The problem of preprofessional students was not considered at this time.

The Assistant Chief of Staff G-1 concurred to the extent of approving the commissioning of third and fourth year medical students, as prospective officers, but he recommended strongly against going further to include freshmen and sophomores. He stated that since the Selective Service Act expired in 1945 no student should be accepted by the military who would not graduate by 1943, to allow for 1 year in internship and 1 year of service before the end of the draft. He added that in his opinion the question of the total production of doctors was a national one, not coming within the province of the War Department, and that if the Selective Service Act endangered medical education it should be revised, rather than resort to the subterfuge of insuring deferment by means of granting semimilitary status.[128] The commissioning of junior and senior medical students only was authorized on 26 May 1941.[129]

---

[126] Memo, Robert P. Patterson, UnderSecWar, for Gen George C. Marshall, 1 May 41. AG: 210.1 Med-Res (5-1-41).

[127] Memo, Maj Gen James C. Magee, for ACofS G-1, 10 May 41. AG: 210.1 Med-Res.

[128] Memo, ACofS G-1 for CofS, 14 May 41, sub: Deferment of medical students. AG: 210.1 Med-Res (5-1-41).

[129] Ltr, TAG to all CA and Dept Comdrs, 26 May 41, sub: Deferment of medical students. AG: 210.1 Med-Res (5-1-41).

In January 1942 the Federal Security Administrator asked the War Department to reconsider its decision against commissioning first and second year medical students, though no additional reasons were given.[130] Again The Surgeon General supported the request, and this time dental and veterinary students were specifically included in his recommendations.[131] The Adjutant General again disapproved such action, stating that it would grant certain students deferment for as long as 5 years,[132] but his advice was rejected, and on 11 February 1942 the War Department announced that any accepted male matriculant in a medical school could be given an inactive commission.[133] Reference to dental students and preprofessional students was again omitted, though the provision for enrolling any "accepted matriculant" might have covered premedical students under certain conditions.

Dentistry had been declared a critical occupancy nearly a year before [134] and in April 1942 the Federal Security Administrator (acting as the Director of the Office of Defense Health and Welfare Services) again recommended that the privilege of accepting inactive MAC commissions be extended to dental and veterinary students.[135] He stated that the seriousness of the situation had been called to his attention by the Health and Medical Committee of the Office of Defense Health and Welfare Services, the Procurement and Assignment Service, and officials of the professional organizations. He noted that Selective Service boards were still refusing to defer professional students in some instances, and emphasized the need to delay the induction not only of actual enrollees in medical, dental, and veterinary schools, but of men preparing for those schools as well. The requests of The Surgeon General and of other bodies responsible for assuring a steady supply of replacements in the health services apparently had some influence on the War Department, and the Assistant Chief of Staff G-1 recommended to the Chief of Staff that the Army authorize the commissioning in the Reserve of dental and veterinary students and of students holding acceptances for dental or veterinary schools.[136] Approval of the Secretary of War was obtained on 14 April and the necessary orders were issued on 17 April 1942.[137] The interpretation of "students holding acceptances for dental or veterinary schools" was not specific, and it has been claimed that, in some cases at least, deans "accepted" enough high school gradu-

---

[130] Ltr, Paul V. McNutt to SecWar, 6 Jan 42. AG : 210.1 Med-Res (1-6-42).

[131] Ltr, Maj Gen James C. Magee to TAG, 15 Jan 42, sub : Granting commissions to medical students in the Medical Administrative Corps. SG : 210.1-1.

[132] 1st ind, 28 Jan 42, SG : 210.1-1. TAG to ltr cited in footnote 131.

[133] Ltr, TAG to all CA and Dept Comdrs (except the Philippine Dept), 11 Feb 42, sub : Commissions for medical students. On file AG central files as Tab A to ltr, Brig Gen J. H. Hilldring, G-1, to CofS, 6 Apr 42, G-1/16455-25, sub : Commission of medical and dental students. AG : 210.1.

[134] See footnote 108.

[135] Ltr, Paul V. McNutt to SecWar, 2 Apr 42. AG : 210.1.

[136] Ltr, Brig Gen J. H. Hilldring to CofS, 6 Apr 42, sub : Commission of dental and veterinary students. AG : 210.1 (4-6-42).

[137] Ltr, TAG to all CAs and Dept Comdrs (except the Philippine Department), 17 Apr 42, sub : Commissions for dental and veterinary students. AG : 210.1 (4-6-42).

ates just starting predental training to assure adequate entering classes 2 years later.[138] It has already been noted that Selective Service did not grant deferment to predental students until December 1942, and then only to men who had completed the first year of training.

In anticipation of the inauguration of the Army Specialized Training Program, the granting of new MAC commissions was discontinued in February 1943.[139] A majority of the 5,383 students already holding Reserve commissions later resigned them to accept active duty in the Enlisted Reserve under ASTP, but a few retained their commissions until graduation. Best information now available indicates that approximately 1,059 MAC graduates were taken on active duty in 1943, 111 in 1944, and 16 in 1945, for a total of 1,186 officers.[140]

The Army Specialized Training Program for Dental Undergraduates

(The Army Specialized Training Program, in its general aspects, has been discussed at length in a report by Col. Francis M. Fitts, M. C.[141] The present discussion will therefore be limited mainly to those phases of the program having special significance for dental education. Much of the material used is from Colonel Fitts' work; his documentation is not repeated.)

In December 1942 the Armed Forces announced a plan to give military status to students in training for certain essential occupations and to continue their education at Government expense.[142] The reasons which impelled the Army and Navy to take a direct part in medical education are not clearly documented, but the following were probably most pertinent:

1. It has already been noted that agencies responsible for the health care of the nation during the emergency were not assured that Selective Service could be relied upon to permit continuous education in the health services during the war. In spite of Selective Service advice to the local boards the latter sometimes hesitated to consider deferment for students when they were compelled to send other young men to combat. It was also felt that Selective Service policies were subject to revision on short notice and that they could not be depended upon in establishing long-term commitments.[143]

2. The Armed Forces wanted to have sufficient prospective professional

---

[138] Info given to author by Maj Ernest Fedor, who was in the Mil Pers Div, SGO, during a large part of the war.

[139] WD Memo W150-3-43, 8 Feb 43, sub: Discontinuance of appointments in the Medical Administrative Corps of accepted matriculants in medical, dental, and veterinary schools and the disposition of those officers previously appointed as such. SG : 210.1-1.

[140] Data computed by Lt Col John Brauer, DC, from statistics furnished by the Procurement Branch, SGO; the Appointment and Induction Branch, AGO; the Classification and Assignment Branch, AGO; and the Resources Analysis Division, SGO.

[141] Fitts, F. M.: Training in medicine, dentistry, and veterinary medicine, and in preparation therefor, under the Army Specialized Training Program, 1 May 43 to 31 Dec 45. HD : 353 ASTP.

[142] SOS Cir 95, 18 Dec 42, sub: Establishment of the Army Specialized Training Program.

[143] See footnote 125, p. 133.

replacements actually under military control to assure the use of these with certainty and without delay as soon as their training was completed.

3. It was feared that students themselves would not be content to remain in school as civilians, even if deferment were assured. Nearly 2,000 former dental students served with the AEF, alone, in World War I, so depleting the schools that only 906 men graduated in 1920, compared with 3,587 in 1919.[144]

4. It was probably felt that if professional students were to be relieved from the obligation to serve in hazardous assignments, the opportunity to attain student's status should not depend upon individual ability to pay the rather heavy costs of university training. Under ASTP the son of a laborer, or a soldier already inducted, would in theory have the same opportunity to get a dental education as the son of a wealthy family.

Details of the new program were released in April 1943 as follows:

1. Professional students already enrolled in the Enlisted Reserve were to be called to active duty under ASTP. Students who held Reserve MAC commissions could resign them and be placed in the Enlisted Reserve for subsequent call to active duty, though they were not obligated to do so.

2. Acceptable dental students not in the Reserve (MAC or enlisted) could volunteer for induction and transfer to the Enlisted Reserve under ASTP.

3. Predental students would be selected from men already enrolled in predental classes who volunteered for induction in the Enlisted Reserve, or from qualified individuals already in the Army who requested transfer to ASTP. Students not already in predental training would be accepted only if they (a) had an Army General Classification Test score of 115 or better, (b) passed an aptitude test for the medical professions, and (c) were approved by an interviewing board representing both the Army and the dental schools. Another board had to approve advancement from predental training to a dental school. Since the ASTP was necessarily started with men already enrolled in the schools, and since the dental phase was largely terminated after 1 year, very few new students were actually selected under the above provisions.

4. Preprofessional training for all the medical sciences was to be given in a common course of five terms of 12 weeks each. The first two terms were devoted to a general course prescribed for all ASTP beginners, medical and nonmedical. The remaining three were consumed in a special preprofessional course drawn up by ASF with the assistance of representatives of the medical, dental, and veterinary schools. The entire 60 weeks of preprofessional training included the following required subjects:

English	8 semester hours
Physics	8 semester hours
Organic chemistry	8 semester hours
Biology	8 semester hours

[144] Dentistry as a professional career. Chicago, American Dental Association, 1946, p. 11.

5. Dental schools were to continue to give their regular wartime undergraduate courses, which had been shortened in January 1942.[145] Individual schools were to determine their own criteria for passing grades, examinations, and the general maintenance of professional standards.

6. On graduation, students were to be commissioned in the Army Dental Corps and called to active duty.

It was planned to utilize 35 percent of the capacity of the dental schools for the Army, starting about 970 new students every 9 months. With an estimated 15 percent attrition, this would provide about 825 potential dental officers every 9 months. Maximum enrollment was reached in March 1944 when 6,143 students in dental schools were enrolled in ASTP. The Navy was expected to take an additional 20 percent of total capacity, to provide 475 dental officers every 9 months, so that the Armed Forces, together, were to account for 55 percent of the capacity of the dental schools. In October 1943, however, the 7,775 students enrolled by the Army and Navy amounted to nearly 90 percent of the total of 8,888 students in the dental schools.[146] Since 5,883 dental students had held Reserve commissions in February 1943, and since only 6,143 were enrolled in ASTP at its maximum, it is clear that the majority of the dental ASTP enrollees were men who had already been deferred as members of the MAC Reserve.

It was also planned to start an average of 130 preprofessional students, earmarked for the dental ASTP, each month. It was expected that this number would provide 110 new students monthly for the dental schools.

The dental ASTP was activated in the period from May through July 1943. All dental schools in the United States, totalling 39, participated, including Meharry and Howard Universities for Negro students.

By 1944 the need for additional young manpower to push the war to a successful, early conclusion became critical and the Army began to consider a reduction in long-term training programs. In March 1944 it was announced that the entire ASTP would be cut back from 145,000 men to 35,000, though no reduction in the medical or dental programs was anticipated at that time. A few days later, however, the director of the Military Personnel Division advised The Surgeon General that it seemed doubtful that men then in preprofessional training would ever be used by the Army in view of changes in the general war situation.[147] He reflected only current confusion on the propriety of the Armed Forces concerning themselves with medical education for civilian needs when he noted that the Army should not be placed in the position of agreeing to an interruption of medical education, even when gradu-

---

[145] In January 1942 the Council on Dental Education, ADA, had recommended that the dental course during the war be continuous (no summer vacation) and that it be cut to three years instead of four. This recommendation was accepted by all schools. See Acceleration of the dental school program. J. Am. Dent. A. 29 : 287–288, Feb. 1942.

[146] 7,775 out of 8,888 in dental schools are in armed services. J. Am. Dent. A. 31 : 164, 15 Jan 44.

[147] Memo, Lt Col Durward G. Hall for SG, 28 Mar 44, sub: Medical section, Army Specialized Training Program. SG : 353.9–1.

ates would not be available until after the emergency, but that the responsibility properly lay with Selective Service, and that in his opinion the latter would not act as long as the military were in the field. He recommended that further procurement for entering classes be terminated. There is no indication that this advice had any direct influence on the subsequent curtailment of the dental ASTP, but it is of interest as revealing the trend of thought among officers charged with personnel responsibilities in the Office of The Surgeon General.

On 18 April 1944 ASF announced that the Army's share of the classes entering dental schools after 1 January 1945 would be 18 percent instead of 35 percent, and that no commitments would be made covering classes to start in 1946.[148] At this time the Dental Corps was approaching its maximum authorized strength (see chapters III and IX), and efforts of The Surgeon General to have a significant number of older dental officers replaced with younger men were meeting with little success; as a result it was impossible to commission the ASTP graduates of June and early July 1944, and they had to be unconditionally released by the Army,[149] causing much adverse comment from dental officers and civilians. On 2 June 1944 the director of the Strategic and Logistic Planning Unit advised The Surgeon General that a demand for continuation of the dental ASTP could no longer be supported on the basis of military requirements,[150] and in drawing up recommendations for future ASTP training in the medical sciences The Surgeon General recommended, on 9 June 1944, that the dental and veterinary programs be dropped. On the protest of the Director of the Dental Division, however, this request was withdrawn on 27 June and resubmitted to provide for a continuation of dental training. In reply, The Surgeon General was advised on 1 August 1944 that the War Department General Staff had definitely decided to drop the dental ASTP.[151] This statement came as an anticlimax, however, since the termination of the dental ASTP had already been announced by the War Department on 18 July 1944.[152] Under the terms of this latter directive all senior students, numbering about 1,175 men, were to be allowed to complete their courses, when they would be commissioned in the Dental Corps. Dental students not in their final year (about 4,810 men), and predental students who would complete their preliminary training at the end of the current term and who held acceptances for dental courses beginning prior to 31 December 1944,

---

[148] Memo, Brig Gen W. L. Weible for SG, 18 Apr 44, sub: War Department policy governing training in medicine and dentistry under ASTP. SG: 353.9–1.

[149] Ltr, Col J. R. Hudnall to Comdt, 3930 Service Unit, ASTU, University of Southern California, Los Angeles, Calif., 1 Jul 44, sub: Disposition of senior dental ASTP trainees on date of graduation. SG: 000.8 (University of S. Calif.) W.

[150] Memo, Lt Col Durward G. Hall for Deputy SG, 2 Jun 44, sub: Demand schedule for ASTP graduates. SG: 353.9–1.

[151] 3d Ind, Brig Gen Russel B. Reynolds, 1 Aug 44, on Ltr, Col J. R. Hudnall to CG ASF, 9 Jun 44, sub: Requirements for ASTP graduates for last nine months of 1944 and the year 1945. SG: 353.9–1.

[152] Ltr, Maj Gen M. G. White, ACofS G–1, to CG, ASF, 18 Jul 44, sub: ASTP dental program. SG: 353.9 (Med).

were to be discharged from the Army at the end of the term, to continue their education at their own expense. Students who could not meet these requirements (about 722 men), or who could not pay for their own schooling, were to be transferred to the Medical Department as enlisted men. The dental ASTP was thus limited to senior students in July 1944 and it came to an end with the classes graduating in April 1945.

Cost of the Dental ASTP. It is difficult even to estimate the cost of the dental ASTP since such unknown factors as the expense of providing medical care for trainees and the potential cost of veterans' benefits following the war were involved. Some of the more important items, calculated to 12 October 1945, have been reported as follows: [153]

Academic cost per student per month (tuitition, books, instruments)	$64.90
Housing (at institutions)	9.04
Housing (on commutation)	37.50
Food (at institutions)	31.50
Food (on commutation)	54.00

The monthly cost for academic expenses, food, and housing thus varied from $105.44 for students housed and fed under contract, to $156.40 for students granted commutation for housing and food obtained on their own responsibility. To this amount must be added at least $50 per month for salary, plus an unknown amount for overhead, including the salaries of military administrators, hospitalization, travel, et cetera. Money received from the resale of books and equipment after the termination of the program reduced the above cost for academic expenses by about $8.00 per month.

Results of the Dental ASTP. The following tabulation summarizes the results of the Dental ASTP:

Number of dental schools participating	39
Number of months in operation	26
Total dental students enrolled	7,734
Disposition of 7,734 enrollees:	
Graduated	2,458
Discharged to continue at own expense at end of program	4,651
Failed	472
Dropped for other reasons	101
Transferred to Medical Department as enlisted men	52
Disposition of 2,458 graduates:	
Commissioned in the Dental Corps	1,914
Discharged for lack of vacancies, June and July 1944	113
Commissioned by Veterans Administration, mainly in June and July 1944	36
Commissioned by Navy, same period	269
Disqualified for physical or other reasons	126
Predental students enrolled	1,407
Completed predental training	499

---

[153] Statistics relating to the dental ASTP program. Published by the Training Contracts Section, Production and Purchases Div, ASF, undated. HD: 314.

Discussion, Dental ASTP. The Dental ASTP was bitterly criticized almost from its inception until long after it had gone out of existence, indicating the need for a careful evaluation of the objectives and policies involved in order to avoid similar difficulties in any future emergency.

Probably the most fundamental criticism was based on claims that there was actually no need for the military to venture into the unfamiliar field of undergraduate professional education. The profession, the schools, and the public were of course interested in maintaining an adequate flow of dental graduates and in keeping the dental schools operating in a healthy condition. It has already been pointed out that various professional and governmental agencies, which apparently did not have full confidence in Selective Service's intentions, had repeatedly requested the Armed Forces to give students inactive military status to insure their deferment. But the professional agencies, at least, vigorously opposed the more detailed involvement of the Army and Navy in the administration of dental education, even though the actual instruction was left to the established schools. As early as May 1943 the position of the ADA was stated as follows:[154]

> ... recalling vividly the awkward blunder of the administration of the Student's Army Training Corps in World War I, which, but for the providential Armistice in November 1918, would probably have led to the collapse of higher and professional education, we have hoped profoundly that dental education might be spared military regimentation during this war. With every wish to see competent dentists provided promptly and unhesitatingly for the Army and the Navy, as they happily have been, and, we believe, will continue to be, we are concerned about the working out of a system of dental education "by contract" with the Army and Navy. We gravely question whether the common end to be gained, about which there is no debate, may not be accomplished more economically, more expeditiously, with sounder educational procedure, with greater assurance of a steady supply of new entrants to dental practice to meet civilians as well as war service needs with greater safety for the future of the profession, by the conduct of the dental schools free from the inevitable effects of Army and Navy regimentation. . . .
>
> After all this military machine does its work, it will transpire, we predict, that there was really no occasion or necessity for doing anything. What more do the Army and Navy want than a steady flow of well-trained dentists to meet their replacement needs? The dental schools could have gone on and would have gone on cheerfully without any overlordship or regimentation, and, indeed, without any financial aid. . . . All the Government needed to do was to establish a sensible working scheme for the deferment of enough bona fide high school and liberal arts college students to sustain the present enrollment in dental schools. . . .

In justification of the Armed Forces' decision to place dental students on active duty, it should be noted that the opinion that professional trainees would be content to remain in school if they were assured of deferment was not universally accepted. Even the Secretary-Treasurer of the American Association of Dental Schools reported that "the average student of the desirable type took a rather dim view of deferment while other young men of his age were in

---

[154] Dental education in wartime. J. Am. Dent. A. 30 : 741–749, 1 May 43.

uniform," and he stated that "assignment [to the Armed Forces], as a principle, appeared to be the most desirable, although uneconomic procedure." [155] The feeling that if young men were to be given deferment from dangerous duty to remain in school the Armed Forces should select those to be given that opportunity, and that those selected should be paid so that such preferred treatment would not be based on economic status, has already been mentioned. By the time the dental ASTP was inaugurated, however, it was already reasonably clear that no general voluntary exodus from the professional schools need be anticipated in World War II, and that deferment would in itself be sufficient stimulus to keep a sufficient number of dental students in training. Enrollment in the dental schools had, in fact, actually increased from 7,184 in 1937 to 9,014 in 1943, when it was higher than at any time since 1928.[156] The contention that any qualified individual should have equal opportunity to obtain deferment for professional education, regardless of ability to pay, was a plausible theory, but in practice the ASTP had to be set up with students who had, for the most part, already been pursuing their courses for from 1 to 5 years, and who were presumably already assured that they would be able to pay the necessary costs. Thus it was found, when the dental ASTP was terminated in 1944 and students were forced to continue at their own expense, that only a little over 1 percent had to drop out. Whether the professional student was entitled not only to deferment in time of war, but to the salve to his feelings which was provided by the fact that he was placed in uniform, is at least open to question.

The belief that the personnel needs of the Dental Services of the Armed Forces could not be met unless dental students were placed under military control has also been challenged. When ASTP was first being considered, in the fall of 1942, the Army Dental Corps was faced with a procurement objective of over 7,000 officers for 1943, and there is every indication that some difficulty in getting this number of dentists was anticipated. (See chapter III.) Selective Service had shown its inability to draft dentists in significant numbers, and it was apparently felt that dental students should be required to make themselves available for immediate military service on graduation in return for the privilege of deferment. The Director of the Dental Division stated in August 1944 that:

> The Dental Corps at one time had an anticipated procurement objective of at least 25% more than the maximum level reached. . . .
> It has been stated that the Army could have attained all the dental officers desired without the ASTP, and that the dental schools could have produced just as many officers for the Army. This statement in all probability is true, but the fact is that the procurement objective for dentists was never reached in many of the states. There was no mechanism whereby dentists could be drafted except through the normal channels of Selective Service. That many dentists refused commissions in

---

[155] Personal Ltr, Dr. John E. Buhler to Col William Wilson, 11 May 48.
[156] Horner, H. H.: Dental education and dental personnel. J. Am. Dent. A. 33: 872–888, 1 Jul 46.

the Army is a fact that nearly every State Dental Procurement and Assignment chairman can testify. Many dentists . . . preferred to have the other fellow go. These facts, and those associated with the potential military needs, caused the War Department to include dentistry in the ASTP.

After the war the Director of the Dental Division noted that:

> . . . when the ASTP was initiated said program was justified for the reason that it was impossible to predict the length of the war and available dentists in civilian life were limited. It is believed, however, that the Army Dental Corps needs could have been satisfied without the AST Program.[157]

The ASTP predental training was criticized by dental educators who felt that the five-term course was inadequate. At the invitation of The Surgeon General representatives of the professional schools met in January 1943 to advise on the premedical, predental, and preveterinary courses. This committee, which included three dental educators, recommended a common program for all branches of medical science and they advised that six semesters of 12 weeks each be allowed for preprofessional schooling. It recommended further that the course include the following minimum requirements:[158]

English	6 semester hours
Physics	6 semester hours
Biology	6 semester hours
General chemistry	8 semester hours
Organic chemistry	4 semester hours

An additional 30 hours were to be selected from optional technical subjects, depending upon the facilities of the school and the desires of the student. The curriculum finally approved by ASF has been described in paragraph 4, page 137.

The charge that dental educators had not been consulted is certainly open to question, though one dental representative on the committee stated later that they had accepted the final plan in an effort to make the best of a program which they had personally thought ill-advised, but which had been definitely decided upon by the War Department.[159]

The effect of the ASTP on the morale of other military personnel was unfavorable, but difficult to evaluate in respect to degree. The young men who had been taken from a school of business administration and sent to New Guinea could not always understand why the able-bodied boy next door was continuing his dental education as before, except that now the Government took care of his expenses and paid him a salary. The paratrooper's pride in his skill as a fighting man was apt to be dampened when he heard that college students at home were wearing uniforms which the general public could not distinguish from the one he was currently wearing in a foxhole on the wrong side of the Rhine. This type of "discrimination" was regrettable but unavoid-

---

[157] See footnote 9, p. 107.
[158] Ltr, SG to Dir ASTP, 2 Jan 43, sub: Premedical and medical education. SG: 353.9-1.
[159] Army specialized training program. J. Am. Dent. A. 31 : 1149–1154, 15 Aug 45.

able if there was to be no break in the training of replacements for vital occupations, but the opinion was widely held and expressed that the Army had done enough when it guaranteed deferment for professional students, without subsidizing them and giving them the status of soldiers.

Probably the most bitter criticism of ASTP came from dental officers of the Armed Forces, especially when it was announced in 1944 that recent graduates would be released to civil life. Dental officers on military duty were not always in full possession of all the facts concerning the ASTP, and the fairly common belief that dental students had been educated at Government expense and then released to enjoy the lucrative practice at home is understandable, if not entirely justified. Actually, no dental student received all, or even a major part, of his schooling under ASTP. Juniors entering the program in 1943 received up to 2 years of education at Government expense; others received a maximum of about 1 year since only seniors were continued in the course after July 1944. Also, in spite of the Army decision to release graduates in June and July 1944 only a small proportion entered civil practice. The lack of vacancies at that time was temporary, and all qualified men graduating from July 1944 until ASTP ended in April 1945 were given commissions in the Army Dental Corps. All but 113 of the physically qualified graduates of the dental ASTP eventually entered the Army, Navy, Veterans Administration, or the Public Health Service.[160] (For a discussion of the reasons why ASTP graduates were not commissioned in the summer of 1944 see chapter III.)

Even a considerable number of the critics of ASTP held that once it had been established it should have been kept in operation until the end of the war, both to assure continued replacements for civilian practice and to provide dental officers when it became necessary to demobilize veteran dentists after the end of hostilities. Colonel Fitts states in his report that:

> It is extremely interesting to note that the curtailment and termination of both the dental and veterinary training programs have proved to have been premature and ill-advised. The lack of replacements for dental officers has required the retention of dentists in the active military service for periods in excess of those required for emergency medical officers, with resulting criticism and dissatisfaction. The dental ASTP trainees who were discharged in order to continue their studies as civilians have upon graduation been under no obligation or compulsion to enter the military service either as enlisted men or officers. Efforts at the recruitment of volunteers as replacements among this group have proved completely futile and on 24 May 1946 the War Department placed a special call on Selective Service for the draft of dentists.

Though the Director of the Dental Division and The Surgeon General had advised against the termination of the dental ASTP, the War Department appeared to feel that it could not justify the program when the Dental Service was refusing to accept graduates for lack of vacancies. At the time the dental ASTP was terminated the demand for combat troops was so critical that

---

[160] Memo, Brig Gen J. J. O'Hare, Chief, Manpower Control Group, to Gen Willard S. Paul, ACofS G-1, 8 May 46, sub: Dental ASTP program. SG: 353 (Student training).

PERSONNEL AND TRAINING 145

partially trained pilots were being transferred to the infantry, and medical units overseas were being stripped of able-bodied enlisted men, who were replaced with untrained, limited-service personnel. It may or may not be held that the action taken was unjustified, but it cannot be argued that the reasons which motivated the War Department were trivial. (See also the discussions of this problem in chapters III and IX.)

The Deferment of Instructors in Dental Schools

The question of maintaining the faculties of the dental schools during the war did not at first receive the attention given the maintenance of their student bodies. Some increase in the load carried by individual instructors was possible, and as a group the teachers were less likely to be subject to induction under Selective Service because of age. The problem eventually assumed important proportions, however, and its solution involved the Armed Forces, Selective Service, PAS, and various other organizations and agencies.

Instructors were not mentioned in the first bills introduced in Congress to provide for the deferment of dental students. A modification of the earlier Murray bills, introduced in the Senate in February 1941, directed the exemption of professional instructors, but this legislation, and later similar acts, met the same fate as the various bills to defer students.[161] Selective Service also omitted consideration of instructors in its early directives concerning occupational deferment, but on 20 June 1941 all State Directors were advised that serious consideration should be given to the exemption of individuals found necessary for the instruction of students in critical occupations.[162]

Early in 1943, PAS became interested in this problem and conducted a survey to determine the actual situation.[163] Thirty-eight dental schools were found to have 2,000 instructors, of whom 1,200 were declared to be essential by the schools themselves. Fifty percent of the instructors were under 45 years of age, and 40 percent were under 40 years of age, but no attempt was made to obtain more detailed information on eligibility for induction under Selective Service. The medical schools were found to vary greatly in the proportion of instructors declared essential, from a minimum of 10 percent to a maximum of 98 percent; similar figures were not given for the dental schools, but comparable variation was reported to exist. PAS recommended that 12 instructors be allowed for the first 100 students in professional schools, and that 9 instructors be authorized for each additional 100 students, but it was found that few schools approached the calculated ideal. Individual institutions varied from a minimum of only 40 percent of the recommended total of instructors to a maximum of 206 percent. PAS appealed to the schools to adhere to the proposed ratio, but the results of this effort, if any, are unknown.

---
[161] See footnote 100, p. 129.
[162] See footnote 107, p. 130.
[163] Minutes of Committee on Dentistry, PAS, 13 Feb 43. Natl Archives, PAS files.

The professional press carried numerous discussions of the shortage of dental instructors, but factual data on this subject, beyond that reported by PAS, have not been revealed. After the war the Secretary-Treasurer of the American Association of Dental Schools advised that in any future emergency it was essential that professional schools be assured an adequate complement of trained teacher personnel, either by deferment or by assignment from the military forces after being taken on active duty.[164]

Summary, Dental Undergraduate Education, World War II

In spite of outspoken criticism of many aspects of the handling of professional students during World War II it is clear that the primary objective, to maintain the dental schools and to provide a continuing flow of graduates, was attained. Shortly after automatic deferment was ended in July 1941, over 80 percent of all dental enrollees were already being deferred by their local boards on an occupational basis. More vigorous action by Selective Service in late 1941 and in 1942, and the granting of inactive military status by the Armed Forces, not only maintained enrollment, but increased it by 1943 to the largest figure since 1928. Average registration in the dental schools in the 5 war years, from 1941 through 1945, was 8,416 students, compared with an average of only 7,354 students in the 9 years from 1932 through 1940.[165]

It would seem that World War II policies in respect to the deferment of professional students cannot be criticized for impeding dental education; it is not equally certain that they should not be criticized for actually increasing the number of students registered in professional schools in wartime. The need for a long-term augmentation of training in the medical sciences cannot be denied, but the propriety of a major increase in enrollment in dental schools in a time of national emergency, when the desire for deferment from dangerous military service was presumably a strong motive for seeking a professional education, is at least open to question. Students who were already enrolled in the dental schools, or who had begun their general university preparation with the specific purpose of entering dental training, were of course above suspicion in this respect, but since average enrollment during the war exceeded the prewar average by more than a thousand men it is difficult to escape the conclusion that a considerable number of men of military age took up the study of dentistry for reasons directly or indirectly connected with the war. To the extent that these men were motivated by a desire to escape military duty, rather than by a strong desire to enter the profession of dentistry, their deferment could hardly be a cause for satisfaction, either to the profession or to the public. It would seem that agencies responsible for the exemption of professional students should, by voluntary agreement if possible, limit such exemption to a number consistent with average normal enrollment.

---

[164] See footnote 155, p. 142.
[165] Enrollment data from 1932 through 1945 obtained by author from the Washington office of the ADA, 26 May 48.

It is true that the end of ASTP in 1944, and the simultaneous termination of Selective Service deferment for predental students, would have resulted in a serious situation if the war had not come to a close in a short time. In October 1945 only 1,197 freshmen dental students were enrolled, compared with 2,496 the year before,[166] and it was estimated that as a result there would be only about 1,000 graduates in 1948.[167] It is highly probable that both the actions which led to this situation were based on a reasonable belief that hostilities would not be prolonged after 1944, but the ensuing rapid reduction in freshmen enrollment emphasized the need for assuring continuous predental education if the dental schools are to continue their operations.

The ideal mechanism for providing deferment for students in essential occupations was not found during World War II. Attempts to attain that end through legislation failed because they conflicted with the basic concept, accepted by Congress, that no group should be granted blanket preferred consideration under the Selective Service law. Any exception to that policy would probably result in strong political pressure to have the privilege extended to an ever-widening population. Even if blanket deferment of dental students were authorized, the administration of such a policy would entail serious difficulties; if no restrictions were prescribed the schools would soon be flooded with applicants who were interested mainly in exemption from military duty, and if the number to be deferred were limited, the question of determining which men should be accepted would involve knotty political and administrative problems.

The Selective Service System was of course charged with formal responsibility for determining which individuals should be inducted and which should be allowed to continue in training for essential occupations, and it actually authorized most deferments of dental students until the Armed Forces started granting inactive Reserve commissions in late 1941 and early 1942. Selective Service was again left to carry almost the entire burden of exempting dental students after the Armed Forces abandoned their dental undergraduate programs in 1944, and during all this period a considerable number of professional students who were not eligible for, or who did not desire, military status continued their education under Selective Service policies. It has been pointed out, however, that in spite of this record many dental educators, members of the profession, and even governmental agencies responsible for national health, had serious misgivings concerning Selective Service's willingness and ability to follow a consistent course which would insure the regular operation of the schools. Selective Service was committed to a policy of placing heavy responsibility on the local boards, on the theory that they were most familiar with circumstances which affected individual priority for induction, and critics appear to have felt that the local boards lacked the technical background for

---

[166] See footnote 120, p. 132.
[167] See footnote 156, p. 142.

selecting dental students and that they could not be relied upon to follow the general policies recommended by national agencies which were familiar with larger aspects of the problem of continuing training in the health services. This fear does not seem to have been supported by the facts since enrollment in the dental schools increased steadily from 1940 through 1943, though it was reported that individual boards refused to defer professional students.

The suitability of Selective Service as the agency to defer professional students may be questioned on more fundamental grounds. The entry of the military into the educational field minimized Selective Service's problem by the time it became necessary to choose large numbers of new students, and it will be seen later that Selective Service actually delegated much of its nominal authority to the dental schools. If it had retained full responsibility in this matter during the entire war it would ultimately have been faced with the necessity for finding acceptable answers to such problems as the following:

1. How many students should be granted deferment each year to take up the study of dentistry?

2. How should students be allocated geographically and according to schools? Should state quotas be determined? Rural and urban? Racial? Should wartime quotas attempt to correct longstanding peacetime imbalances in the distribution of dentists? How assure that state universities would accept a reasonable proportion of students from adjoining states having no dental schools?

3. How coordinate the actions of local boards which had no way of comparing the qualifications of their applicants with those appearing before other boards?

4. How select approximately 2,000 students each year from some 10,000 applicants so as to insure deferment for those who were most likely to succeed in school and in the practice of the profession? Could this selection be left to the schools without risking charges of favoritism? Should Selective Service set up agencies for investigating scholastic records, giving aptitude tests, and otherwise determining the relative eligibility of thousands of would-be dental students?

5. Should ability to pay for a dental education be a deciding factor in the selection of students for deferment in time of war?

6. How eliminate applicants who were interested in deferment rather than in the practice of dentistry?

A similar situation arose very early in the war when it became apparent that Selective Service alone could not handle the problem of procuring physicians, dentists, and veterinarians, on the basis of individual liability for military service, without endangering the health services of the nation. In this instance the Procurement and Assignment Service of the War Manpower Commission was established to render expert advice, though cooperation between the two agencies sometimes left much to be desired. It is possible that with the assistance of some such body of professional experts, either in or out of its own organization, Selective Service could have handled the question of deferring students with reasonable satisfaction, but it seems probable that a purely lay body would have been on unfamiliar ground had it attempted to administer such a highly technical matter unaided.

It is noted above that during the period when it was nominally responsible for the deferment of dental students Selective Service actually delegated most of its responsibility to the schools. Students already enrolled were generally continued in their studies without question by the Selective Service boards, and the deferment of new applicants was normally based on acceptance for admission to a dental school. For all practical purposes, therefore, the deans of the professional schools had the final decision in determining which applicants would be accepted to continue their education and which would be rejected and inducted into the Armed Forces. It is clear, from published criticisms of the Army and Navy programs, that the dental schools preferred to select their own students, and that they wanted nothing from any governmental agency but deferment of the men chosen.[168] The Armed Forces entered the situation before the results of this policy could be fully determined in World War II, and there is no evidence that the deans of the dental schools did not choose applicants as impartially as possible, on the basis of their desirability for the profession as interpreted by the deans themselves. It is possible, however, that with the best intentions in the world both the schools and Selective Service would ultimately have come in for serious criticism if the matter had not been largely taken from their hands by the inauguration of the Army ASTP and the Navy V-12 programs.

In the first place, it is doubtful if dental educators, as individuals, were any better fitted than Selective Service to answer such questions as the following:

1. How many students should be admitted? During the war the capacity of the school was apparently the deciding factor in most cases, and it appears that the schools and the profession escaped criticism for the resulting great increase in enrollment only by sheer good luck.

2. Should students be selected purely on the basis of individual qualifications, or should some effort be made to apportion vacancies on a geographical basis? If the latter, how?

3. How could a dental school supported by state funds resist strong political pressure to limit deferment to citizens of that state, so as to provide for students who normally came from adjoining states with no dental schools of their own? If vacancies were to be reserved for out-of-state students, how should they be apportioned among the many schools which might be called upon to accept such students? Who would enforce such apportionment?

---

[168] See footnote 154, p. 141.

4. If questions of the fair allotment of vacancies could be solved by voluntary cooperation between schools, how could accepted policies be implemented through Selective Service, which alone could grant actual deferment?

5. How select a few thousand new students from the many thousands of applicants each year? Educators were presumably best fitted to determine the scholastic qualifications of applicants, but even the opinions of experts in this field are notoriously fallible. During World War II the problem was further complicated by the fact that in order to insure his deferment until he could complete predental requirements, a dean often had to "accept" a dental student soon after graduation from high school, long before his capacity to absorb highly technical university training had been established. The increasing reliability of aptitude tests also suggests that in the near future trained personnel administrators may be able to select prospective dental students with greater accuracy than educators relying upon their own impressions and upon scholastic records, but neither personal impressions nor aptitude tests will eliminate the opportunist who is interested in draft deferment rather than in the practice of dentistry.

Such problems can be solved only by an agency which has full information on national as well as local needs, which has close liaison with the Armed Forces, with Selective Service, with other interested governmental activities, and with the professional organizations; and which has sufficient official authority to insure adequate consideration for its recommendations.

Potentially at least, the greatest objection to leaving the deferment of students to dental educators is probably the degree of personal responsibility involved. It has already been pointed out that wartime enrollment in the dental schools exceeded normal peacetime registration by more than a thousand men, and that Selective Service boards openly charged that the universities were "havens for slackers." [169] So far as is known the corollary charge, that the schools were using the national emergency to swell their own income, was never made, but the possibility that it would be was constantly present. It seems highly probable that most deans were influenced only by a sincere desire to provide needed personnel for the profession, but the administration of any policy having to do with exempting individuals from dangerous duties in wartime inevitably and properly receives close scrutiny from Congress, the public, and the press, and the opportunity for misunderstanding is enormous. The objections to allowing any private individual or organization to select men to receive such a fundamental privilege as exemption from military service are obvious. It is probable that if the deans had carried this heavy responsibility during the entire war they would ultimately have become targets for such vigorous criticism, and such political and personal pressure, that they would have welcomed the intervention of some official or semiofficial agency roughly similar to the Procurement and Assignment Service.

---

[169] See footnote 96, p. 126.

The military were probably least qualified of all agencies to select new professional students, and it is difficult to find theoretical or practical justification for the Army and Navy becoming involved in such extraneous matters in a national emergency. The Armed Forces initiated their World War II training programs with men already enrolled in dental schools or in predental preparation, and had the assistance of dental educators in selecting new applicants during the short time they were directly concerned with dental undergraduate instruction, but this field was so remote from military activities that it would seem more appropriate to leave it to other agencies. Much can also be said for the early contention of the War Department that the military should not involve itself with any phase of professional education beyond the minimum steps necessary to insure sufficient trained replacements, and that questions of deferment of professional students to meet the needs of the civilian population should properly be the responsibility of Congress, Selective Service, the Federal Security Agency, the War Manpower Commission, and other nonmilitary organizations. The fact that at least some of these agencies considered it necessary to request the Armed Forces to assume such an unfamiliar role in World War II emphasizes the need for a clear and enforceable policy on student deferment at the start of mobilization.

The statement of the Director of the Dental Division after the war, that Army requirements for dental officers could have been met without recourse to the ASTP, seems well substantiated.

AUXILIARY DENTAL PERSONNEL

Period Before World War II

Soon after contract dentists were first authorized it was provided that each would have an enlisted assistant detailed from members of the Hospital Corps and that these assistants would be under full control of dentists during duty hours.[170] As early as 1904, Dr. Marshall reported to The Surgeon General that it was difficult to obtain enlisted assistants, and that competent men became dissatisfied with the long hours, confining work, and lack of opportunity for advancement incident to assignment to the Dental Service.[171]

In World War I, about 5,000 enlisted assistants were on duty with 4,620 dental officers. These men were detailed from Medical Department enlisted personnel and were largely trained by the officers with whom they worked.

In the period between World Wars I and II, dental auxiliary personnel continued to be obtained from the Medical Department though provision was made in Army regulations for special detail of enlisted men to the Dental Service.[172] Men so detailed, on the authority of The Surgeon General, were

---
[170] Manual for the Medical Department, 1906. Washington, Government Printing Office, 1906, p. 40.
[171] Ltr, Dr. John S. Marshall to SG, 16 Feb. 04. Natl Archives: 70760-27.
[172] AR 40-15, 28 Dec 42.

to be more directly under the control of dental officers for training and duty than would those merely *assigned*, and it was believed that this provision would ensure a more stable source of auxiliary dental personnel. In practice few men were ever so assigned and the merits of the plan were never determined. It was abandoned completely in May 1943.[173]

Before World War II, it was generally believed by enlisted men of the Medical Department that duty with the Dental Service meant long hours and loss of opportunity for promotion. Dental officers spent months training laboratory technicians and chair assistants, knowing all the while that the best grade they could offer in their relatively small clinics would be that of private first class or corporal, and that as soon as these men had sufficient service to be considered for promotion they would have to transfer to the surgical service or medical supply. The alternative was to accept those misfits who had no ambition or hope for advancement. Seldom could the Dental Service offer grades comparable to those available in other, larger departments. Further, when the enlisted man of the Dental Service was examined for promotion he was questioned on general medical subjects in which men assigned in other services had the obvious advantage. As a result, service in the dental clinic came to be regarded as a dead end on the road to promotion. There was very little change in this situation until the start of World War II.

Auxiliary Personnel, World War II

Mobilization for World War II brought considerable improvement in the adequacy and status of auxiliary personnel provided the Dental Service. In June 1941, only 1,488 enlisted men and a limited number of civilians were on duty with dental installations.[174] In September 1943, 13,851 enlisted men and 2,441 civilians were so engaged,[175] and by January 1944 the number had increased to 15,585 enlisted men and 2,410 civilians.[176] The percentages of men in the various grades and a comparison with grades held by enlisted men of the Medical Department as a whole were as follows:

Grade*	Dental Service (Total Army)	Dental Service (Continental US)	Medical Dept. (Continental US)
	Percent	Percent	Percent
Master sergeant	0.06	0.09	0.50
Technical sergeant	0.48	0.61	1.50
Staff sergeant and technician 3/c	4.36	3.84	5.00
Sergeant and technician 4/c	13.60	12.72	11.70
Corporal and technician 5/c	44.01	39.19	17.80
Private first class	20.35	23.56	23.10
Private	17.11	19.96	40.90

*308 Wacs in unknown grades are not included in above percentages for the Dental Service.

[173] AR 40–15, C 1, 10 May 43.
[174] History of the Army Dental Corps, Personnel, 1940–43. HD: 314.7–2.
[175] Ibid.
[176] Annual Rpt, Dental Div SGO, 1945. HD.

It is apparent that the enlisted man of the Dental Service had a poor chance of reaching the top three grades, but he had a better chance than the enlisted man of the Medical Service to reach the grades of sergeant and corporal.

By June 1944, enlisted personnel were being replaced somewhat by civilians and the number of enlisted men on duty had dropped to 14,859 while that of civilians had increased to 3,446. These figures remained substantially unchanged until the start of demobilization.[177]

When initially assigned to the Dental Service all enlisted assistants had completed from 8 to 17 weeks of basic military training; many had no other experience in the duties they would have to perform.

Dental Laboratory Technicians. One of the first problems to be solved by the Dental Service in World War II was a severe shortage of dental laboratory technicians. When the dental requirements for induction were considerably relaxed in October 1942, the disqualification rate for dental reasons sharply decreased and by the end of 1942 it reached the level of 0.1 percent. It remained at about that level for the remainder of World War II.[178] To meet the needs of the hundreds of thousands of men who would previously have been considered unfit for military duty, the Army was eventually to construct over two and a half million dentures, requiring a mobilization of laboratory facilities on a scale not foreseen in early planning.

To meet this need for increased laboratory facilities, the Army could count on inducting only a fraction of the required personnel. A survey by the Dental Laboratory Institute of America and the American Dental Association showed that in 1942 there were only a little over 12,000 trained dental technicians in the entire United States.[179] Many of these were ineligible for induction because of age or dependency, and when it is noted that about one-third of all men actually called by Selective Service during World War II were rejected for physical and mental reasons, it is apparent that but a few laboratory men could be taken from the civilian reservoir. It should be noted that civilian demand for dental prosthetic appliances also increased greatly during the war because of the rapid rise in general income levels. A sample group of laboratories questioned early in 1942 reported that they had lost about 18 percent of their technicians.[180] If this proportion held throughout the country the Armed Forces inducted about 2,200 laboratory workers from this source.

To make the situation worse, many of the dental technicians taken into the Armed Forces during the first part of the war were lost to the Dental Service.[181] The test group of laboratories previously mentioned reported that only 44

---

[177] Unpublished data from the files of the Dental Division. Abstracted by Lt Col John C. Brauer, DC, Dent Div SGO.

[178] Unpublished data from the Medical Statistics Div, SGO.

[179] Complete survey of dental laboratory technicians to be undertaken by committee. J. Am. Dent. A. 29 : 2060, 1 Nov 42.

[180] Ibid.

[181] Proceedings of The Surgeon General's Conference with Corps Area and Army Dental Surgeons, 8-9 Jul 42, p. 11. HD : 337.

percent of their inducted laboratory men were sent to duty with the Dental Corps. Some were assigned from the reception centers to nonmedical units, probably on the basis of mechanical ability; others were assigned as chair assistants because Army classification procedure at first failed to distinguish clearly between laboratory and assistant functions.[182] The latter mistake was readily correctible, except when technicians taken from Zone of Interior laboratories were assigned as chair assistants to units going overseas, in which case they were often irrevocably lost to the prosthetic service.

On 23 November 1942, on the advice of the Director of the Dental Division, the chief of the Personnel Service, SGO, asked Army Service Forces to take steps to insure that dental laboratory technicians would be assigned to the Medical Department, and requested further that the forces in the United States be combed for technicians who had already been assigned to other branches.[183] At about the same time the ADA and the Dental Laboratory Institute of America cooperated to make the survey of laboratory manpower which has already been mentioned and to furnish the Dental Division, SGO, with the names of inducted technicians so that a check could be made of their current assignments. In January 1943 the Dental Division also requested that the practice of assigning laboratory men to chair assistants' duties be stopped.[184]

In February 1943 it was reported that The Adjutant General was taking the following steps:[185]

1. Directing an Army-wide report on dental technicians performing other duties.

2. Requesting from the Surgeon General's Office a list of vacancies for dental technicians.

3. Notifying reception centers to send all inductees with laboratory experience to the nearest Medical Department replacement training center for assignment.

While few dental technicians were assigned outside the Medical Department after the spring of 1943, another critical situation soon arose when ASF directed that personnel fitted for general overseas assignment would not be retained in service commands in the United States. Some laboratory men were of course required overseas, but in April 1943 the Director of the Dental Division complained that Zone of Interior installations were being stripped of dental mechanics who were subsequently being assigned to tactical units as dental chair assistants.[186] He strongly recommended to ASF that dental laboratory men be assigned only to those organizations having prosthetic facilities. Two

---

[182] AR 615-26, 15 Sep 42.
[183] Ltr, Chief, Pers Serv, SGO, to Dir, Mil Pers, ASF, 23 Nov 42, sub: Dental technicians. SG: 221 (Technologists).
[184] Memo, Dental Div. SGO for Pers Serv, SGO, 28 Jan 43. SG: 221 (Technologists).
[185] Memo, Dir Tng Div, SGO, for Pers Serv, SGO, 26 Feb 43, sub: Dental laboratory technicians (067). SG: 221 (Technologists).
[186] Ltr, Chief, Pers Serv, SGO, to Dir, Mil Pers, ASF, 7 Apr 43, sub: Dental laboratory technicians (Dental Mechanics). SG: 221 (Technologists).

PERSONNEL AND TRAINING   155

days later The Adjutant General authorized The Surgeon General to make his own arrangements to that end with the individual service commands concerned. On 14 April 1943 The Adjutant General notified The Surgeon General that a separate personnel category (SSN 067) had been reserved for dental technicians, to distinguish them from dental chair assistants (SSN 855), paving the way for a clear definition of the two types of duty in drawing up tables of organization.[187] The new classifications were published in a memorandum from The Adjutant General's Office (AGO), dated 13 May 1943.[188]

These measures did much to prevent the waste of laboratory men in routine jobs. In January 1944, however, the whole matter was again thrown into confusion when ASF placed laboratory men in the "scarce" category and directed that they would not be assigned to *any* overseas organization.[189] [190] This action was apparently designed to prevent the misuse of such personnel, but it overlooked the fact that a limited number of technicians were needed in theaters of operations, and the Director of the Dental Division immediately recommended modification of the order. A letter was subsequently prepared for the Commanding General, ASF, listing the specific units in which the assignment of laboratory men was essential,[191] and the misunderstanding was corrected in a War Department circular of 4 April 1944.[192] A supplementary order of 29 May 1944 directed that dental technicians would be used only in the duties for which they had been trained.[193]

Steps to improve the utilization of laboratory personnel proved generally effective, but they did not prevent a minor loss of technicians to other duties. Hospitals sometimes reclassified dental technicians as chair assistants to avoid an excess of this category over the numbers permitted by tables of organization, but in such cases the individual usually continued to perform his old duties as long as he remained with the unit. If he were transferred, however, he was likely to be assigned on the basis of his specification serial number. In other cases the authorization for laboratory technicians was revoked for certain units, and the men holding laboratory ratings were sometimes reclassified under such circumstances to prevent their loss to the organization. Keeping dental technicians assigned to their proper duties was a continuing problem for the Dental Service throughout the war.[194]

A defect of the broad classification of "dental technicians" was that it failed to specify individual special skills or degrees of experience. Both Army and civilian laboratories normally function on a "production line" basis, with

---

[187] Memo, TAG for SG, 14 Apr 43, sub: Dental laboratory technicians. SG: 221 (Technologists).
[188] AGO Memo W 615–45–43, 13 May 43, sub: Revision of specification serial numbers—AR 615–26. SG: 221 (Technologists).
[189] ASF Cir 26, 24 Jan 44.
[190] ASF Cir 50, 16 Feb 44.
[191] Ltr, Chief, Oprs Serv, SGO, to CG, ASF, 3 Mar 44, sub: Dental laboratory technicians (067). SG: 300.5–5.
[192] WD Cir 130, 4 Apr 44.
[193] WD Memo W 615–44, 29 May 44, sub: Critically needed specialists.
[194] History of the Army Dental Corps, 1 Apr 44–1 May 1944. HD: 024.10–3.

each man carrying out a limited operation. The technician who is qualified to perform all duties in a laboratory with equal competence is therefore rare. Under the Army classification a hospital which needed a man to set up teeth was likely to receive a replacement whose specialty was polishing dentures.

Even in peacetime the number of trained technicians entering the Army from civilian life had been negligible, and the Medical Department had conducted training for this category of personnel since the founding of the Army Dental School in 1922. An average of 18 men had graduated from the 4-month course each year in the period 1935–1938.[195] The training emphasized laboratory work, but it also included some instruction in administration, x-ray technique, and chair assisting. The course was expected to be increased to a full year beginning with the class of September 1939, but the outbreak of war caused this class to be graduated in July 1940, and thereafter the period of instruction was reduced to 3 months.

The wartime 3-month course for laboratory technicians was really a combined course for laboratory men and chair assistants, though most time was spent on laboratory procedures. It included instruction in dental anatomy and tooth carving, dental materials and metallurgy, dental records, dental roentgenology, dental hygiene, inlays and crowns, chair assisting, impressions, clasps, full and partial dentures, and actual work in the laboratory. It also included instruction in the care and maintenance of equipment.[196] Applicants were required to have the equivalent of a high school education and must have completed basic military training. The course given at Fitzsimons General Hospital in 1942 was as follows:

Organization		2 hours
Basic dental instruction		40 hours
Dental assisting		47 hours
Chair assisting		9 hours
Army dental records		6 hours
X-ray		25 hours
Fractures		5 hours
Mailing dental materials		2 hours
Prosthetics:		
Upper partial dentures	42 hours	
Lower partial dentures	78 hours	
Full dentures	128 hours	
Acrylic splints	35 hours	
Total		283 hours
Crown, bridge, and inlay:		
Metallurgy	12 hours	
Posterior bridge	92 hours	
Anterior bridge	28 hours	
Total		132 hours

---

[195] Annual Reports . . . Surgeon General, 1935–38.
[196] ASF Manual M3, 25 Apr 44. HD.

The first month was devoted to didactic instruction and the last 2 months to actual work in a laboratory under supervision. It was recognized that competent dental technicians could not be trained in 3 months and the course was expected to establish a basis for the individual's further progress at his home station. The rating of SSN 067 was conferred at the schools only on the best qualified graduates (40 percent at Fitzsimons General Hospital, 1943). More often it was given later, on recommendation of the unit dental surgeon after the student had improved his knowledge by "on-the-job" training. Those who showed little aptitude for laboratory work remained SSN 855's (chair assistants).

The dental technician training program soon outgrew the Army Dental School and courses were given in six general hospitals in 1940. Nine schools were in operation during fiscal 1943 and over 5,000 students were enrolled during that year. Maximum authorized capacity was 600 men a month. Many of the schools operated double shifts during 1943 to accommodate the augmented classes without additional equipment. The program fell off sharply in the latter part of 1944 and only a handful of students remained after March 1945.

Results of the training program for dental technicians are listed in the following tabulation: [197]

Fiscal year	Enlisted men enrolled	Wacs enrolled*	Enlisted men graduated	Wacs graduated*
1940	13	0	13	0
1941	295	0	121	0
1942	1,012	0	843	0
1943	5,438	0	3,691	0
1944	3,361	103	3,791	69
1945	1,007	396	1,550	346
Totals	11,126	499	10,009	415

*In the entire program, from July 1939 through January 1946, 511 Wacs enrolled in the dental technicians schools of whom 473 graduated.

The percentage of failures from July 1939 through January 1946 were as follows: [198]

Type	Enlisted men	Wacs	All students
	Percent	Percent	Percent
Scholastic	4.7	2.2	4.6
Other	4.8	5.3	4.8
Totals	9.5	7.5	9.4

[197] See footnote 79, p. 126.

[198] The percentages of failures quoted here were calculated from figures of the Training Division, SGO, which show 541 scholastic failures and 573 other failures out of a total enrollment of 11,847. Of the entire enrollment, 10,713 men were graduated through April 1946 (men enrolled in January did not graduate until April). Since 20 enrollees of the total number are not accounted for in the numbers reported for failures and graduates, it may be that these students did not complete the course during the February–April 1946 period. However, if these 20 were to be considered as failures, the total percent would only be changed from 9.4 to 9.6.

Since graduates of the technicians' schools were seldom given specialist's ratings until they had served for some time at their own stations it is not known exactly how many became laboratory workers and how many remained chair assistants. In July 1945, 2,494 men, or 17.6 percent of the 14,191 enlisted men with the Dental Service, were rated SSN 067.[199]

The Director of the Dental Division stated in 1945 that the 3-month course had been too short for dental laboratory workers, though he felt that it was adequate for chair assistants. He recommended a minimum course of 6 months for technicians, to be extended to one year if possible.[200]

Use was made of civilian laboratory technicians to replace enlisted men where possible but civilians were never employed in this work to the extent that they were as assistants and hygienists, probably due to difficulties of procurement. By August 1943, 144 civilian laboratory men were on duty with the Army, but this number declined through 1944.

Prosthetic Supply Clerks. Beginning on 20 March 1944, six enlisted men of the Dental Service were given 4 weeks of training at Binghamton Medical Depot to prepare them for duty as prosthetic supply clerks. The scarcity of personnel capable of handling the many sizes, shapes, and shades of porcelain teeth stocked in laboratories and depots made this small but important course necessary.[201]

Dental Assistants. With mobilization it became necessary to staff large numbers of clinics with assistants in a very short time and more emphasis was placed on training for this category. In the paragraph on dental technicians it is explained that the dental technicians' course was a combined project, including instruction in both laboratory procedures and the duties of a chair assistant. Those men who did not show mechanical aptitude for laboratory work eventually went to duty as chair assistants (SSN 855). It is not known exactly how many graduates of Army schools became dental assistants because the final rating as technician or assistant was often made at the home station. In July 1945, 11,697 men, or 82.4 percent of a total of 14,191, were rated as SSN 855.[202] Since only 11,625 enlisted personnel attended the Army schools through fiscal 1945, and since the enlisted auxiliary personnel of the Dental Service numbered over 15,000 men at its maximum, we can assume that not more than two-thirds of the chair assistants had formal school training. The equivalent of a high school education and completion of basic military training were prerequisites for training as a dental assistant.

In January 1943, the Director of the Dental Division recommended approval of a request from Camp Pickett for 100 WAC personnel for duty as

---

[199] Information from the Strength Accounting Branch, AGO, given the author on 11 Dec 46.
[200] See footnote 9, p. 107.
[201] A report of the schooling of enlisted personnel, Medical Department, 1 Jul 39 to 30 Jun 44. *In* the history of training in the Army Service Forces for the period 1 Jul 39–30 Jun 44, vol IV, p. 109. HD: 314.7-2.
[202] See footnote 199, p. 158.

dental assistants, and at the same time recommended that women be used to replace male assistants in all large clinics.[203] The Surgeon General approved this request and forwarded it to the Director of the Women's Army Corps for action. In June 1943, The Surgeon General estimated, on information from the Dental Division, that 1,519 Wacs could be used in Army dental installations.[204] Training courses for Wac dental technicians were established at Army-Navy, Brooke, Fitzsimons, Wakeman, and William Beaumont General Hospitals and at Fort Huachuca, and a total of 473 female dental technicians, including 9 Negro Wacs, were trained from September 1943 to January 1946, most of these (335) at Wakeman General Hospital.[205] Three hundred and eight Wac assistants were on duty in January 1944. By June the number had increased to 462.[206] It is not known how many ultimately went to duty with the Dental Service but the figure was certainly far short of the 1,519 which it had been estimated could be used.[207]

The fact that wider utilization was not made of Wac dental assistants was due mainly to inability to obtain them. There were, however, certain disadvantages in using women for such work. Requirements for quarters were more difficult to meet, their sickness rate was higher, and they could not be assigned to some types of tactical units. Another objection to Wac assistants was that male clinic personnel had to assume additional work in connection with heavy clinic maintenance. In many places the Wacs scrubbed floors and worked on an almost equal basis with the men, but there was a feeling among the males that they were given additional work when a considerable number of women assistants were assigned to a clinic. On the other hand, the Wac assistants were not subject to the strict limitations on hours and type of work which applied to salaried civilian women assistants.

For some years civilian dental assistants had been used in a few large clinics. As enlisted assistants became harder to replace an effort was made to obtain a substantial number of civilians for this duty in fixed installations in the United States. In July 1942 The Surgeon General specified conditions under which female civilian assistants could be hired.[208] Civilian dental assistants were to be given the Civil Service grade of SP-3, paying $1,440 yearly. They were required to have a minimum of 6 years grade school education and at least 1 year of experience as a dental assistant. They provided their own uniforms. Civilian dental assistants were to conform to the rules of conduct prescribed for Army nurses. In January 1943 the additional grade of "Junior Dental

---

[203] Memo, Dir Dental Div, SGO, for General McAfee, 5 Jan 43, no sub. SG : 322.5 (Camp Pickett).
[204] Ltr, SG to CG, ASF, 2 Jun 43, sub : Technical training of WAAC personnel. SG : 322.5-1.
[205] See footnote 79, p. 126.
[206] Ltr, Capt Emily Gorman to Mr. Frank Rand, 11 Oct 44, no sub. SG : 221 (Technicians).
[207] It is extremely difficult to get information on the personnel on duty with the Dental Service during the war since all enlisted men and women were assigned only to the Medical Department; they were placed on specific duties by local surgeons and might be shifted on short notice. Strength returns from installations did not specify the services to which personnel were assigned.
[208] SG Ltr 75, 27 Jul 42.

Assistant," SP–2, paying $1,320 yearly, was established.[209] The position of Junior Dental Assistant was to be filled by persons with limited experience and was considered temporary until additional training had been completed in the dental clinic. By June 1944, 2,909 civilian dental assistants were on duty in the United States and 15 had been hired overseas. (None were sent overseas from the United States during the actual combat period.) Later figures are not available, but it is probable that the strength given for June 1944 represents about the maximum number on duty during the war as the percentage of the Army on duty overseas increased rapidly after this time and civilian assistants were not sent abroad.

The use of civilian assistants released a large number of men for other duties. In general, they were superior to enlisted men in the handling of patients and in the care of instruments and small equipment. On the other hand, they worked limited hours and were not available for emergencies. They could not be called upon to clean floors and do major maintenance work in the clinic, and the rate of absence was generally thought to be higher than for enlisted men, though there are no statistical data bearing on this matter. The use of both enlisted and civilian personnel in the same clinic sometimes resulted in friction as the women received twice as much pay for shorter hours. Also, unless janitor service was provided, the enlisted man was required, after the close of the day's operations, to clean not only his own operating room but also that of the civilian assistant. In general, the service rendered by civilian assistants justified their use, but best results were obtained when civilian and enlisted personnel in clinics were mixed as little as possible.

Dental Hygienists. Before the war civilian dental hygienists were on duty in only a few of the larger clinics. Training in this work was given enlisted men in the Army Dental School course and oral prophylactic treatments were generally given by enlisted men or by dental officers. With mobilization it was decided to make wider use of civilian hygienists and the conditions of employment were prescribed in July 1942.[210] The position of dental hygienist was rated as SP–4, and paid $1,620 yearly. The applicant was required to (1) be a graduate of a course of at least 2 years at a recognized school of oral hygiene, (2) have a license from a state or territory, and (3) have practiced 2 years in a clinic or office of a private dentist. In July 1943 this last requirement was waived.[211] The position of senior dental hygienist, SP–5, was authorized in clinics where five or more hygienists were on duty, or under certain other circumstances involving increased responsibility. The pay of a senior hygienist was $1,800 yearly. In January 1944, over 500 hygienists were on duty, a figure which was approximately the maximum during the war.[212] Soon after the declaration of war four civilian dental hygienists were

---

[209] SG Ltr 1, 1 Jan 43.
[210] See footnote 206, p. 159.
[211] SG Ltr 117, 1 Jul 43.
[212] See footnote 177, p. 153.

sent overseas with their organizations and they were allowed to remain until returned to the United States under routine, established policies. No additional female hygienists were permitted to leave the Zone of Interior, however, and their places were taken by enlisted men prior to embarkation.

The status of dental hygienists during the war was the cause of considerable dissatisfaction on the part of hygienists' organizations. Difficulty was first encountered when dental assistants were occasionally promoted to the grade of hygienist, SP–4. Such promotion was never authorized, but occurred with sufficient frequency to make necessary a specific prohibition against the practice in July 1943.[213] The Dental Division agreed with hygienists' organizations that, except for military personnel trained by the Army itself, the scaling and polishing of teeth should be limited to persons who had completed the prescribed course of instruction in authorized schools. With the inauguration of the Women's Army Corps, requests were made for the incorporation of dental hygienists as officers in that organization. This request was opposed by both the Medical Department and the Dental Division because of rigid regulations affecting the utilization of WAC personnel. These regulations provided that Wacs could not replace civilian employees and would replace male officers in the ratio of one Wac for one male officer. It was therefore feared that commissioning of hygienists in the WAC would entail the loss of an equal number of dental officers.[214]

Late in 1942 the Medical Department sponsored a bill (H. R. 3790, S. 839) to provide commissions for female dietitians and physiotherapists. This step was made necessary by difficulties encountered when organizations employing these essential civilians were shipped overseas. The Dental Division called attention to the fact that hygienists would probably remain a permanent part of the Army Dental Service and recommended that they also be included in the pending bill, but this recommendation was returned with the penciled notation "not now," signed by the executive officer of the Surgeon General's Office. Organizations representing the hygienists made a vigorous presentation of their cause in congressional committee hearings, however, and finally succeeded in having a clause incorporated authorizing the President to provide commissions for other "technical and professional female personnel in categories required for service outside the continental United States." [215] But since the bill did not specifically mention hygienists the Medical Department later held that their services were not required outside the United States and that it was not necessary to invoke the provisions of the bill in their interest.[216]

In July 1944, the Director of the Dental Division called attention to difficulties in obtaining dental hygienists and assistants and noted that the Army

---

[213] See footnote 211, p. 160.
[214] Ltr, Maj Gen Norman T. Kirk to Hon Harve Tibbott, 2 Sep 43. SG: 231 (Dental Hygienists).
[215] 56 Stat 1072.
[216] Ind, Brig Gen Larry B. McAfee to IAS to SG from TAG, 6 Apr 43, sub: Dental hygienists not included in Public Law 828, 77th Congress. SG: 231 (Dental Hygienists).

had no installations with five hygienists where the grade of SP–5 could be authorized.[217] He recommended creation of the position of "Senior Dental Assistant," SP–4, and a corresponding increase of rating for hygienists to SP–5 and SP–6, the latter to pay $2,000 yearly. At the end of the war no action had been taken on this recommendation. In September 1944 the Director of the Dental Division again recommended the establishment of a Hygienist's Corps, on the basis of 0.3 officers per 1,000 strength of the Army. He recommended that hygienists be limited to the grade of captain, unless dietitians and physiotherapists were to be granted higher grades, in which case it was recommended that hygienists be placed on an equal status. In 1945 he again recommended the commissioning of hygienists, but advised that only graduates holding a bachelor of science degree in oral hygiene be accepted.[218] No action had been taken in this direction at the end of the war. (In 1943 the Navy offered commissions in the WAVES to hygienists who were graduates of courses of at least 2 years. Hygienists with less than this minimum training were accepted as pharmacist's mates.)[219]

Informal Training, Auxiliary Personnel. One of the most important aspects of the training of auxiliary personnel was the daily informal instruction which such personnel received while performing their duties in dental installations. New men were placed on duty in operating clinics, learned their work under the supervision of dental officers, and in turn helped teach other men or were incorporated into cadres to form the nucleus of new organizations. This training was continuous during the war and accounted for the only instruction (other than basic training) that at least one-third of all dental enlisted men received.

Course on Care of Equipment. Early in 1942, a course of instruction in the care and minor repair of dental equipment was initiated by a large dental manufacturer. The course lasted 2 weeks and representatives of other manufacturers were invited to lecture on their particular products so that a wide coverage of the field was obtained. Approximately 180 enlisted assistants received this training.[220]

Summary, Auxiliary Personnel

Over 18,000 auxiliary personnel were used in the operation of the Dental Service by 15,000 dental officers. In wartime, dental officers should not waste their efforts in work which can be done by less specialized personnel, and considerably more than the above number of auxiliary assistants could have been used efficiently if they had been available. It has been estimated that the

---

[217] Memo, Maj Gen R. H. Mills for Pers Serv, SGO, 24 Jul 44. SG: 231 (Dental Hygienists). (This communication accompanies a memo to Col George Kennebeck from Brig Gen Rex McDowell (no subject), 16 Mar 45, same file.)

[218] See footnote 9, p. 107.

[219] Capt Robert S. Davis discusses problems of Navy Dental Corps. J. Am. Dent. A, 31:587–589, 15 Apr 44.

[220] Report of the Dental Division, SGO, for fiscal 1942. HD: 319.1–2.

services of a full-time dental assistant will increase the output of a dentist from 30 percent (U. S. Public Health Service) to 63 percent (U. S. Navy), but the wartime ratio of 1.2 auxiliary personnel per dental officer did not permit assignment of a full-time dental assistant to each officer after provision had been made for hygienists, x-ray technicians, clerical workers, and laboratory technicians.[221]

Shortage of manpower in time of war makes necessary the wide use of female auxiliary personnel, including civilians.

In a mobilization, competent laboratory technicians will not be available in sufficient numbers from among inducted men, and a program for their training must be anticipated. Every precaution must be taken to insure that inducted laboratory technicians are assigned to appropriate duties in the Army.

A course of 3-months duration is not adequate for the training of laboratory technicians, but will provide a sufficient basis for further "on-the-job" training in a dental laboratory.

It is evident that there was considerable waste effort involved in giving laboratory training to nearly 10,000 enlisted personnel when over 80 percent ultimately served as chair assistants. The whole period of training was not entirely wasted for this group, however, since the course included some work important to dental assistants as well as to the laboratory technician. There is also some need, especially in time of peace, for assistants who can "double in brass" to carry out minor laboratory procedures at smaller stations having no assigned technicians. But in the opinion of senior dental officers the training for chair assistants in a time of emergency could profitably be cut to 1 or 2 months and separated from that given prosthetic workers. During World War II it was necessary to send a large number of men to the technician's schools to obtain the few who could acquire the needed special skills, but aptitude tests developed during the latter part of that war should make it possible in the future to select candidates for laboratory training with a much higher degree of accuracy. When it can be predicted with fair certainty that students chosen for technician training will be able to complete the course successfully it will probably be more economical of time and effort to shorten the period of training for assistants and to eliminate from the already overcrowded laboratory course all instruction intended for them.

It was the general opinion of dental officers that the Dental Service exercised inadequate control of its enlisted auxiliary personnel. The most serious difficulties were:

1. Clinic personnel were under the direct command of the medical detachment commander, acting for the surgeon. They could be, and were, taken from their duties in the clinic for training or other nondental work. When such withdrawals were moderate in number and made on adequate notice, they were annoying but unavoidable. When they were made in large numbers on short

---

[221] Army-Navy Register, 21 Sep 46, p. 11.

notice they were disastrous in a service which had to schedule its work weeks ahead.

2. The fact that auxiliary personnel were not permanently assigned to the Dental Service was directly responsible for some inefficiency in operation. Months of training were required to qualify a competent dental assistant, and when a skilled man was transferred to other duties because he felt that life was easier in the surgery, or to increase his chance for promotion, both the Dental Service and the Army suffered.[222]

3. The fact that promotion of enlisted assistants was in the hands of medical officers was widely believed to have resulted to the disadvantage of dental auxiliary personnel. This belief is not wholly confirmed by comparison of the grades held by dental and medical enlisted men in the United States. Medical officers did have the authority to promote or demote dental personnel without consultation with the dental officers in charge of clinics, however, and though this action was rarely taken, the results, when it did happen, were inevitably detrimental to efficiency and morale.

The following changes were among those most commonly recommended by dental officers:

1. Permanent assignment of enlisted personnel to the Dental Service, with transfer only for significant reasons which would normally justify transfer between other corps of the Army.

2. Adequate provision for promotion of outstanding enlisted men within the Dental Service so that competent men could plan a career in that service without jeopardizing their chances of arriving at the higher grades.

3. Correction of the system whereby dental personnel were examined for promotion in purely medical subjects, in competition with men who had been engaged in medical activities in their daily work.[223]

---

[222] See footnote 9, p. 107.
[223] Ibid.

CHAPTER V

Dental Equipment and Supply[1]

EARLY SHORTAGES OF DENTAL SUPPLIES

The critical shortage of dental equipment and supplies was probably the most serious difficulty faced by the Dental Service during the first 2 years of mobilization. There is ample evidence of the extent of this shortage. The Committee to Study the Medical Department of the Army reported, about November 1942, that "there are serious deficiencies in certain critical items of equipment and supplies. Dental officers . . . have been handicapped by an appalling lack of certain materials and equipment." A survey of 199 Air Force stations in December 1942 revealed that only 26 were without serious shortages which ranged from instruments to chairs, units, x-ray machines, and field chests,[2] and the following reports were typical of many received in the Dental Division during the early part of the war:

> The July (1941) Report of Dental Service from Camp Davis, N. C., reveals the fact that for some time construction of both DC-1 and DC-2 dental clinics has been completed, and that only four handpieces, all of which were borrowed from other stations, were available. This means that at this station, where twenty dental officers are on duty with the station complement, the services of only four can be utilized in a professional capacity at one time. This situation has existed at Camp Davis for many months. . . .[3]
>
> The dental clinic No. 1 at Camp Livingston, La., has not been activated due to the lack of cabinets, sterilizers, handpieces, and lights. Requisition was made for these items in December 1940. (This report was made in October 1941.)

Overseas, where the shortages were further aggravated by delays and losses in shipping and by difficulties of storage and distribution, the situation was for a while even worse.[4] The dental surgeon of the European Theater of Operations (ETO) reported in November 1942 that 30 percent of the dental officers in England had no equipment.[5] In December 1942, 39 dental officers in the Middle East theater had a total of 6 field sets, 2 units and chairs, 1 incomplete laboratory, and a few miscellaneous items purchased locally.[6] In

---

[1] A general discussion of the organization and operation of the medical supply service has been written under the title, "The Procurement and Distribution of Medical Supplies in the Zone of the Interior during World War II," by Capt Richard E. Yates. This chapter deals only with aspects of the supply problem which were of particular concern to the Dental Service. HD.

[2] Memo, Col George R. Kennebeck for Brig Gen David N. W. Grant, 11 Jan 43. SG: 444.4-1.

[3] Memo, Brig Gen Leigh C. Fairbank for Finance and Supply Div, SGO, 29 Aug 41. SG: 444.4-1 (Camp Davis)C. (At the time of this report there were about 15,000 men at Camp Davis.)

[4] Medical supplies for Europe waited in the channel for as long as four months while high priority munitions were being unloaded. See History of the Dental Division, Headquarters, ETOUSA, 1 Sep-31 Dec 44. HD: 319.1-2 (ETO).

[5] Personal ltr, Col William D. White to Brig Gen Robert H. Mills, 2 Nov 42. HD: 730.

[6] Personal knowledge of the author who was dental surgeon of the Middle East theater in December 1942.

December 1942 the North African theater was short 37 percent of its authorized MD Chests No. 60.[7] [8] In January 1943 the Director of the Dental Division, SGO, stated: "We have no chests 60 at all, it seems, to issue to troops in this country." [9]

Serious deficiencies of supplies and equipment involved shortages of the following important items:

Burs. The War Production Board (WPB) reported in 1943 that stocks of dental burs in the hands of civilian dealers averaged only 33 percent of prewar levels, and that 88 percent of all dentists complained of difficulty in obtaining this essential item.[10] Total output in 1943 was estimated at 48 million, while total requirements were placed at over 93 million, of which 52 million were requested by the Armed Forces.[11] In spite of the fact that the Army was given only 15 million in 1943 instead of the 35 million requested, final allocations to the Armed Forces still totalled more than half of all production for the year.[12] As late as November 1944 WPB considered construction of a new bur factory at Government expense, though the project was dropped when it became apparent that low output was due more to the lack of materials and labor than to inadequate capacity.[13]

Heavy clinical equipment. Production of units, chairs, x-ray machines, and other large clinical items had naturally been small in peacetime since they could be classed as capital goods which required replacement only after many years of use. In 1940, civilian dentists purchased only about 2,000 units and 2,500 chairs.[14] In 1943, however, the Army alone required about 5,500 units and 5,000 chairs.[15] The production of individual companies manufacturing these items was increased from 50 to 300 percent [16] but capacity was severely strained. In April 1943, delivery of 1,697 units, of 8,359 contracted, caused certain manufacturers to be classed as "delinquent." [17]

Dental field chests. During the early part of the war many units were sent overseas without field dental equipment, or with chests which were incom-

---

[7] Ltr, Col Egbert W. V. Cowan to Chief Surg, NATOUSA, 13 Mar 43, sub: Dental needs in the Theater of Operations. On file as incl to pers ltr, Col William D. White to Brig Gen R. H. Mills, 7 Apr 43. HD: 730.

[8] Personal ltr, Brig Gen R. H. Mills to Col William D. White, 18 Jan 43. HD: 730.

[9] See this chapter, p. 180 for contents of M. D. Chest No. 60.

[10] Special problems discussed at War Service Committee meeting. J. Am. Dent. A. 31: 445–450, 15 Mar 44.

[11] Memo, Col Clifford V. Morgan, Chief of Materials Br, Production Div, SOS, for SG, 6 Jan 43, sub: Dental burs—production and requirements. SG: 444.4–1.

[12] Memo, Col F. R. Fenton, Resources and Production Div, SOS, for SG, 24 Feb 43, sub: Dental burs—proposed allotment. SG: 444.4–1.

[13] Ltr, Senator Harold Burton to Mr. Highland G. Batcheller, Vice Chairman of Operations, WPB, 10 Nov 44. SG: 444.4–1.

[14] Info, Medical and Health Supplies Section, Consumer Programs Branch, WPB, for Col C. F. Shook, 18 Sep 42. The original of this letter cannot be located. The source of the figures given was said to be the American Dental Trade Association.

[15] Ltr, Maj J. E. Rice to Chief, Reqmts Br, Resources and Production Div, Hq, ASF, 5 Apr 43, sub: Allocation of dental operating units and chairs. SG: 444.4–1.

[16] Annual Report of the Army Medical Procurement Office, fiscal 1944. HD: 319.1–2.

[17] Incl to memo, Lt Col C. G. Gruber for Chief, Health Supplies Section, Production Div, ASF, 10 Jun 43, sub: Report on dental supplies. SG: 444.4–1.

plete in essential items.[18] This particular deficiency was one of the most critical encountered since it was extremely difficult to make any informal arrangement for obtaining dental care in the areas first occupied by American troops.

Handpieces. The production of handpieces, especially of the contra-angle type, was such a specialized operation that expansion of facilities was slow and for many months output lagged behind wartime needs. In many otherwise fully equipped clinics the dental officers could perform only the operations possible with the simpler straight handpiece. At times, in early 1943, dental officers scattered over thousands of miles of desert in the Middle East theater had only a single contra-angle handpiece per dentist, and there was not one replacement in the theater.

These shortages resulted from a number of factors among which the following were most important:

1. The Armed Forces took nearly one-third of the Nation's active dentists. In addition to providing these men with complete outfits, adequate reserve stocks had to be assembled for future operations as the loss of dental supplies was inevitably high under combat conditions. (The dental surgeon of the ETO reported that 40 complete field outfits were lost while in shipment to his area.)[19]

2. The Supply Division, SGO, suffered from a lack of officers trained in dental supply. The director of that division stated in September 1942 that "The dental supply program has been materially retarded due to shortage of personnel capable of negotiating contracts for the Medical Department." [20] The Director of the Dental Division, SGO, noted that difficulties encountered had been "in part due to the inexperience of supply personnel in evaluating dental needs and requirements." [21]

3. Requirements for lend-lease aggravated shortages in some of the most critical items. Late in 1942 when units were being shipped without their dental field chests, the British Army was supplied with 200 of these scarce items under previous commitments.[22]

4. In peace, the United States had depended to a considerable extent on imports of dental items from European countries. For instance, American industry had produced only from 60[23] to 70 percent of the 33 million burs used each year prior to World War II. With the outbreak of hostilities these imports were immediately cut off not only to the United States, but to its allies and to South and Central America.

---

[18] Personal ltr, Col William D. White to Maj Gen Robert H. Mills, 22 Oct 43. HD: 730.

[19] See footnote 4, p. 165.

[20] 3d ind, Assistant Chief of the Supply Div, SGO, 19 Sep 42, on Ltr, Lt Col James P. Holliers. SG: 444.4–1.

[21] Final Report for ASF, Logistics in World War II. HD: 319.1–2 (Dental Division).

[22] Personal Ltr, Brig Gen R. H. Mills to Col William D. White, 28 Nov 42. HD: 730 (ETO).

[23] President J. Ben Robinson discusses personnel and supply problems arising out of the war. J. Am. Dent. A. 30: 163–166, 13 Jan 43.

5. High wartime wages swelled the demand of the civilian population for dental care which it had not received in the years of depression preceding World War II.

6. The threat of future shortages probably resulted in some hoarding of dental supplies. At a conference of dental manufacturers in September 1942 the representative of one firm noted that his company alone was under contract to provide 261,000 instruments for the Army, and he expressed doubt that such a number was actually required.[24] The Director of the Dental Division immediately pointed out the elimination of many dental items from the supply lists of the Army, and claimed, in turn, that the Navy had ordered as many burs as the Army though it had only one-fourth as many dentists.[25]

In December 1942 a representative of the Supply Division, SGO, claimed that large quantities of surplus burs were in the hands of the schools, supply houses, and the profession, and asked the Association of Dental Manufacturers of America to attempt to collect these for military use. The Association issued a bulletin to its dealers asking that customers be impressed with the need for turning in excess stocks as an alternative to a complete "freeze" on sales to civilians, but this action produced more criticism than burs. The president of the ADA protested vigorously, both at the supposed threat of a "freeze" on civilian sales, and at the implication that civilian dentists were guilty of what was delicately called "anticipatory buying."[26] The Supply Division, SGO, replied that it had never intended to hint that hoarding had occurred, and that its action had really been expected to impress the manufacturers with the need for intensive efforts to increase production.[27] In any event, the attempt to collect burs from civilian sources produced only about 2,100 packages, and the effort was soon dropped.[28]

It is difficult to deny, however, that hoarding of scarce supplies was practiced both by civilian and military users. The chairman of the Medical Supplies Commission, Army and Navy Munitions Board, reported that civilian purchases of burs in 1941 had been 70 percent higher than in any previous year, in spite of the number of dentists and patients in the Armed Forces.[29] In 1943 total requirements for burs were placed at nearly 94 million, compared with an average prewar demand for about 33 million burs. The Army, alone, asked for over 35 million burs in that year, or more than the normal total peacetime requirement, and combined requests of the Armed Forces totalled 52 million burs.[30] The clashes reported above, between the Army, Navy, civilian practi-

---

[24] Memo, Col C. F. Shook for Col F. C. Tyng, 3 Sep 42. HD: 444.4–1 (Dental).
[25] 2d ind, Dir. Dental Div, to Memo cited in footnote 24, 16 Sep 42. HD: 444.4–1 (Dental).
[26] (1) Ltr, Dr. J. Ben Robinson to Col F. C. Tyng, 29 Dec 42. SG: 444.4–1. (2) See footnote 23, p. 167.
[27] Ltr, Col F. C. Tyng to Dr. J. Ben Robinson, 10 Jan 43. SG: 444.4–1.
[28] Ltr, Dental Manufacturers of America to Col F. C. Tyng, 29 Jan 43. SG: 444.4–1.
[29] Ltr, Lt Col C. F. Shook to Hon Leslie C. Arends, 23 Jan 42. SG: 444.4–1.
[30] Info memo, Safety and Technical Equipment Division, Health Supplies Committee, WPB, 5 Jan 43. SG: 444.4–1.

tioners, and the manufacturers, are significant mainly because they show that users tend to overestimate their needs when supplies are uncertain, and because they indicate the need for disinterested control of distribution when production is inadequate to meet all demands.

In the final analysis, wartime shortage of dental supplies was due primarily to increased demand rather than to defects in production. In spite of the difficulties noted in obtaining labor and materials, the output of dental items soon exceeded peacetime rates. The manufacture of burs, for instance, tripled between 1937 and 1944.[31] A representative of The Surgeon General stated that wartime production of dental supplies reached 3½ times normal peacetime levels.[32] It is apparent that in time of war the production of dental supplies for civilian needs can be reduced very little if at all, and that any reduction in the output for civilians will be more than balanced by the increased demands of the Armed Forces.

ACTION TAKEN TO IMPROVE THE DENTAL SUPPLY SITUATION

Improvement in the dental supply situation depended mainly on an increase in civilian production, and this phase of the problem was largely out of the hands of the Dental Division. The latter did cooperate, however, in a number of steps to assure the most effective use of the available stocks and raw materials, of which the following were the most important:

Simplification of Dental Items

Early in the war the Armed Forces, governmental agencies, manufacturers, and the civilian profession cooperated to reduce the number of types, and to simplify the design, of many items produced for dental use. As early as February 1942 the Dental Division had voluntarily suggested that for the duration of the war 81 items, including 33 sizes of burs, be dropped from Army supply tables. A total of 134 items were eventually recommended to be dropped, and most were actually removed from the tables. The requisition of nonstandard items was also discouraged.[33]

In June 1942 WPB issued a "general limitation order" restricting the production of dental burs to 42 of the most used sizes.[34] In November 1942 delegates from the Armed Forces, the ADA, the American Dental Trade Association, and WPB, agreed on methods for simplifying other dental items, particularly chairs and units.[35] Wood and plastics were to be substituted for metals

---

[31] See footnote 10, p. 166.
[32] Testimony, Maj Gen George F. Lull before the Senate Subcommittee on Wartime Health and Education. *In* Hearings before a Subcommittee of the Committee on Education and Labor, United States Senate, Seventy-eighth Congress. Washington, Government Printing Office, 1944, pt 5, p. 1672.
[33] SG Ltr 2, 8 Jan 42.
[34] WPB General Limitation Order 139, Schedule 1, pt 1254. *In* Federal Register, 26 Jun 42.
[35] Memo, Col C. F. Shook for Col F. C. Tyng, 26 Nov 42, sub: Dental Equipment Advisory Committee for the WPB. SG ˆ34.8–1.

wherever possible, and the production of units was to be limited to the smaller, simpler types similar to the Ritter "Tri-dent." These units provided only the basic essentials: a dental engine, cuspidor, bracket table, warm water syringe, hot and cold compressed air, and operating light. The amount of brass and copper used was to be drastically reduced.

With the aid of a committee appointed by the ADA, and with the advice of all interested parties, the Bureau of Standards also drew up "simplified practice recommendations" aimed at eliminating minor and nonessential variations of standard articles. Steps recommended by this agency, such as the reduction in the number of sizes and types of hypodermic needles produced, were generally accepted voluntarily by manufacturers, though had they not it would have been possible to enforce them through WPB's control over the allocation of materials.

Improved Distribution of Dental Supplies

In the early part of the war supply officers with experience in handling dental items were scarce, resulting in occasional poor distribution of even the minimum stocks then available. An especially frequent defect was failure to balance the equipment sent to each station; one post might receive all its units and no chairs, while another received all its chairs and no units. Angle handpieces were furnished which did not fit the particular straight handpieces issued. To improve this situation the Director of the Dental Division recommended in March 1941 that a dental officer be assigned to the Supply Division, SGO.[36] Such an assignment was actually made in November 1942, but it was terminated in March 1943. Subsequent improvements in the allocation of dental supplies resulted mainly from the increasing experience of medical supply officers.

In July 1941 The Surgeon General directed that stations with excess stocks of dental items would report them for redistribution where more urgently needed.[37] Stations were also directed to turn in any handpieces in excess of one per operator, plus a 25 percent station reserve.[38]

In January 1943 WPB issued a general limitation order controlling the production and sale of dental units, chairs, x-ray machines, and sterilizers,[39] and governmental agencies were thereafter given first priority in the purchase of such items. Stocks of new equipment already in the hands of jobbers and dealers had to be reported, and 54 chairs and 109 units were obtained for the Army from this source.[40]

The storage and issue of porcelain teeth, involving hundreds of molds, sizes, and shades, offered considerable difficulty in most supply depots. In

---
[36] Memo, Brig Gen Leigh C. Fairbank for Supply Div, SGO, 17 Mar 41. SG: 210.31.
[37] SG Ltr 75, 25 Jul 41.
[38] SG Ltr 83, 25 Aug 41.
[39] WPB General Limitation Order L-249, pt 3172, 20 Jan 43. In Federal Register, 21 Jan 43.
[40] Ltr, Maj Robert E. Hammersberg to Purchase Div, Army Medical Procurement Office, 26 Feb 43. SG: 444.4-1.

March 1944 each base medical depot was authorized two dental prosthetic clerks who were qualified to handle artificial teeth.[41] [42] In England, teeth were first stocked in 18 separate depots for convenience in distribution, but without skilled personnel the supply soon became badly mixed. Also, since each depot could keep only a small stock, the supply of any individual mold might run out quickly, necessitating a canvas of other depots to locate additional quantities. To eliminate these difficulties a single depot was finally designated to handle all procelain teeth, and an expert was brought from the United States to supervise their distribution.

It has already been noted that in the early part of the war units were shipped overseas without their authorized dental field chests. This situation was due primarily to the serious shortage of this item, but it was aggravated by the policy of shipping personnel and equipment on different transports, in the mistaken belief that if the equipment failed to arrive promptly the dentists could readily draw new chests from theater supplies. This difficulty had been encountered in the First World War, and a dental officer was finally assigned to the New York Port of Embarkation with specific instructions to make sure that no dentist left the United States without his dental equipment.[43] Similar action was taken in November 1942,[44] but improvement in this situation was slow until overseas depots were finally stocked with dental field outfits which could be issued promptly on arrival. The difficulties encountered in both World Wars indicate that every effort should be made to have dental equipment accompany dental officers as part of their personal baggage.

Purchase of Used Equipment

During the period when supply shortages were most acute The Surgeon General was deluged with proposals that he purchase used dental equipment for Army clinics. In particular, large numbers of dental officers who were paying for items lying idle in storage, and who noted the scarcity of these same items at the stations where they reported for duty, urged that the Army solve both problems by purchasing or leasing such equipment. Widows of dentists, and finance companies, were also eager to unload dental outfits for which the market was poor at a time when dentists were entering the military service in large numbers. Late in 1942 WPB made a preliminary investigation which indicated that some 11,000 each, chairs and units, could be obtained from dentists entering the Army or Navy; and on the basis of this information it even recommended, for a while, a complete suspension of the manufacture of the

---

[41] For training given enlisted men to qualify them as prosthetic supply clerks, see ch IV, p. 158.
[42] T/O & E 8–187, C 1, 24 Mar 44.
[43] The Medical Department of the United States Army in the World War. Washington, Government Printing Office, 1928, vol III, p. 624 (cited hereafter as The Medical Department . . . in the World War.)
[44] See footnote 22, p. 167.

larger dental items during the war.[45] In January 1943 ASF also urged all its agencies to make maximum use of secondhand equipment.[46]

Superficially, the proposal to purchase the equipment of dentists entering the service appeared to have considerable merit. The attitude of The Surgeon General, however, was one of caution, typically expressed by Brig. Gen. C. C. Hillman, assistant to The Surgeon General, in September 1942:

> It appears to this office that medical and surgical supplies now in the possession of civilian physicians might better be used to continue the care of the civilian population than to be acquired for the Army. For military use a certain degree of standardization is essential. You can well imagine the difficulties that the Medical Supply Division would encounter if they attempted to gather up generally supplies and instruments from civilian physicians and with them supply our military hospitals.[47]

A later statement by Col. C. F. Shook was even more specific:

> It is possible that dental units may be acquired in this manner, but the number is questionable. The plan is an Utopian plan, but it would require more personnel than The Surgeon General's Office has at its disposal, and in many instances [it] would rob professional schools and recent graduates of the equipment they need in their profession.[48]

Under pressure of the great need for dental equipment, however, The Surgeon General did make an effort, beginning in the fall of 1942, to acquire secondhand items. In October 1942 he reported that where suitable used equipment was found it was being purchased,[49] though such procurement was certainly on a small scale, apparently by local supply officers.[50] On 30 October 1942 questionnaires were sent to 3,000 new dental officers, asking if they owned suitable equipment, and if they would sell it to the Army at a suggested price of original cost, less 5 percent for each year of use. (Instruments were not to cost over 80 percent of original price.)[51] Of the 3,000 officers questioned, only 496 were willing to sell any equipment. Of this latter number, only 184 had items which the Army considered suitable. The remaining equipment was old, was manufactured by firms which had gone out of business, or was otherwise undesirable. It appeared that men with modern outfits were not anxious to sell. The equipment offered was also scattered over 41 states, so that a con-

---

[45] Ltr, WPB to Col C. F. Shook, 18 Sep 42. SG: 444.4-1.

[46] Memo, Maj Gen Lucius D. Clay for Chiefs of Supply Services, SOS, 25 Jan 43, sub: Used equipment and supplies in the hands of jobbers, dealers, and users. SG: 400.139-1 (St. Louis Medical Procurement District) M.

[47] Ltr, Brig Gen C. C. Hillman to editor, Journal of the American Medical Association, 7 Sep 42. SG: 400.139-1.

[48] 2d ind, Col C. F. Shook, on ltr 16 Sep 42, to SG from the surgeon, Camp Adair, Oregon, 1 Oct 42. SG: 440.1 (Camp Adair) C.

[49] Ltr, Col C. F. Shook to Mrs. Edna Francis, 29 Oct 42. SG: .400.139-1.

[50] Formal authority to purchase used dental equipment without the usual advertising for bids was not granted until January 1943. See Ltr, Col M. E. Griffin to CO, New York Medical Department Procurement District, 21 Jan 43, sub: Purchase of second-hand dental equipment from dentists in the Army. SG: 400.139-1 (St. Louis Medical Department Procurement District) M. This requirement appears to have been ignored by local purchasing agents, however.

[51] Ltr, SG to all newly commissioned officers, 30 Oct 42, sub: Acquirement of dental equipment. SG: 444.4-1.

siderable administrative organization would have been required to inspect it and advise on acceptance or rejection.

In spite of these unfavorable developments The Surgeon General directed medical depots, on 12 February 1943, to purchase used items when such action seemed justified by sound business judgment.[52] Results were poor, however, and in April 1943 The Surgeon General reported that the amount of equipment being obtained did not justify further expenditure of time by military personnel. He stated further that the replies to his questionnaire were being turned over to WPB for use in its program of procurement for civilian needs. WPB, in turn, followed up 100 offers as a test, and quickly decided to abandon the whole project, leaving the purchase and resale of used equipment to established dealers.[53] The Army-Navy Medical Procurement Office reported that only 45 used chairs and 25 units were purchased by medical depots in 1943, and all of these were obtained from dealers.[54] It is probable that a few secondhand outfits were purchased locally, by medical supply officers of camps or hospitals, but the number was certainly small, and played a very minor part in meeting total requirements. By September 1943 all prospective sellers were being referred to civilian agencies.

WPB sponsored a voluntary collection of instruments, as a test, in the vicinity of St. Louis in October 1942, but the drive netted more scrap than useable supplies.[55]

Some of the causes for failure of the used equipment program were the following:

1. Dental officers were reluctant to sell equipment without ironclad guarantees that they would be able to purchase the same or corresponding items at the end of the war. However, World War I experience had shown that excess dental items had not been available for sale until 2 years after demobilization and the Army was therefore in no position to give prospective sellers the assurance they required.

2. Much of the newer equipment offered was encumbered with liens which so complicated purchase that the Legal Division, SGO, advised against any attempt to procure such items.[56]

3. The attempt to use miscellaneous types of secondhand equipment involved serious problems of maintenance. Isolated posts could not conveniently obtain the parts needed for the repair of older items which might break down in use.

---

[52] Ltr, SG to COs of all medical depots, 12 Feb 43, sub: Procurement by depots—purchase used equipment. HD: 314 (Code R-3).

[53] See footnote 30, p. 168.

[54] 1st ind, Col M. E. Griffin, 3 Jun 46, on ltr, Brig Gen Thomas L. Smith to Army-Navy Medical Procurement Office, 24 May 46, sub: Purchase of dental units and chairs. SG: 444.4-1.

[55] Ltr, CO, St. Louis Medical Procurement District, to SG, 23 Oct 42. SG: 400.139-1 (St. Louis Medical Procurement District) M.

[56] Memo, Legal Div, SGO, for Col C. F. Shook, 1 Feb 43, sub: Purchase from Army officer of secondhand dental chairs and equipment subject to liens. SG: 400.139-1.

4. Inspection of items offered for sale involved long trips by dental officers, and only a small proportion of the outfits offered proved suitable for purchase.

5. Used equipment was actually more expensive to the Government than new. One officer inspecting an outfit in New York reported that the price was reasonable by retail standards, but that the old chair would cost more than the Army regularly paid for a new one, and that the small unit would cost more than the quantity price for a new senior unit.[57] Equipment was often offered to the Army only because it was hoped that an even better price would be obtained than in what soon became an inflated civilian market. Also, the depots could not issue used items until they had been reconditioned, and such reconditioning, with transportation charges, often cost almost as much as new equipment.[58]

6. With the productive capacity of manufacturers strained to the limit to meet military needs it was felt that the purchase of used equipment by the Army would result in a critical shortage of items urgently needed by civilian dentists. It was believed, further, that the sale, maintenance, and repair of miscellaneous used equipment could better be handled by established dealers than by the Armed Forces, and that such nonstandard items were better suited to civilian needs, especially after the WPB stopped production of new equipment for civilian use in January 1943.

The easing of the supply situation in 1943 permitted the Medical Department to withdraw from a program which had originally been undertaken, as an emergency measure, with strong misgivings.

Local Procurement of Dental Supplies

World War I attempts to obtain dental supplies by local purchase had not been encouraging. The American Expeditionary Forces contracted for some French equipment in 1918, but the French Government was soon forced to limit sales to items totaling not over 1,000 francs per month to prevent a threatened exhaustion of the civilian market. A considerable amount of laboratory supplies was then purchased in London, but the British War Office quickly prohibited further procurement from that source.[59] It was apparent that local markets, geared to peacetime needs, could not furnish any significant proportion of the supplies needed by a major force.

In World War II, medical supply officers in the Zone of Interior were authorized to make emergency purchases of small items not obtainable from medical supply depots, and this privilege was sometimes extended to include dental units or chairs. The amount of material obtained by such means was not an important factor in the overall supply situation in the United States.

---

[57] Ltr, Lt Col H. T. Marshall to SG, 14 Jan 43, sub: Purchase of secondhand dental equipment. SG: 400.139–1.

[58] Ltr, Brig Gen R. H. Mills to Dr. McCarthy, 29 Sep 42. SG: 444.4–1.

[59] The Medical Department . . . in the World War (1927), vol II, p. 115.

In overseas areas local purchase was restricted only by the need and by the availability of stocks, and local procurement played a more important part in supplying equipment required to establish initial dental installations. Cabinets, lathes, cuspidors, and angle handpieces were obtained in Australia; burs, porcelain teeth, and acrylic resin in Palestine, and general dental supplies through reverse lend-lease in England. The Chief Surgeon of the European theater claimed that all the dental burs needed by the United States forces in England in 1944 could be obtained through local purchase.[60] The British Army also loaned field chests to the United States Army units arriving in the Middle East without dental equipment in 1942 and 1943. Supplies procured abroad were important at a time when equipment was not plentiful, but in general they did not go far to meet the total needs of the United States forces overseas. Production in the less industrialized nations was often negligible, and stocks on hand were quickly reduced to a point where civilian dental care was threatened. In Cairo, for instance, a single representative of a United States aircraft plant practically cleaned the shelves of the few dental supply houses, and acrylic resin disappeared into the black market for the remainder of the war, where it sold for approximately $20 a unit.[61] Except in those rare instances where a highly industrialized nation could assume full responsibility for supplying one or more items, local procurement was little more than an expensive and ineffective measure to meet emergency needs pending arrival of standard Army supplies.

Measures to Insure the Maximum Use of Available Items

In April 1942 Brigadier General Huebner, AGF inspector for training, reported that large numbers of men in the field were unable to chew the Army ration because of dental defects.[62] Since deficiencies in dental treatment at that time were due mainly to lack of supplies, the Director of the Dental Division, SGO, was forced to take radical action to insure full use of the limited equipment then available. He recommended that outfits in critical locations, especially in replacement training centers, be used for from 15 to 24 hours a day, by the employment of 2 or 3 shifts of dental officers.[63] It is not known exactly how many dental officers were used on night shifts during this period, but 916 additional dentists were requested at the time the system was initiated, and it is believed that most of this number were so used, at least temporarily. The use of double shifts could only be regarded as an emergency measure, however. The output of dental officers at night was less than during daylight hours, the proportion of broken appointments was nearly doubled,[64] and patients were

---

[60] Cable, Brig Gen Hawley to SG, 26 Oct 43. SG : 444.4-1.
[61] See footnote 6, p. 165.
[62] Memo, Dir, Mil Pers, SOS, for SG, 27 Apr 42, sub: Dental supplies in the field. SPGAP/10282-14 (G-1).
[63] Memo, Brig Gen R. H. Mills for Exec Off, SGO, 27 Apr 42. SG : 703.1.
[64] Annual Report of the Medical Service, Camp Claiborne, La., 1944. HD : 319.1.

tired and hard to handle after a full day's work. It was also difficult to arrange meals and transportation for both dentists and patients at irregular hours. The operation of multiple shifts did accomplish its primary purpose, which was to increase the total amount of work completed in the face of a crippling shortage of supplies.

In the field the contents of a single M. D. Chest No. 60 were often divided so that two officers could utilize one set of equipment. One officer might devote his time to operative procedures while the other handled extractions, gingival diseases, and emergencies. The multiple shift system was also used to a limited degree in some theaters until adequate supplies arrived.[65]

Conservation of Scarce Supplies

Every effort was made to conserve critical items during the war. After December 1942, dull burs were saved and returned to depots for resharpening under contracts with civilian firms.[66] Wax was collected, sterilized, and reused in the larger laboratories, and scrap amalgam returned to depots for recovery of the mercury and silver content. Items of rubber, brass, lead, tin, or other scarce materials were saved for salvage.

In 1942 about 180 enlisted men were sent to dental manufacturing plants for intensive 2-week courses in the maintenance and minor repair of dental equipment.[67]

In September 1944 The Surgeon General published a technical manual covering the care, lubrication, and repair of dental handpieces.[68]

The repair of unserviceable handpieces was undertaken on a large scale. At first it was anticipated that manufacturers would assume responsibility for the reconstruction of their products, but they proved reluctant to use their overburdened facilities for this purpose and the medical supply service had to take over the program. Two shops equipped to rebuild handpieces were established in the United States in 1944 but shortages of equipment and personnel hampered early operations so that only 3,500 handpieces were returned to service that year. By early 1945, however, most of the previous difficulties had been overcome and in February these shops together reconstructed a total of 2,500 handpieces. Since only about 700 handpieces were received for repair each month this capacity permitted a rapid reduction of the large backlog of defective handpieces which had accumulated over the past months.[69]

---

[65] In the Middle East theater and in England, RAF dentists sometimes used their outfits in the mornings and early afternoons, lending them during the late afternoons and evenings to U. S. Army Air Force dentists stationed nearby.

[66] SG Ltr 176, 8 Dec 42.

[67] Report of the Dental Division, SGO, for fiscal 1942. HD: 319.1-2.

[68] TM 8-638, 23 Sep 44.

[69] The problem of the repair of dental handpieces. Bulletin of the U. S. Army Medical Department, 89: 25 June 1945.

Substitution of Critical Items

The Army, like the civilian profession, made wide use of substitutes for critical items of dental supply. Acrylic resin was substituted for vulcanite, though this inevitable change was only hastened by the shortage of rubber. The alginates were used in impression materials in place of scarce agar compounds. Various substitutes for tinfoil were evolved. An attempt to use silver in place of nickel for plating instruments was unsuccessful, however, as the coating tended to pit and was subject to attack by mercury particles. Very early in the war diamond points were made available, to conserve dental burs. Items of copper were almost eliminated from dental supply tables. In general, no item made of critical materials was purchased for the Dental Service unless diligent research failed to reveal any acceptable substitute.

PACKING AND SHIPPING DENTAL SUPPLIES

General principles for the packing and shipping of dental supplies were no different from those for other items, and the handling of dental material offered few unique problems. Early in the war considerable breakage of heavy equipment, especially of dental x-ray machines, was reported, but this situation was remedied as the depots gained experience in preparing medical items for shipment under wartime conditions.[70] The handling of gold offered some difficulties. It was found that unless such materiel was placed in the custody of a responsible ship's officer, to be delivered only to an authorized agent on arrival, it was often "misplaced" either en route or at the docks were it was unloaded.[71]

EFFECTS OF CLIMATE ON DENTAL SUPPLIES

Considering the wide variations of climate encountered by the United States troops it is surprising that complaints of damage from extremes of temperature were relatively few. Cements, especially the silicate cements, set so rapidly in the hotter areas that their manipulation offered some difficulty; when the humidity was high it was impossible to cool glass slabs to the desired 70 degrees without precipitation of moisture. In the tropics the softer brands of waxes and impression compounds proved unsatisfactory, but materials specifically designed for use in such areas gave no trouble. Anesthetic solutions and x-ray film deteriorated rapidly when they could not be stored in cool locations, necessitating care to use oldest stocks first and to avoid accumulating quantities which could not be utilized in a reasonable time.[72] Small

---

[70] For additional data on packing problems see annual reports of the Supply Division, SGO, for fiscal years 1943 and 1944. HD: 319.1–2.

[71] Personal Ltr, Dental Surgeon of the China-Burma-India theater, to Maj Gen R. H. Mills, 1 Jul 44. This letter has been seen by the author but it was not made a permanent record.

[72] See Essential Technical Medical Data Reports for China-Burma-India theater, 1943 and 1944. HD: 350.05.

carpules (ampules) of anesthetic solution were reported to be undamaged by freezing in the Arctic, though later investigations indicated that the rubber plugs sealing such carpules might be pushed out by exposure to extreme cold.[73] In general, standard items on the supply tables proved satisfactory under any conditions where dental treatment was practicable.

ZONE OF INTERIOR AND COMMUNICATIONS ZONE EQUIPMENT

Prior to World War I it was planned that in a mobilization only portable equipment would be issued to dental officers, in the Zone of Interior as well as overseas. By the fall of 1917, however, it was apparent that this policy was not economical because dental officers could not operate as effectively with equipment which had been designed primarily for portability as with the more convenient chairs and units used routinely in civilian offices. Standard chairs, wall-bracket engines, cabinets, instruments, and laboratory equipment were therefore issued to all Zone of Interior training camps and to base and general hospitals (fig. 4).[74] Teams of 10 dentists, with base equipment, were also organized for use in favorable locations overseas.

Prior to World War II it was recognized that field units would require outfits which were easily portable and could be used well forward in the combat zone; on the other hand, it was clear that dentists outside the combat area should not be required to use equipment designed to be set up in a tent or dugout. It was therefore planned to provide standard base items in the Zone of Interior and in fixed and semifixed installations in the communications zone. (For establishments in that zone, it was expected that minor modifications, such as substitution of a mobile engine and cuspidor for the dental unit, could be effective.) This policy was actually carried out in the Zone of Interior, where dentists generally worked with equipment similar to that in their own offices. Zone of Interior camps and hospitals had units, chairs, cabinets, operating lights, x-ray machines, air compressors, and instruments which met normal civilian standards for convenience and reliability.[75] In the summer of 1942, however, lack of shipping space became so acute that drastic restrictions were placed on equipment for overseas use.[76] The large hospitals and dispensaries of the communications zone were thereafter allowed only the dental field chests, augmented with essential laboratory and surgical tools and equipment,[77] though many installations were later able to obtain captured base outfits or to purchase chairs and engines locally.

---

[73] Ltr, Dr. J. Edward Gilda to Maj Ernest Fedor, 21 Jul 47. This letter was seen by the author but not entered in permanent files.
[74] See footnote 43, p. 171.
[75] U. S. Army Medical Department Supply Catalog, 1942.
[76] Personal Ltr, Brig Gen R. H. Mills to Lt Col Richard F. Thompson, 18 Jul 42. HD: 730.
[77] Memo, Brig Gen R. H. Mills for chm, Medical Department Supply and Equipment Board, SGO, 25 Sep 43. SG: 444.4-1.

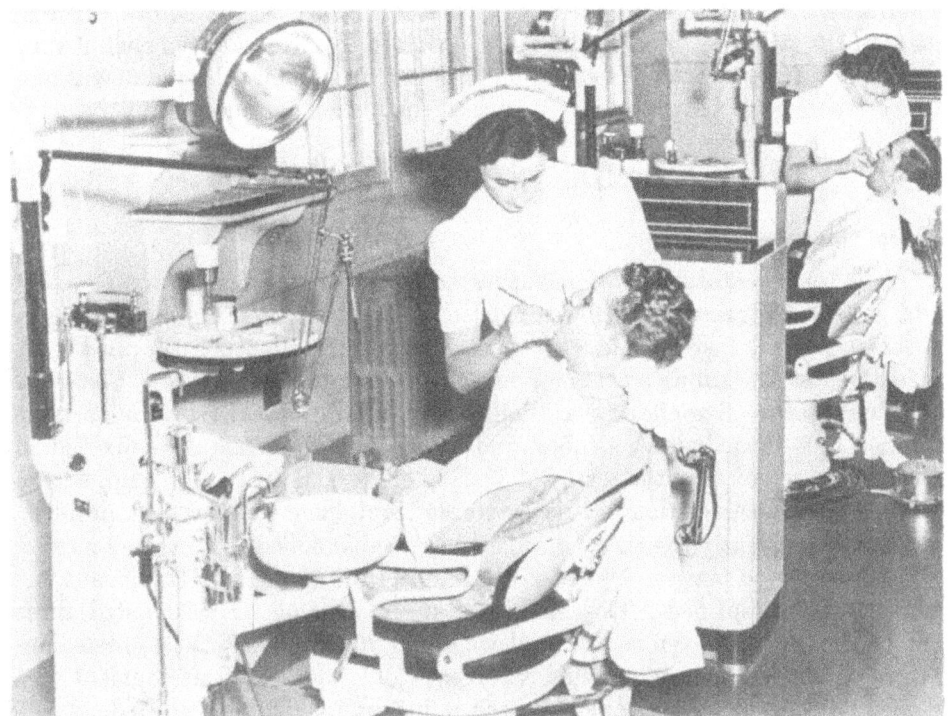

Figure 4. Zone of Interior dental equipment.

The primitive character of the communications zone equipment was soon the target of much unfavorable comment. The Chief Surgeon of the European theater asked that hospitals and general dispensaries in his area be given at least a minimum of base equipment.[78] Another senior medical officer, returning from an overseas inspection trip in November 1943, reported that "Field observations and the opinions of qualified dental officers in the Southwest Pacific Area indicate the need for revision of equipment lists for fixed installations to provide electric engines (portable), wall-bracket operating lamps, and portable cuspidors, small type. It is recommended that the Dental Division be consulted with reference to this matter." [79] The Dental Division had already requested reconsideration of the restricting order in September 1943, but the recommendation had been disapproved. A new request for authority to ship mobile dental engines, operating lights, and cuspidors overseas was now made, and this time approval was granted.[80] Until then the

---

[78] Ltr, Capt F. J. Reynolds, Overseas Supply Div, NYPOE, to SG, 2 Nov 42, sub: Dental equipment. SG: 444.4–1.

[79] Report of Col William Wilson on inspection trip to the Southwest Pacific theater. Quoted in: Memorandum to the chairman, Medical Department Supply and Equipment Board from Maj Gen R. H. Mills, 2 Nov 43. SG: 444.4–1.

[80] Ltr, Capt M. H. Kannal to Overseas Supply Officer, NYPOE, 13 Nov 43, sub: Dental equipment. SG: 444.4–1.

small amount of base equipment which had arrived overseas before enforcement of the embargo, or which had been obtained locally, had been spread very thin, over a few important installations. Fixed and semifixed units now began to receive items which materially increased their efficiency and output.

DENTAL FIELD EQUIPMENT

Dental Operating Chests

The basic dental field equipment issued in the First World War was bulky and difficult to transport. It was packed in six chests, containing an engine, a chair, a desk, instruments (two chests), and miscellaneous supplies.[81] A seventh chest containing a cuspidor was added in September 1917.[82] For overseas use another five chests were added, containing an oil stove, a portable table, a box of medicines, alcohol, and additional supplies. As delivered in France the complete outfit occupied 39.28 cubic feet of space and weighed 775 pounds.[83] Transportation of this "portable" equipment was always a problem, and not infrequently the entire outfit had to be abandoned in a hurried move.[84]

In the period between World Wars I and II the dental field equipment was considerably simplified. The Medical Supply Catalog of 1928 listed three chests, occupying 8.7 cubic feet, and weighing 209 pounds.[85] The chests contained a foot-engine, chair, and instruments and supplies. Development of a dental field outfit which could be packed in a single, standard, Medical Department chest had been going on at the same time, however, and this same 1928 catalog listed, for the first time, the new M. D. Chest No. 60, which was essentially the item used during World War II. (Figs. 5 and 6.)

The M. D. Chest No. 60 occupied 5 cubic feet, and weighed from 157 to 187 pounds, depending upon variations in the constituent items.[86] Total cost was approximately $305. This chest contained a wood, aluminum, or steel folding chair, a foot-engine, an alcohol sterilizer, and routine operative and surgical instruments and supplies to a total of about 160 different items. It contained no prosthetic equipment as such supplies were packed in other chests not available to the smaller units. Issued to the dental officers of each tactical command allocated dental facilities, it provided the minimum equipment

---

[81] Manual for the Medical Department, 1916, Washington, Government Printing Office, 1916 (cited hereafter as Manual . . . Medical Department).

[82] Manual . . . Medical Department, C dated 29 Sep 17.

[83] See footnote 43, p. 171.

[84] The Annual Report of The Surgeon General for 1919 states that "The transportation of dental equipment and supplies has ever been a source of irritation to division commanders, transportation officers, and division surgeons. . . . Much loss of equipment and consequent loss of dental service in several divisions has resulted thereby. The First Division, moving into combat area in May 1918, was forced to abandon their entire dental equipment through lack of transportation facilities. . . . At that time it required the entire resources of our Medical Supply Depot No. 3 to resupply emergency equipment for this division after its arrival in the new area." *In* Annual Report of The Surgeon General, U. S. Army, 1919, vol II, Washington, Government Printing Office, 1920.

[85] AR 40–1710, 23 Apr 28.

[86] See footnote 75, p. 178.

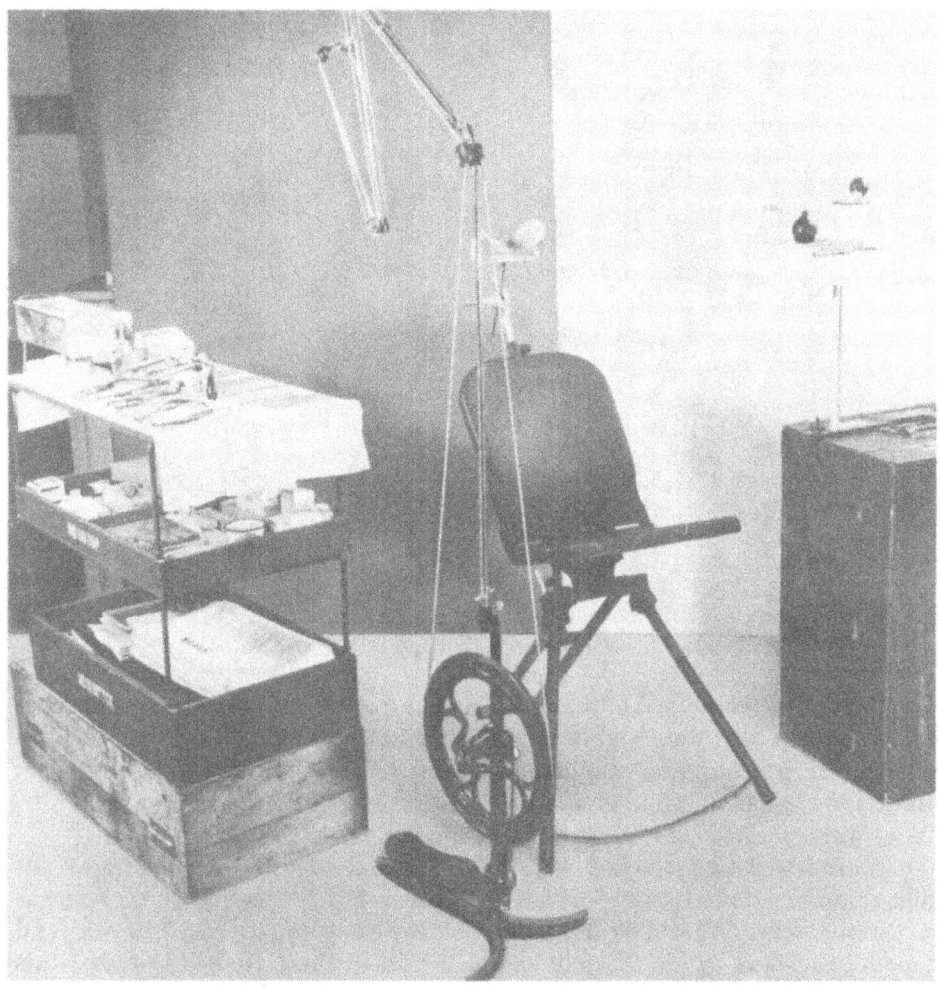

Figure 5. Dental field operating equipment, M. D. Chest No. 60, 1941.

needed for operation of a dental service where mobility was essential. When restrictions were placed on the shipment of more elaborate outfits overseas, Chest 60, augmented, was also supplied to general and station hospitals and general dispensaries of the communications zone. It lacked many of the refinements which made for convenience in operation, but contained the basic elements needed to meet routine needs in the combat zone. Patients requiring major oral surgery or prosthetic replacements had to be sent to more fully equipped installations, such as hospitals or mobile prosthetic teams.

Thousands of dentists who had always enjoyed every convenience in their civilian offices soon found themselves operating with dental field chests on tropical islands or at the edge of arctic glaciers. It is not surprising that their

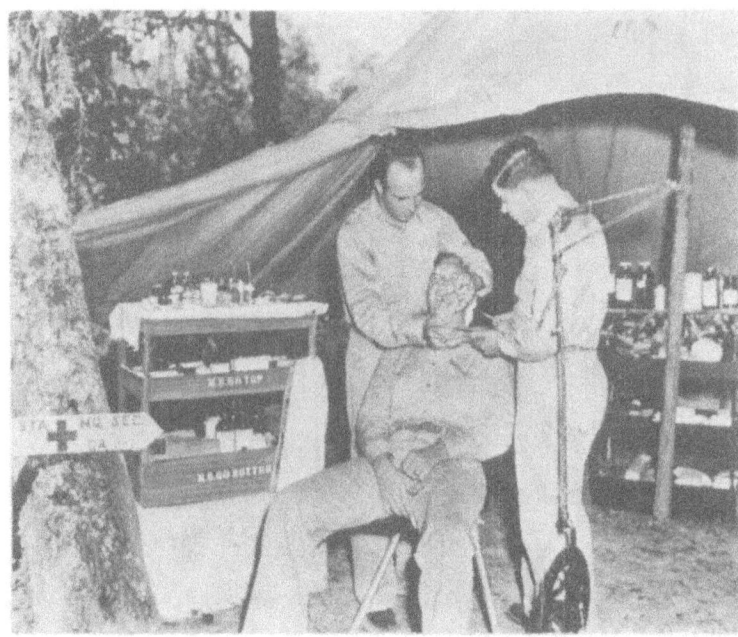

Figure 6. Field dental clinic using M. D. Chest No. 60.

equipment was the subject of much thought and criticism. Many recommendations from the field were highly impractical, failing as they did to consider the realities of procurement, maintenance, and transportation in time of war; others were based on sound observation and suggested changes which were ultimately incorporated into the outfit as the war progressed.

Addition of an Electric Dental Engine. Older dentists who had operated foot-engines had no difficulty with the engine in M. D. Chest No. 60. Younger men mobilized in World War II had not had such experience, however, and generally refused to use the foot-engine.[87] The Dental Division resisted this trend at first, and as late as September 1943 stated that "The addition of a small electric engine is not recommended. It is no great hardship to operate a foot-engine and it can be used under most any condition. If at fixed or semifixed installations an electric engine is considered necessary, a requisition can be submitted for item 52530, Engine, electric, portable."[88] It was found, however, that dental officers either used their assistants to pump the foot-engine, making them unavailable for their normal duties, or they obtained some type of improvised motor for attachment to their engines. Shops wasted valuable time and materials devising weird contraptions to mechanize this equipment. It was also

---

[87] Personal knowledge of the author confirmed by numerous photographs in the files of the Signal Corps Photographic Library. In no photograph is a dental officer shown pedaling his own foot-engine. Dentists either improvised engines or had the assistant operate the foot-engine.

[88] Memo, Dir, Dental Div, SGO, for Oprs Serv, SGO, 3 Sep 43, sub: Proposed plan for dental service in an Armored Division. SG: 703.1.

found that modern warfare required electric current in a surprising number of locations, even in the field. In March 1944 the Dental Division therefore reversed its policy and recommended development of a motor which could be attached to the foot-engine.[89] Issue of a conversion unit for use on existing foot-engines was authorized in November 1944.[90]

Addition of Operating Lamp. Dentists in the field usually had to work under cover, often in dark buildings or tents. Natural light under such circumstances was completely inadequate for dental operations. In February 1944 the Dental Division requested development of a dental operating light which could be packed in M. D. Chest No. 60,[91] and issue of this item was authorized in June 1945.[92]

Reduction in Weight of M. D. Chest No. 60. Chest 60, weighing something over 167 pounds, was too heavy to be hand-carried long distances in rough terrain or in jungles. In November 1944 a project was started to divide the contents of the field chest between two smaller containers weighing about 100 pounds each.[93] Plans were being made at the same time to pack other medical Department outfits in smaller chests, and progress on the dental equipment was held up pending development of a basic container, so that little had been accomplished on this development at the end of the war.[94]

Reduction in Weight of the Dental Field Chair. An aluminum field chair had originally been authorized for the dental field chest, but when quantity production was started the critical shortage of that metal forced the substitution of steel.[95] As a result the chair supplied during most of the period of hostilities was too heavy for convenient use in a portable outfit. Aluminum did not become available again until near the end of the war, and since the chair could not be placed in production in time to be of much use in the current conflict it was decided to redesign the entire item before resuming manufacture.[96] This project was commenced in October 1944, but had not been completed at the end of the war.

Minor Changes in Contents of M. D. Chest No. 60. During the war a number of minor changes were made in the contents of Chest 60. In May 1941 the old glass syringe designed for use with a fresh anesthetic solution made from tablets was replaced with a cartridge-type syringe using prepared car-

---

[89] Memo, Dir, Dental Div, SGO, for Oprs Serv, SGO, 15 Mar 44. SG: 700.2.

[90] Medical Supply Catalog, ASF, C 2, Med 6, November 1944. Washington, Government Printing Office, 1944 (cited hereafter as Medical Supply Catalog).

[91] Memo, Col Rex McK. McDowell for Inspections Br, Oprs Serv, SGO, 29 Feb 44. SG: 350.05–1.

[92] Medical Supply Catalog, C 5, Med 6, June 1945.

[93] Ltr, Brig Gen R. W. Bliss to Dir, Medical Department Equipment Laboratory, 7 Nov 44, sub: Item 9502500—Chest M. D. No. 60, Complete. SG: 428 (Carlisle Barracks) N.

[94] Monthly Status Report on Medical Department Research and Development Projects for Period 1–31 May 1945. HD: 700.2.

[95] The Corps Area Dental Surgeons' Conference. The Dental Bulletin. 13: 254, October 1942.

[96] Ltr, Brig Gen R. W. Bliss to CG, ASF, 6 Oct 44, sub: Chair, dental, field, folding—development project on. SG: 444.4–1.

pules of solution,[97] making it much easier to maintain sterility of anesthetic solutions in the field. Early in 1945 the alcohol burner for the sterilizer, for which it had been difficult to obtain fuel, was replaced with a gasoline burner.[98] A bone-file, rongeur forceps, and m-o-d matrix retainer were added at about the same time.[99]

Army Air Forces Operating Chest

In May 1944 the Army Air Force approved a special dental field chest for use by its units. Complete, this chest weighed only 2 pounds more than the *empty* M. D. Chest No. 60. Reduction in weight was accomplished partly by using lighter materials, and partly by omitting certain heavy items, particularly the dental field chair, for which a headrest attachable to an ordinary chair was substituted. The foot-engine was replaced with an electric dental engine. Only 50 of these chests were produced since later modifications in the regular Chest 60 made it better adapted to Air Force needs, and nonessential modifications of standard items were discouraged in the interests of maximum output.[100]

Prosthetic Field Chests

At the start of the First World War dental replacements were authorized only for teeth lost traumatically in line of duty. Some laboratory equipment was issued to base installations, but no field outfit was provided, and even at Zone of Interior camps the dental surgeon had to draw teeth or gold for each individual case. In March 1918 this policy was liberalized somewhat to authorize the replacement, in time of war, of any teeth needed for mastication, and thereafter a dental field laboratory set, weighing over 200 pounds, packed in a single chest, was issued to each division.[101] World War I prosthetic service was supplied on a relatively small scale, however, and nearly three times as many cases were completed overseas in the single month of October 1944 (35,-657)[102] as were completed in France during the entire period of hostilities in the First World War (13,000).[103]

The World War II field laboratory set consisted of 2 chests (M. D. Chests Nos. 61 and 62, figs. 7 and 8), which occupied 10 cubic feet of space with a combined weight of 332 pounds. The cost of the complete outfit was about $600. This equipment included a casting machine, a hand-operated lathe, an assortment of teeth, and all the supplies needed for fabricating or repairing

---

[97] SG Ltr 47, 22 May 41.
[98] New items of dental equipment. Army Medical Bulletin, No. 88, May 1945.
[99] Ltr, Brig Gen R. W. Bliss to CG, ASF, 24 May 45, sub: Stock No. 9502500, Chest M. D. No. 60, Complete; Stock No. 9502600, Chest M. D. No. 61, Complete. SG: 444.4-1.
[100] Memo, Col George R. Kennebeck for Plans and Services Div, Office of the Air Surgeon, 3 Jul 46. SG: 428.
[101] See footnote 84, p. 180.
[102] See footnote 67 for fiscal 1945. HD: 319.1-2.
[103] History of the Army Dental Corps, 1941-43, Equipment and Supply Section, p. 15. HD: 314.7-2.

the ordinary types of bridges or full or partial dentures.[104] It could be set up well forward in the combat zone where it helped dental officers reduce emergency evacuations for prosthetic treatment, but was not adequate for routine quantity production because such conveniences as good lights, electric lathes, handy benches, and well-arranged plaster bins could not be furnished in such an outfit. The limited amount of expendable supplies included was also insufficient to maintain continued high output.

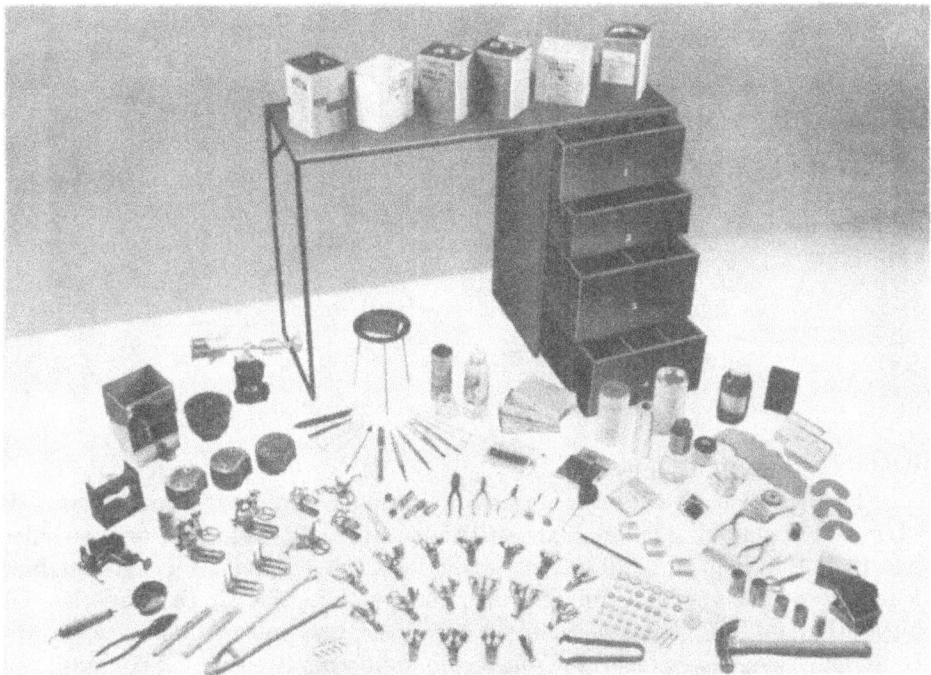

Figure 7. Contents of dental field laboratory, M. D. Chest No. 61.

The Chests 61 and 62 were at first supplied to field hospitals, evacuation hospitals, surgical hospitals, the prosthetic teams of auxiliary surgical groups, convalescent hospitals, general and aviation dispensaries, and to the medical battalions of divisions. The later withdrawal of laboratory equipment from most of these units, and its results, are discussed in the chapter on the operation of the Dental Service overseas. The most important change in the Chests 61 and 62 was the substitution, in February 1945, of a motor-driven lathe for the hand-driven type which required two men, working in relays, to operate. Since it had become apparent that electricity would be available in most locations where dental laboratories could function, the wisdom of this move was obvious.

---

[104] See footnote 75, p. 178.

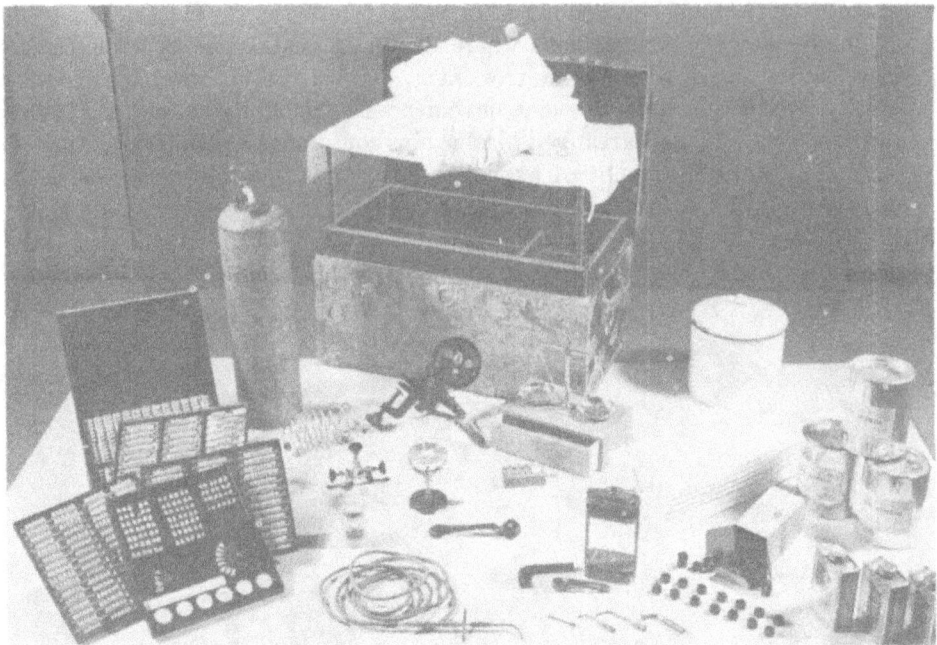

Figure 8. Contents of dental field laboratory, M. D. Chest No. 62.

Dental Pack Chests "A" and "B"

The dental pack chests contained operating equipment to meet the needs of mounted units. The 2 chests, which occupied 6 cubic feet and weighed less than 100 pounds, made a convenient load for 1 animal. They contained a little over 100 items, compared with 160 items in the M. D. Chest No. 60, but with a folding chair, foot-engine, sterilizer, and routine instruments they could be used to perform the most common operations.[105] No significant changes were made in them during the war, but in a mechanized Army their use obviously became more and more limited.

Dental Officer's and Assistant's Kits

The dental officer of each tactical unit was supplied 1 large shoulder pouch, and his assistant carried 2 smaller pouches, containing instruments for emergency use in combat when M. D. Chest No. 60 was not available. The 3 pouches were supplementary to each other, and together included items required for the relief of pain, simple extractions, emergency treatment of maxillofacial injuries, and temporary fillings. These kits were also useful during the movement of large units, when regular equipment was crated, and for that reason were frequently issued to general hospitals and other installations having base dental outfits. They were also used by dental officers serving with ski troops or paratroops. The only important change in them was the

---

[105] See footnote 75, p. 178.

DENTAL EQUIPMENT AND SUPPLY

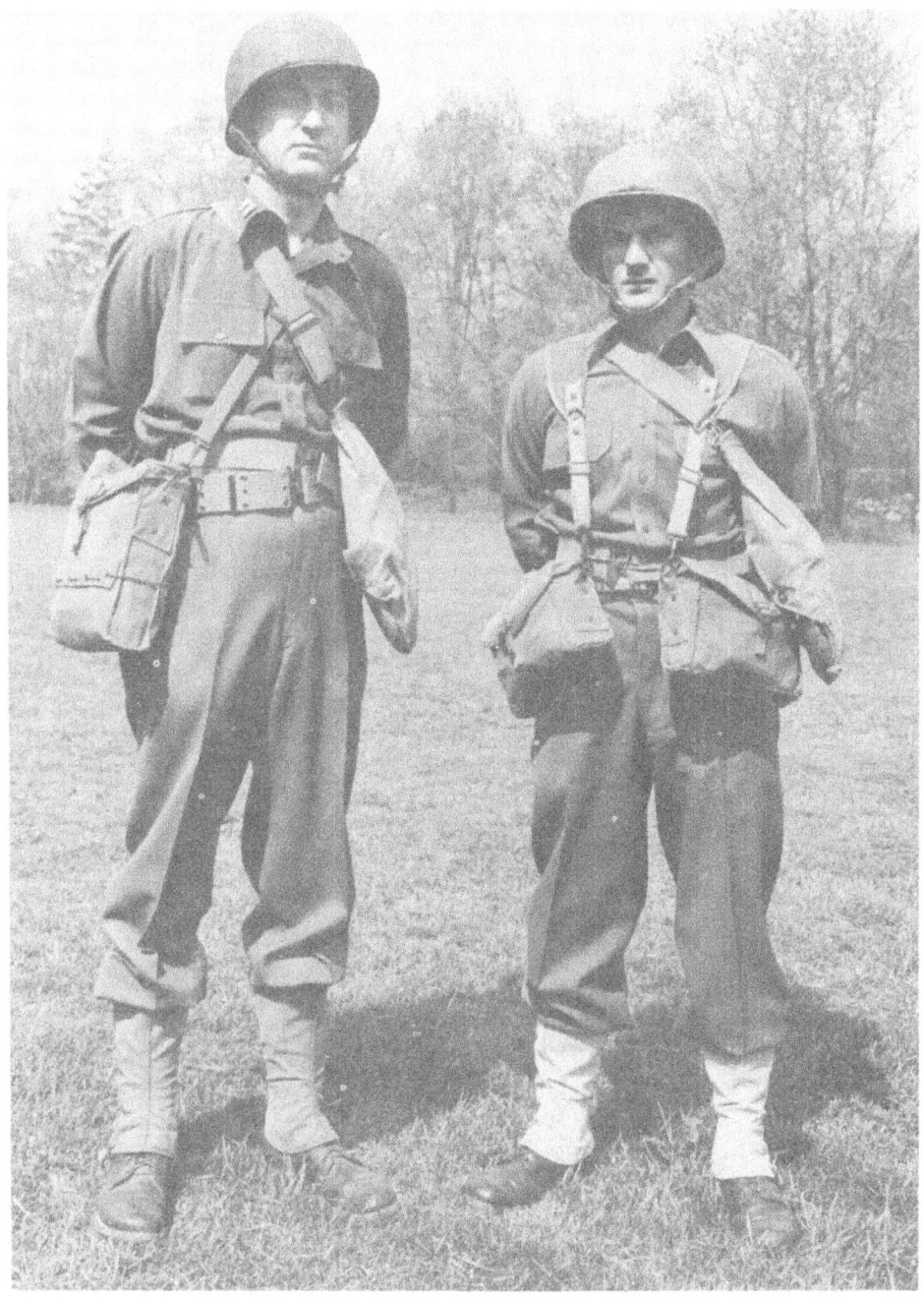

Figure 9. Dental officer and assistant with field kits.

replacement, in May 1941, of the glass-barrelled anesthetic syringes with cartridge-type syringes. Contents of kits could be augmented or changed at will to meet the individual ideas of dental officers. It was reported that very little dental work was attempted in combat, and that dental officers often carried kits of medical supplies in addition to, or in place of, the dental sets (figs. 9, 10, and 11).[106]

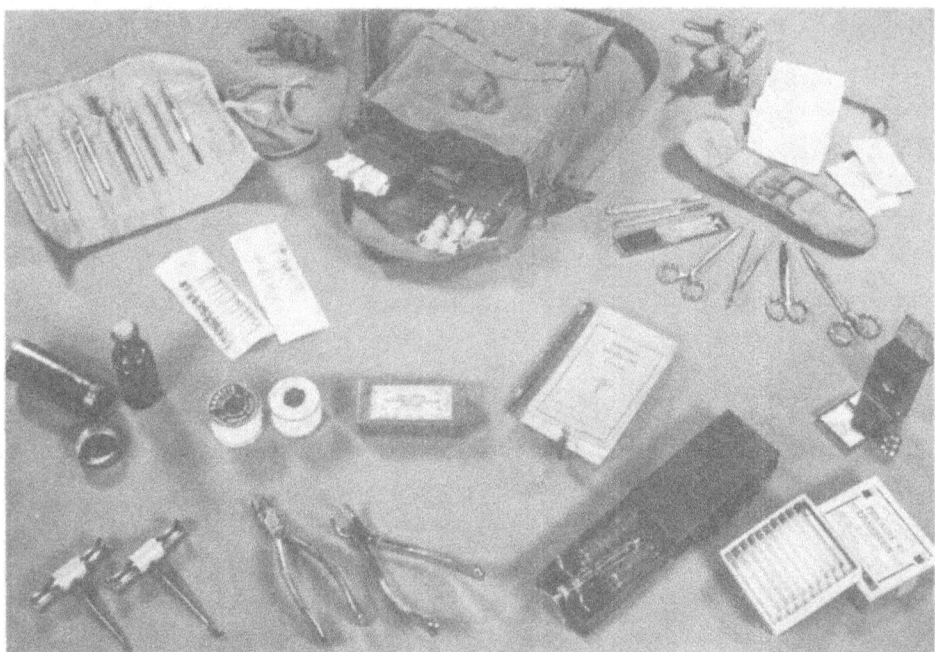

Figure 10. Contents of dental officer's kit.

Maxillofacial Kit

The maxillofacial kit which provided the highly specialized instruments needed for the care of wounds of the oral structures was designed for use by the dental member of a maxillofacial team.[107] It contained forceps, elevators, rongeurs, chisels, hemostats, lances, wire ligatures, and anesthetic syringes. The principal change in this set during the war was the introduction of the cartridge-type anesthetic syringe (fig. 12).

The Mobile Dental Laboratory

(The complete story of the development of this important item is told in a monograph by Lieutenants John B. Johnson and Graves H. Wilson.[108] Much

---

[106] History of the Dental Division, Headquarters, ETOUSA, 1 Sep–31 Dec 44. HD: 319.1–2.
[107] See footnote 75, p. 178.
[108] Johnson, J. B., and Wilson, G. H.: History of wartime research and development of medical field equipment. HD: 314.7–2.

DENTAL EQUIPMENT AND SUPPLY 189

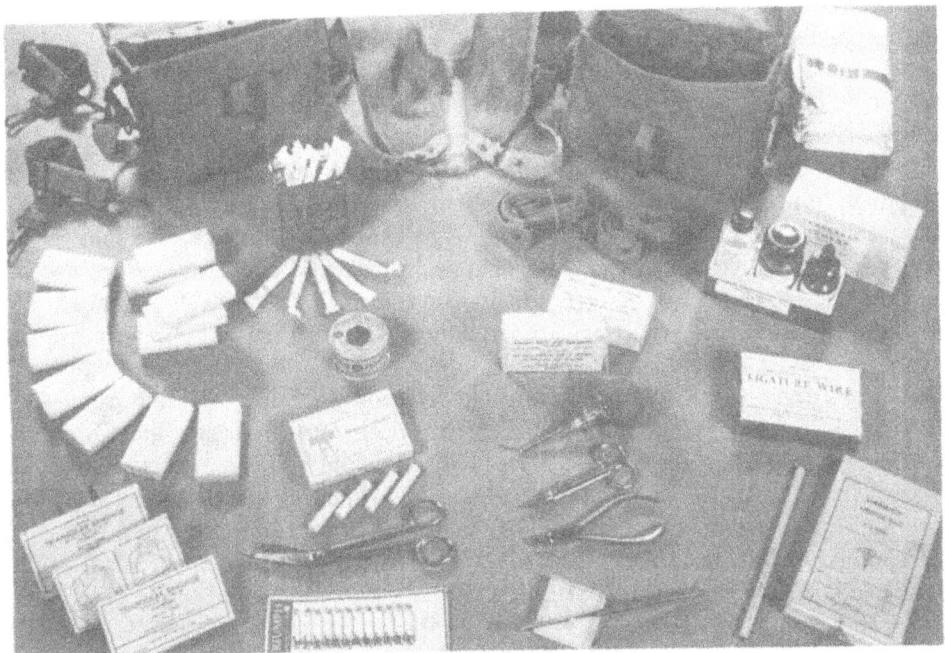

Figure 11. Contents of dental assistant's kit.

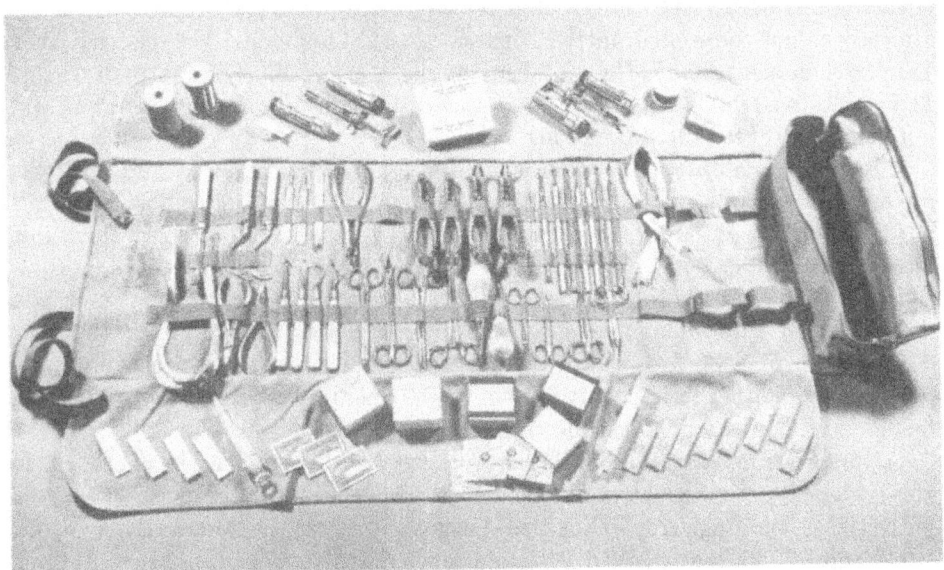

Figure 12. Contents of dental maxillofacial kit.

of the material presented here has been taken from that monograph, and its extensive documentation is not repeated.)

The need for improved dental laboratory facilities was based on a number of considerations, some of which are discussed in greater detail in the chapter on the operation of the Dental Service overseas. In brief, it was generally agreed that prosthetic equipment had to be taken to the soldier whenever possible, to prevent his evacuation to a rear area for the construction of dental replacements. For tactical units this meant that laboratory service had to be provided well forward in the combat zone, where frequent moves were necessary. The laboratory with such a unit had to be highly portable, it had to be put in operation quickly after a move, and it had to turn out a maximum of work in a short time when the opportunity was presented. M. D. Chests Nos. 61 and 62 were portable, but they failed to meet the other two requirements; it took considerable time to find shelter and set them up in a new location, and with no source of water, fuel, power, or light the only equipment which could be used was wasteful of manpower and did not encourage the most accurate work. Further, the two small chests could not contain enough supplies for prolonged operation in an emergency. The Dental Division therefore recommended, as early as May 1939, that development of a more satisfactory, truck-mounted outfit be initiated.[109]

For reasons which are not clear this project proceeded very slowly. Approval was not granted until December 1941, and a pilot model, constructed with the aid of $18,000 contributed by the manufacturers of precious metal alloys, was not completed until February 1943. This model was tested in the Tennessee maneuvers of May and June of the same year. The first delivery of 11 vehicles was made in March 1944, and distribution in foreign theaters did not begin until near the end of 1944.

As finally adopted, the mobile dental laboratory (figs. 13 and 14) was mounted on a 6-wheel drive, 2½-ton chassis, capable of maneuvering in all but the roughest terrain. It carried a 1½-KW generator, 50-gallon water tank, electrically heated boiling-out and curing apparatus, acetylene tanks, a folding dental chair, a dental engine, an electric lathe, a full assortment of teeth, and all other equipment and supplies for completing or repairing ordinary dentures or bridges. A small trailer was later supplied for carrying the generator and other bulky equipment. It was operated by 1 officer and 3 dental technicians, one of whom was also the driver.

Numerous improvised mobile laboratories had been placed in operation in foreign theaters while the standard truck was being developed. Constructed on vehicles ranging from captured German trailers to 30-passenger buses, these units had already given valuable service, so it was no surprise that the new trucks were highly commended from the start. A typical report was that

---

[109] Memo, Brig Gen Leigh C. Fairbank for SG, 11 Sep 41, sub: Field dental laboratory. SG: 322.15–16.

DENTAL EQUIPMENT AND SUPPLY

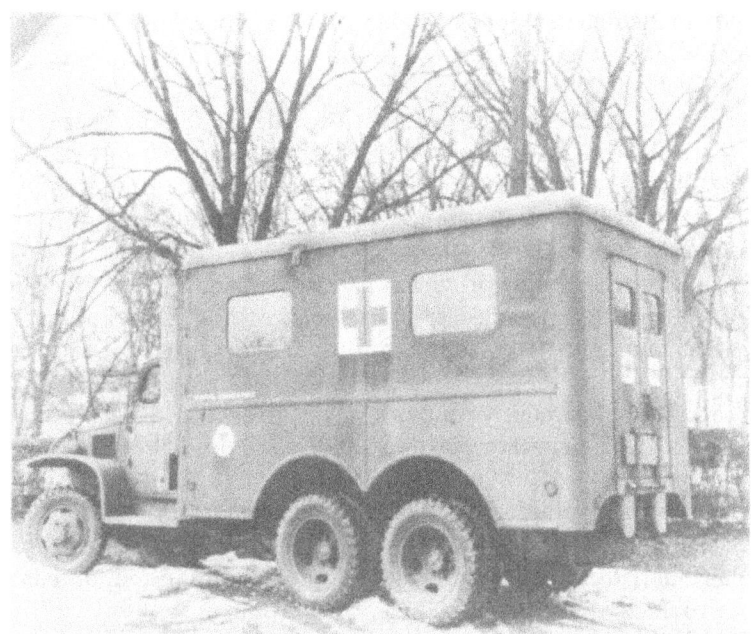

Figure 13. Mobile dental laboratory.

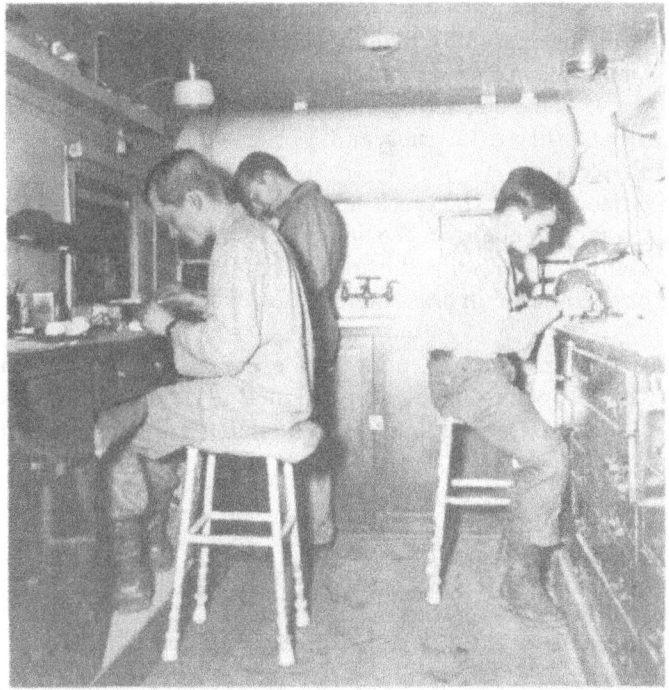

Figure 14. Interior, mobile dental laboratory.

from a division which saw combat in both North Africa and Italy, stating that "The mobile laboratory has proved to be the only answer to the division's prosthetic problem." [110] Minor defects were reported, however, as follows:

1. While the mobile laboratory provided shelter for the operators in poor weather it was badly crowded when the chair was set up inside for taking impressions. In practice the chair was usually set up in an adjoining building or tent, and when time and circumstances permitted some of the laboratory equipment was removed as well.

2. In bad weather, some provision had to be made for waiting patients.

3. The laboratory was tied to its vehicle, so that no transportation was available for picking up supplies and mail, or for carrying water for the storage tank.

4. When the truck required repairs it was necessary to close the laboratory.

5. The 1½-KW generator proved inadequate, and a 2½-KW model had to be substituted.

6. The single dental lathe was not sufficient, and another had to be authorized.

7. The small tanks of acetylene were quickly exhausted, and larger ones had to be provided.

8. Trouble was experienced in obtaining "white gas" (i. e. without a leaded additive) for the burners.

The most fundamental defects were those noted in "3" and "4." These might have been eliminated by placing the laboratory in a trailer, pulled by a truck which could also be used for other transportation. This possibility was considered, but it was rejected because:

1. Maneuverability of a truck and trailer would be considerably reduced in unfavorable terrain.

2. It was feared that the truck might be commandeered in an emergency, making it necessary to abandon the entire laboratory.[111]

The mechanical defects noted were quickly corrected, and the mobile laboratory was an important aid in bringing effective laboratory service to the forward areas.

A total of 107 laboratory trucks were ordered, and the last was delivered in October 1945. It cannot be determined at this time just how many of these units were shipped overseas, though the distribution authorized in December 1944 was as follows:

European Theater of Operations	30
Southwest Pacific Area	15
Pacific Ocean Area	5
China-Burma-India theater	4
South Pacific Base Command	4
North African theater	2

---
[110] Dental Service with a Division in the Army. J. Am. Dent. A. 32: 1475–1476, Nov–Dec 45.
[111] Statement of Col Rex McK. McDowell to the author, May 1946.

It has already been noted that many theaters had improvised large numbers of mobile laboratories in addition to those standard trucks authorized by the War Department, and it is probable that the number of these unofficial units considerably exceeded the number shipped from the Zone of Interior.

The Dental Operating Truck

(The history of the development of the dental operating truck has been told in a monograph by Lieutenants John B. Johnson and Graves H. Wilson, to which the reader is referred for greater detail and documentation than will be given here.) [112]

Dental operating trucks, which were not made available until near the end of World War II, had been used to a limited extent in the First World War. In the summer of 1917 the Cleveland Chapter of the Preparedness League of American Dentists suggested a project for the construction of "dental ambulances" which would be presented to the Army in the name of the Red Cross. Plans drawn up by the League were approved by The Surgeon General, and the first two units presented in October 1917.[113] Other chapters of the League cooperated until contracts had been let for a total of 13 trucks, at a unit cost of about $4,000. These dental ambulances were constructed on a standard ambulance chassis, and contained a chair, 6-volt electric engine operated by storage batteries, cuspidor, air compressor and tank, bracket table, sterilizer, and cabinet. Running water was supplied from a storage tank to a small washbasin. The sides of the ambulance opened out and canvas flies were available to cover additional operating space adjoining the vehicle. Four dentists and 1 or 2 assistants could thus operate from each ambulance. Folding chairs and field equipment were provided for the three officers who worked outside the unit.[114] The World War I dental operating truck was therefore a compromise which provided efficient equipment and utilities for 1 dentist and transported the regular equipment of 3 others.

Unfortunately, the dental ambulances constructed in the United States in the First World War never saw service in France. A shortage of transportation held them at an American port of embarkation in spite of urgent requests for their delivery by the dental surgeon of the AEF.[115] Two dental ambulances were presented in France, however, and they were assigned to duty with motor transport troops and with the Air Service, where they rendered very satisfactory service. The chief surgeon of the AEF commented upon these units as follows: [116]

> The need for dental ambulances—mobile dental offices—has been indicated many

---

[112] See footnote 108, p. 188.

[113] Weaver, S. M.: Standardized motor dental car and equipment. J. Am. Dent. A. 5: 3–19, Jan 1918.

[114] Ibid. *See also* Dental ambulances and Christmas roll call. J. Am. Dent. A. 5: 1283–1284, Dec 1918.

[115] See footnote 59, p. 174.

[116] See footnote 84, p. 180.

times during the campaign. . . . The use of dental ambulances with outlying commands or detachments within divisional training areas, in the rear of combat sectors, or with the Air Service, would have proven of great value inasmuch as these mobile units could proceed to the various localities with little loss of time, either in actual transport or in the unpacking and repacking of equipment ordinarily required of dental officers on itinerary dental service.

So far as is known, no effort was made to develop a standard dental operating truck in the period between World Wars I and II. When the Dental Division requested such a project in May 1939 it was rejected within the Office of The Surgeon General, and later numerous requests for a mobile dental unit from overseas theaters did not affect this decision. The Air Force particularly desired such equipment, and in December 1943 it finally undertook development of a dental unit on its own initiative. Johnson and Wilson imply that this action precipitated a sudden change of opinion in the Surgeon General's Office. In any event the Dental Division resubmitted its recommendations; they were approved by the SGO, submitted to the Commanding General, ASF, and accepted as a research project by the end of the month. When the Air Force asked for equipment for 50 dental trucks on 30 December 1943 it was told that a standard model was already being developed, and its model was dropped.[117] The Medical Department Equipment Laboratory completed a pilot model which was tested and accepted as a standard item by 16 March 1944. Contracts were immediately let for 35 trucks, the first of which was delivered in October 1944.

The mobile dental clinic (figs. 15 and 16) was mounted on a 6-wheel drive, 2½-ton chassis, similar to the one used for the mobile laboratory. In a space 13 x 7 feet were installed a unit, chair, cabinet, sink, sterilizer, 50-gallon water tank, hot-water heater, and an operating light. Equipment included all items needed for extractions, operative procedures, and for taking impressions for dentures. A 2½-KW generator supplied electric current. No x-ray machine was provided. One hundred and thirty-eight operating trucks were purchased, at a unit cost of about $9,000, including equipment. It is not known how many trucks were actually shipped overseas, but the allotment authorized in December 1944 was:

European Theater of Operations	33
North African theater	18
China-Burma-India theater	18
Southwest Pacific Area	15
Pacific Ocean Area	5
South Pacific Base Command	4

The standard operating truck was not available soon enough to receive extensive testing under combat conditions and estimates of its performance are based

---

[117] Ltr, Col Gustave E. Ledfors, Chief of Supply Div, Air Surgeon's Office, to SG, 30 Dec 43, sub: Requirements of equipment to be installed on mobile dental units. SG: 444.4–1. See also 1st and 2d inds to above, 30 Dec 43 and 11 Jan 44.

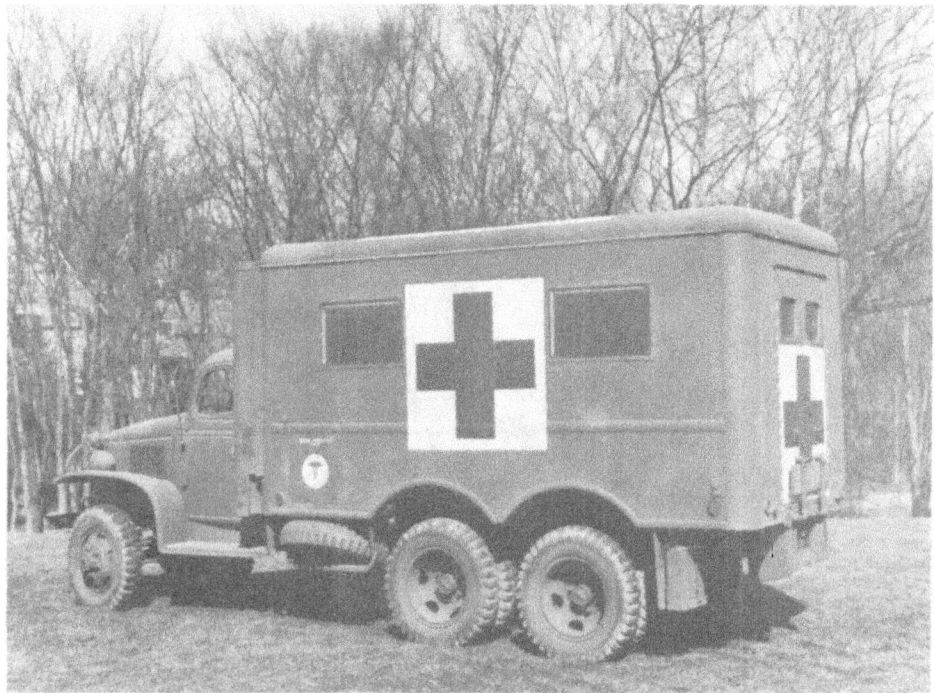

Figure 15. Mobile dental clinic.

mainly on reports on similar improvised units which had been used in almost every theater since early in the war. There was little doubt, however, that this item met an important need. The Director of the Dental Division stated in 1945 that "The success of the mobile operating units in the several theaters, especially in Italy, warrants the conclusion that such units are essential to modern warfare." On the other hand, he did not consider that the final word had been written on the subject. He especially recommended that further thought be given to a possible combination of a light trailer and truck.[118] A German trailer of this type had been towed by a United States unit from the Rhine to Pilsen in Czechoslovakia, behind no more powerful a vehicle than a weapons carrier. If practical, a trailer clinic would not tie up transportation needed to carry supplies and would not have to be closed down when the truck needed repairs or maintenance. It would also be unnecessary for the dental operating team to drive a 2½-ton truck to pick up mail or supplies. The objections to the use of a trailer are the same as those enumerated for the laboratory truck; decreased maneuverability and the danger of losing the prime mover in an emergency if it were detachable from the operating equipment.

---

[118] See footnote 21, p. 167.

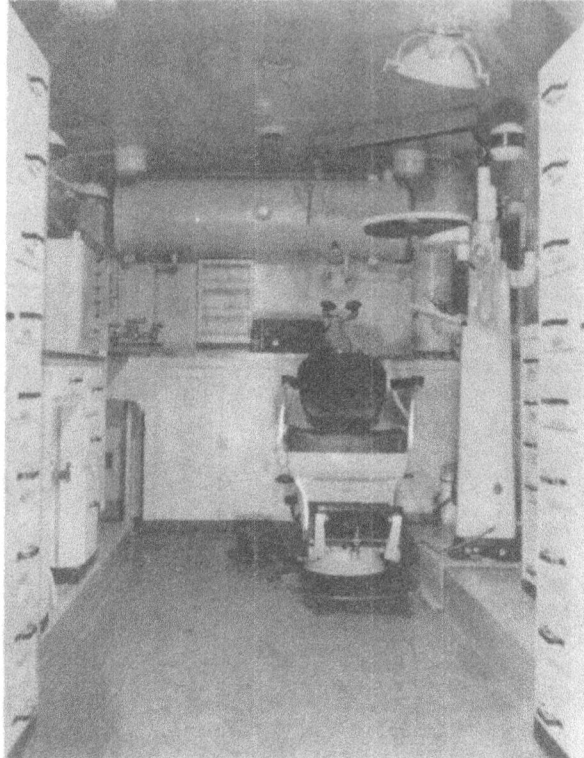

Figure 16. Interior mobile dental clinic.

In spite of the fact that it was not accepted for production, the operating truck developed by the Air Force was believed by officers of that organization to have certain features which should be considered in designing new models. Some of these features were:

1. Provision of a few laboratory items for simple acrylic repairs.

2. Use of a pressure-type water tank located under the body, where it was easily accessible, rather than the gravity-type tank which had to be mounted on the roof.

3. Installation of the unit at floor level instead of about 6 inches above the general floor level, as was necessary in the 2½-ton truck body.

4. More window space, better natural lighting.

Nonstandard Impression Chests

Units equipped only with the dental field chest had no supplies for taking impressions for prosthetic appliances. Normally, prosthetic patients could be transferred to nearby hospitals for this service, but in some circumstances such a procedure meant the loss of a man to his organization for extended periods. To meet this situation the dental surgeon of the European theater assembled chests containing materials and equipment for taking impressions and pouring models which could in turn be sent to a central dental laboratory. A chest would be loaned to an organization for a week or two at a time, and when all prosthetic cases had been cleaned up the chest was returned to a depot for replacement of missing or damaged items and for issue to another unit. Later in the war the mobile laboratory units were often able to bring prosthetic service to these isolated organizations, and the improvised impression chests never became a standard item of issue. At the time they were devised, however, they filled a definite need.

THE DENTAL WARD CART

In hospital practice it was often necessary to provide dental care at the bedside of patients. Personnel who were bedridden for considerable periods of time frequently required definitive treatment which could not be provided with a few instruments carried in a tray, and dentists improvised carts to carry the more essential equipment from patient to patient and from ward to ward. Some of the more elaborate outfits carried a dental engine, operating lamp, sterilizer, air compressor and spray bottles, and drawers of instruments and supplies for most operative and oral surgical procedures. These improvised carts proved so efficient that a project for their development as a standard item was authorized in May 1945.[119] This project was of course not completed before the end of hostilities, but the standard ward cart promised to add to the comfort of patients and the convenience of operators as soon as it should become available.

SUMMARY

Experience in dental supply problems during World War II emphasized the following points:

1. In an emergency calling for the mobilization of many millions of men and thousands of dentists, requirements for dental equipment and supplies will far exceed normal peacetime needs. At the same time production will be hampered by shortages of manpower and materials, and imports are likely to be cut off. Adequate production of such essential items as burs should be insured in advance, and some control of distribution established to prevent such irresponsible buying, by both civilians and the military, as increased the demand for burs from 33 million a year before the war to nearly 100 million in 1943. To insure that minimum needs of the population will be met, plans to stop the production of any item, such as operating units, as nonessential, should be considered carefully and cautiously before being adopted; in many cases it will actually be necessary to increase production to meet new military requirements. It is possible of course, that new types

---

[119] See footnote 94, p. 183.

of warfare will eliminate mass mobilizations, and hence reduce military needs; it is also possible that the manufacture of dental supplies could become one of the casualties of a war for survival. It must be noted, however, that treatment received by the American public in peacetime is far from adequate, and any further reduction, even in time of war, would have serious results which should be weighed carefully before deciding to cut the production of items used by dentists.

2. Availability of supplies and equipment may well prove to be the factor which will determine the rate of mobilization of dental facilities in an emergency. Nothing will be gained by taking dentists on active duty to stand idle at their camps because they have no handpieces or chairs. The procurement of dental supplies in sufficient quantities will therefore be one of the first responsibilities of officials directing the establishment of an emergency Dental Service.

3. A considerable amount of dental equipment in the hands of civilian dentists will become idle when they are taken into the Armed Forces in a mobilization. It is possible that such equipment will have to be purchased or leased for the military. The individual purchase of thousands of outfits, of widely varying types and degrees of serviceability, is in itself no small problem, however, and the cost of using secondhand equipment will generally exceed the cost of purchasing new items. It should not be assumed that large quantities of dental supplies will be available from civilian sources until test projects have shown that such is actually the case.

4. Close cooperation between the Dental Service and procurement agencies is essential, and such cooperation will probably be best obtained by assigning qualified dental officers to major supply installations.

5. Convenient and complete dental equipment should be supplied as far forward in the theater of operations as is consistent with the operational situation. Mobile operating and laboratory units will make it possible to provide efficient equipment within easy reach of the fighting men.

6. In major moves dentists should not be separated from their equipment if their outfits can possibly be forwarded as personal or unit baggage. Too many dentists spent from 1 to 4 months in idleness after their arrival overseas in World War II because their field chests had been shipped on different vessels or in different convoys.

CHAPTER VI

Operation of the Dental Service—General Considerations

DENTAL STANDARDS FOR MILITARY SERVICE

In time of peace the Army tends to establish physical standards for military service which cannot be maintained in time of emergency. This policy is not inconsistent since it ensures that time and money will not be wasted in training poor physical specimens, but when these rigid standards are carried over into a general mobilization difficulties may result.

The dental standards for full military duty which were in effect at the end of the First World War were not significantly altered prior to World War II. The early Mobilization Regulations (MR 1-9, dated 31 August 1940) which established the physical criteria to be used by Selective Service in time of emergency, prescribed dental requirements which were substantially the same as those published in AR 40-105 for the Regular Army in time of peace. Section VII of these regulations reads as follows:

DENTAL REQUIREMENTS

31. Classes 1-A and 1-B.—*a. Class 1-A.* (1) Normal teeth and gums.

(2) A minimum of 3 serviceable natural masticating teeth above and three below opposing and three serviceable natural incisors above and three below opposing. (Therefore the minimum requirements consist of a total of 6 masticating teeth and 6 incisor teeth.) All of these teeth must be so opposed as to serve the purpose of incision and mastication.

(3) *Definitions.*
   (a) The term "masticating teeth" includes molar and bicuspid teeth and the term "incisors" includes incisor and cuspid teeth.
   (b) A natural tooth which is carious (one with a cavity), which can be restored by filling, is to be considered a serviceable natural tooth.
   (c) Teeth which have been restored by crowns or dummies attached to bridgework, if well placed will be considered as serviceable natural teeth when the history and appearance of these teeth are such as to clearly warrant such assumption.

b. Class 1-B. Insufficient teeth to qualify for class 1-A, if corrected by suitable dentures.

32. Class 4.—*a.* Irremediable disease of the gums of such severity as to interfere seriously with useful vocation in civil life.

b. Serious disease of the jaw which is not easily remediable and which is likely to incapacitate the registrant for satisfactory performance of general or limited military service.

c. Extensive focal infection with multiple periapical abscess, the correction of which would require protracted hospitalization and incapacity.

d. Extensive irremediable caries.

(Note: Class I-A was acceptable for full military duty, class I-B was eligible only for limited duty, and class IV was rejected for *any* military service. No registrants found acceptable for limited service were called for military service prior to July 1942.)[1]

These regulations did not specify whether or not teeth replaced on removable bridges would be counted as serviceable natural teeth, and this point was not made clear until March 1941, when Selective Service Medical Circular No. 2 provided that either fixed or removable bridges were acceptable if supported at least in part by the remaining teeth.[2]

When the preceding regulation was published the United States was still more than a year from actual participation in the war. The partial mobilization then in progress was for training purposes only, and fairly strict physical standards were necessary to avoid waste of effort in the instruction of men who might later prove unfit for military service. However, the Dental Division did not expect the criteria of the prewar MR 1-9 to apply in case of actual conflict, for as early as May 1941 Brig. Gen. Leigh C. Fairbank, Director of the Dental Division, stated:

> It is estimated that a large percentage of men, inducted into the Army in the operation of a compulsory draft law, would require extensive dental replacements. The men of military age today will certainly show the [effects of] lack of dental care during the depression years. This condition must not be permitted to constitute a disqualifying factor. . . . However great our desire to maintain high dental standards for military service, we must realize that the safety of our nation depends on trained manpower. If the situation at present indicates a lowered state of dental health among those of military age, we must provide the means for adequate dental service to correct the dental health of drafted men. The entire plan for dental service in time of mobilization has been revised to meet the conditions which we are certain will exist in every Army camp.[3]

The number of men actually disqualified for dental reasons under MR 1-9 far exceeded all expectations. About 8.8 percent of the registrants examined during the period from November 1940 through September 1941 could not qualify for general service. About one-third of these disqualified registrants were classified as IV-F, namely, as totally unfit for military service, and the remainder as I-B, fit for limited service only.[4] Since no registrants with limited service qualification were called for military service during this period, the 8.8 percent was the actual disqualification rate for dental reasons. In addition to those registrants who were disqualified for strictly dental conditions (8.8 percent), about 0.4 percent of the examined registrants were rejected by the local boards for serious pathology of the mouth or gums, and while

---

[1] Teeth, mouth, and gum defects of men physically examined through the Selective Service System, 1940–1944, 28 Dec 45, p. 11. Natl Hq, Selective Service System.

[2] Medical Circular No. 2, Dental, 28 Mar 41. Natl Hq, Selective Service System.

[3] Fairbank, L. C.: Prosthetic dental service for the Army in peace and war. J. Am. Dent. A, 28: 798–802, May 1941.

[4] Causes of rejections and incidence of defects, Medical Statistics Bulletin No. 2, 1 Aug 43, pp. 6 and 9. Natl Hq, Selective Service System.

the proportion disqualified by the induction stations for such pathology is not known it is apparent that about 1 of each 11 registrants examined was disqualified at that time for military service because of dental or oral diseases. These disqualification rates refer to rejections where the dental defects were the principal disqualifying cause. It should be noted, however, that in establishing the disqualification rates, only one disqualifying reason was given as the cause of rejection. Obviously, whenever there was more than one disqualifying defect, an order of precedence was followed in determining the principal disqualifying cause. In this respect, dental defects had a low priority. Therefore, if it were assumed that the frequency of disqualifying dental defects was the same among the registrants who were disqualified for reasons other than dental, it seems that about 1 out of 8 examined registrants would have failed to meet the early dental standards for general service.

During 1940 and 1941, when 89 percent of all dental rejections were made by local boards, dental and oral disqualifications by these boards were based on the following specific conditions: [5]

Defects of the teeth:

	Percentage of all dental rejections		
	Total	White	Negro
Missing teeth, replaced by dentures	23.1	23.8	6.3
Missing teeth, no dentures	64.0	63.6	73.6
Excessive caries	10.0	9.7	16.1
Other defects of the teeth	2.9	2.9	4.0

Defects of the mouth and gums:

	Percentage of all oral rejections		
	Total	White	Negro
Periodontoclasia	71.7	71.4	73.8
Gingivitis	5.1	4.7	8.2
Congenital defects, lips and palate	8.6	9.6	1.6
Other defects of the mouth and gums	14.6	14.3	16.4

For a year and a half after the early MR 1–9 (1 August 1940) was published, changes in dental standards were relatively unimportant. In October 1940 the War Department directed that the provisions of MR 1–9 which had previously applied only to inductees would thereafter also constitute the physical standard for voluntary enlistment in the Regular Army and the National Guard.[6] In March 1941 both Selective Service and the Office of The Surgeon General published circulars of interpretation directing that (1) the specified minimum number of teeth were required to be in occlusion only during movements of the mandible, as long as there was no impingement on soft tissues while the jaw was at rest, (2) missing teeth replaced by either a fixed or removable bridge could be counted as serviceable teeth if at least part of the stress of mastication was carried by the remaining natural teeth, (3) teeth with pyorrhea

---
[5] See footnote 1, p. 200.
[6] WD Cir 110, 4 Oct 40.

pockets would be considered unserviceable if the pockets involved the bifurcation of multirooted teeth or the apical third of single-rooted teeth, and (4) teeth with caries involving the pulp would be considered unserviceable.[7] [8] In May 1941 dental requirements for officers of the Medical Department Reserve and the Chaplains' Reserve were relaxed to authorize commissioning of men with less than the minimum 12 teeth if the missing teeth were replaced by full or partial dentures.[9]

After Pearl Harbor it was apparent that the manpower needed to fight a global war could be obtained only if dental standards for induction were drastically relaxed. The War Department and Selective Service therefore directed, in February 1942, that pending revision of MR 1-9 the following would be acceptable for general military service: [10] [11]

> Registrants who lack the required number of teeth as set forth in paragraph 31a, Mobilization Regulations 1-9, 31 August 1940, when, in the opinion of the examining physician, they are well nourished, of good musculature, are free of gross dental infections, and have sufficient teeth (natural or artificial) to subsist on the Army ration.

This modification, interpreted literally, temporarily authorized the induction of edentulous individuals provided they had procured the necessary dental replacements.

The revised MR 1-9 [12] which was published 15 March 1942 provided for acceptance for general military duty:

> Individuals who are well nourished, of good musculature, are free from gross dental infections, and have the following minimum requirements:
> 1. In the upper jaw—Edentulous, if corrected or correctible by a full denture.
> 2. In the lower jaw—A minimum of a sufficient number of natural teeth in proper position and condition to stabilize or support a partial denture which can be removed and replaced by the individual and which is retained by means of clasps, with or without rests, to stabilize or support the denture.

Malocclusion was a cause for rejection only when it interfered with the individual's health or resulted in damage to the soft tissues. Registrants with less than the required number of natural teeth were to be placed in Class I-B, for limited military service, if the condition was correctible by the construction of dentures. In April 1942 [13] these revised standards were made applicable to graduates of officer candidate schools and, after October 1942,[14] applied to Reserve and National Guard officers.

---

[7] See footnote 2, p. 200.
[8] SG Ltr 26, 28 Mar 41.
[9] SG Ltr 39, 5 May 41.
[10] Memo, Dir, Selective Service System, for all State Directors, No. I-372, 13 Feb 42, sub: Revised physical standards. Natl Hq, Selective Service System.
[11] WD Cir 43, 12 Feb 42.
[12] MR 1-9, 15 Mar 42.
[13] WD Cir 126, 28 Apr 42.
[14] AR 40-105, 14 Oct 42.

In a further revision of MR 1-9 in October 1942, dental requirements for induction were practically eliminated.[15] Thereafter the prospective inductee needed only "at least an edentulous upper jaw and/or an edentulous lower jaw, corrected or correctible by a full denture or dentures." No dental conditions were thereafter to warrant classification for limited service, and the only disqualifying dental defects were "diseases of the jaws and associated structures which are irremediable or not easily remedied, or which are likely to incapacitate the individual for the satisfactory performance of military duty" or "extensive loss of oral tissue in an amount that would prevent replacement of missing teeth by a satisfactory denture." The effects of the relaxed dental standards soon became evident. The available statistics for 1942 (beginning with April) indicate that the disqualification rate for dental reason during that year was around 1 percent. It decreased from 2.9 percent in April 1942 to about 0.1 percent in December 1942.[16] In 1953, the disqualification rate for dental defects fluctuated around 0.1 percent, and it remained practically at that level for the remainder of World War II.[17] Selective Service Headquarters estimated that out of 4,828,000 registrants aged 18-37 who were still classified as IV-F on 1 August 1945, 36,000 registrants were so classified because of dental defects. An additional 12,500 registrants were disqualified by mouth and gum defects. In other words, according to this estimate defects of the teeth accounted for 0.7 percent of the IV-F category, and mouth and gum defects accounted for another 0.3 percent, together amounting to 1.0 percent of the entire IV-F class. These data refer to the entire period since the enactment of the 1940 Selective Service Act.[18]

At the end of hostilities higher dental standards were still maintained for commission in the Regular Army, for divers, for cadets, and for airborne duty; other components, including flying personnel, were subject only to the relaxed provisions of MR 1-9.

Selective Service Regulations of World War II did not at first provide for dentists to serve on induction boards, but the mounting importance of dental defects as a cause for rejection, plus the fact that many men accepted by the local boards were subsequently disqualified at induction stations, led to the decision in March 1941 to include dentists in the local and advisory boards whenever feasible.[19] By 7 December 1941, 8,040 dentists had been officially appointed to this voluntary duty,[20] and a Selective Service memorandum of 1 August 1941 noted that dentists were then available on all local boards.[21] After Febru-

---

[15] MR 1-9, 15 Oct 42.
[16] Unpublished data from the Medical Statistics Division, SGO.
[17] Induction Data, Results of Examination of Selectees at Induction Station, during 1943, Army Service Forces, Office of The Surgeon General, Medical Statistics Division.
[18] Medical Statistics Bulletin No. 4, Natl Hq, Selective Service System, Table 4.
[19] Selective Service Regulations, vol. I, sec V, amendment 12 to par 134. In Selective Service Regulations, 23 Sep 40 to 1 Feb 42. Washington, Government Printing Office, 1944.
[20] Camalier, C. W.: Preparedness and war activities of the American Dental Association. J. Am. Dent. A. 33: 84, 1 Jan 46.
[21] Memo, Dir, Selective Service System, for all State Directors, 1 Aug 41, sub: Dental examination. Natl Hq, Selective Service System.

ary 1942 local boards limited their dental examinations to a gross screening for obviously disqualifying pathology.[22] The more detailed examination necessary to chart all defects and finally determine eligibility for military service was thereafter carried out at Army induction stations.[23]

MISSION AND CAPABILITIES OF THE DENTAL SERVICE

At the start of World War II, available information on the dental condition of young adults of military age was at best fragmentary and often contradictory. Though studies on the dental needs of the civilian population had been conducted by various agencies,[24][25][26][27][28] these had been restricted to small segments of the population which were not representative because of age, economic status, or geographical distribution. No governmental or private agency had attempted the nationwide examination of hundreds of thousands of persons from all income, age, and racial groups, both urban and rural, which alone could have given a complete picture of the dental needs of the American public. However, the one conclusion accepted by all researchers was that the dental attention received by the average citizen during the preceding decade had been anything but adequate. The reasons for this inadequacy were not primarily the concern of the Armed Forces, but since the dental care of the average inductee had not been sufficient to prevent the steady accumulation of serious, preventable dental defects, this accumulation materially complicated the problems of the Army Dental Service during the emergency. Thus in formulating a policy for the dental care of military personnel, the Dental Service had a choice of one of three principal alternatives.

First, it might have continued to furnish only such treatment as the average inductee had received in civilian life. Sporadic attention of this type, limited very often to the relief of intolerable conditions, was being provided the American public with a ratio of only 1 dentist for each 1,850 persons, including infants and the aged.[29] The Dental Corps could have supplied such symptomatic treatment without serious difficulty.

---

[22] See footnote 10, p. 202.

[23] Though induction stations operated under Army supervision they were often staffed with contract civilian medical and dental personnel.

[24] Beck, D. F.: Costs of dental care for adults under specific clinical conditions. Under the auspices of the Socio-economics Committee of the American College of Dentists. Lancaster, Lancaster Press Inc., 1943.

[25] Walls, R. M.; Lewis, S. R., and Dollar, M. L.: A study of the dental needs of adults in the United States. Chicago, American Dental Association, Economics Committee, 1941.

[26] Collins, S. D.: Frequency of dental service among 9,000 families, based on nationwide periodic canvasses, 1928–31. Pub. Health Rep. 54: 629, Apr 1939.

[27] Dollar, M. L: Dental needs and the cost of dental care in the United States. Ill. Dent. J. 14: 185–199, May 1945.

[28] Klein, H., and Palmer, C. E.: The dental problem of elementary school children. Milbank Mem. Fund Quart. 16: 281, Jul 1938.

[29] O'Rourke, J. T.: An analysis of the personnel resources of the dental profession. J. Am. Dent. A. 30: 1002, 1 Jul 45.

Unfortunately, such a low standard of dental health was not acceptable for military personnel. The civilian whose health was being undermined by oral sepsis might conceivably follow his normal sedentary pursuits without noticeable inconvenience, but in the Army he had to function at top efficiency under the most adverse conditions, and disease which would reduce his physical endurance or cause him to be lost to his unit at a critical time, had to be eliminated. Moreover, the soldier had to be able to masticate any rough food which might be available in the field. Disregarding all humanitarian considerations, the Army could expect the most effective service from inductees only if their oral health was maintained at a much higher level than was common in civilian life.

As a second alternative, the Dental Service might have provided only such regular annual care as was essential to prevent further deterioration of the soldier's dental health, ignoring old defects except when treatment became urgently necessary for the relief of pain. It had been estimated, on the basis of the ADA study of 1940, that 267,000 dentists, or a ratio of 1 dentist for each 493 persons, would be able to furnish such attention for the civilian population.[30] This figure was of course not directly applicable to the military population, but it is certain that all regular maintenance care could have been provided Army personnel with the authorized ratio of 1 officer for each 500 men. However, this policy was undesirable because the average inductee as he was received in the Armed Forces was dentally unfit for military service even if the development of new defects could be checked. In addition, it was open to all the objections discussed in the preceding paragraph.

The remaining alternative was for the Dental Service to undertake the complete dental rehabilitation of every inductee, providing not only annual maintenance care, but correcting as far as possible the old defects which had resulted from earlier neglect. In view of the demand for top physical condition in military personnel this was the only objective which could be accepted, but based on fundamental considerations of available dental personnel and supply, it was necessarily a long-term project, not to be achieved in a few months, or even in a year.

The first goal of the Army Dental Service was to correct conditions which might cause a man to become a dental casualty, adversely affect his health, or result in further serious damage to dental structures. The precedence for this care was determined by the following dental classification:[31]

Classification	Treatment required
Class I	Extractions, other treatment urgently needed for the relief of pain or the maintenance of health.
Class I-D	Replacement of missing teeth for the necessary restoration of function.

---

[30] See footnote 27, p. 204.
[31] AR 40-510, 31 Jul 42.

Classification	Treatment required
Class II	Fillings or other routine, preventive care.
Class III	Replacement of missing teeth not urgently required for the restoration of function. Care for chronic conditions.
Class IV	No treatment required.

Though this classification gave some indication of the amount of treatment needed, the information was qualitative rather than quantitative; a man in Class II might have one carious tooth, or a dozen. Nor did it indicate all the types of work required; a single individual might have defects coming under three or more groupings, but only the most urgent classification was reported. Furthermore, different camps reported widely varying dental classification, indicating a lack of uniformity in application of the specified criteria.

Sample surveys of men arriving at three large replacement training centers at different periods from 1942 through 1945 show that they fell into approximately the following categories. These figures are given in round numbers because the available statistics do not justify more detailed conclusions:[32]

Class I	15 percent
Class I–D	5 percent
Class II	40 percent
Class III and IV (combined)	40 percent

It must be noted, however, that a large proportion of the men in Class I eventually required prosthetic replacements; similarly the men in Classes I and I–D often required routine fillings as well.

Treatment was normally rendered while the soldier was in training, and, in any event had to be completed before his departure for an active theater.[33] After urgent work was taken care of the next objective was to provide men destined for a combat area as much routine treatment as possible. By the latter part of 1943 one major theater was able to report that 85 percent of new replacements were in Class IV, requiring no dental attention.[34]

The final goal of the Dental Service was to provide all essential treatment for every soldier, no matter where located. The extent to which this objective was attained is difficult to determine. It is known that the number of men needing the most urgent types of treatment, including the construction of dentures, was reduced from 20 percent on entry into the service to 3 percent at time of discharge; the number requiring routine care was correspondingly reduced from 40 percent to 14 percent.[35] These figures fail completely to reveal the actual improvement in dental health, however, since the man who

---

[32] Calculations based on unpublished data in the files of the Dental Division, SGO, covering the initial classifications of 25,000 men examined at Ft. Sill, Okla., in 1944 and 1945; 5,884 men examined at Ft. Meade, Md., in Jan. 1945; and 5,000 men examined at Camp Robinson, Ark., in 1942. Obviously a high proportion of these men came from the states in which the incidence of caries was low.

[33] Preparation for overseas movement, 1 Aug 43. HD: 370.5–1.

[34] History of the Dental Corps in the Southwest Pacific Area, World War II. HD: 314.7 (Southwest Pacific).

[35] See footnote 32, above. The dental classification of separatees was calculated on data covering 12,000 men discharged at Ft. Dix, N. J., in 1946.

entered the Army with 10 carious teeth and left it with 1 small cavity detected at the time of examination for discharge, would still be recorded as "needing routine treatment," and statistically no change in his dental condition would be noted. It is probable that many of the dischargees listed as still needing dental care fell in this category, but pending a study of individual induction and separation records, it is possible to say only that the average soldier returned to civilian life in much better condition than when he left it.

PERSONS AUTHORIZED TO RECEIVE DENTAL CARE

Military Personnel

During World War II dental treatment was authorized on an equal basis and without cost for all Army personnel on active duty without respect to rank or component.[36] At least once a year, and usually more often, members of each organization were examined in a "dental survey" and placed in the appropriate category as listed on pages 205–206. First priority was given to emergency conditions; other personnel, beginning with those in Class I, were treated in accordance with their classification established on the survey. Retired personnel were authorized dental care when facilities were available, but total requirements for this group were so small that they were a negligible factor in planning the Dental Service.

Civilian Dependents

Prior to the war, dependents of military personnel were authorized dental treatment in Army clinics. Most of this treatment was maintenance care for persons receiving fairly regular attention, but it accounted for about 25 percent of all work completed by the Dental Corps.[37] To have continued this type of treatment for the dependents of the millions of men being taken into the Armed Forces for the emergency would have required a minimum of 5,000 additional dentists, with equipment and housing, at a time when both manpower and supplies were critically short. The Dental Division therefore recommended that treatment for Army dependents be limited to the care of emergencies, and then only when such care would not interfere with the treatment of military personnel.[38]

However, enforcement of the limitations on dental care for dependents sometimes led to considerable embarrassment for dental officers. The Dental Division had recommended that only "emergency care *for the actual relief of pain*" be authorized, and the application of even this provision would probably have required the exercise of a great deal of tact. But through

---

[36] For a detailed list of persons entitled to dental treatment see AR 40–505, 1 Sep 42.

[37] Summary of dental attendance (Dental Corps, U. S. Army, 1939). Dental Bulletin, supp. to Army Medical Bulletin 11 : 128, Jul 1940.

[38] Memo, Brig Gen Leigh C. Fairbank for Exec Off, SGO, 8 Oct 40. SG : 337.–1.

error or intent the published directive merely provided for "emergency treatment," leaving a loophole for strong and continuous pressure for all kinds of care.[39] A wife who lost a bridge-facing on the day before a dinner party had no trouble in convincing herself that hers was an emergency situation, and patients demanded, and sometimes received, permanent fillings, denture repairs, and even the replacement of missing teeth. Some contended that dental care was authorized by Army regulations and that it could not be denied by an emergency directive, but the Legal Division of the SGO decided that medical attention for dependents was "a matter of discretion and not a matter of right."[40]

Even with the above defect rigid application of the directive would have eliminated almost all dental work for dependents since it also prohibited such care when it would interfere with the treatment of military personnel, and very rarely could it honestly be said that any work for dependents would not be at the expense of the troops. But the dental surgeon who tried to refuse civilian dental care on this basis sometimes found that he did not have the support of either the surgeon or the commanding officer. He could legally enforce the restriction, but such action frequently had to be taken on his own responsibility and against the fairly clear wishes of the superiors who made out his efficiency reports, assigned his duties, and approved or disapproved recommendations for promotion. This situation was understandable since officers outside the Dental Service seldom understood the time-consuming nature of dental work. Few realized that the request to "just take a look at this tooth" usually meant at least a half-hour lost from a busy day. Only the dentist knew that in spite of his best efforts some of his men would leave for combat areas with uncorrected dental defects, and that every minute devoted to nonmilitary personnel was taken from a soldier. But the knowledge that he was in the right was very little consolation to a dental officer who had to enforce a regulation which was unpopular with his immediate superiors.

In spite of these deficiencies, the directive against wartime treatment of dependents accomplished its primary purpose fairly well. Only 1.4 percent of all care rendered during 1942–1945, inclusive, went to nonmilitary personnel, and much of that to civilian employees overseas.[41] Its principal defect was ambiguity; a flat prohibition against any care for dependents was enforceable, but a compromise attempt to provide only a little treatment was not. The very fact that only 2 or 3 percent of dependents received any

---

[39] Ltr. TAG to CGs all CAs and Depts and COs of Exempted Stas, 14 Jan 41, sub: Dental service during the national emergency. AG : 703.1.

[40] Memo, Lt E. R. Taylor, Legal Div, SGO, for Col McDowell, 25 Jan 45, sub: Dental attendance for dependents of military personnel. SG : 703.

[41] Data on the treatment of civilians assembled by author from data in the files of the Dental Division, SGO.

dental care at all is in itself evidence that dental surgeons could not provide even the minimal authorized treatment on an equitable basis. The dentist was forced to select a very few patients from the hundreds needing attention, and under such circumstances charges of favoritism were inevitable. Dependents of overseas personnel who had no one to support their requests for assistance, and dependents of men in the lower grades, who could least afford to pay for civilian dental care, generally fared worst of all.

The few dependents who received the scanty treatment authorized were seldom satisfied, while the majority who did not, felt that they had been arbitrarily denied a valuable privilege because they lacked influence or because the dentist was lazy. Wives of Army personnel published lurid accounts of the "run-around" they had experienced, describing graphically how they had waited all day for consultation, only to be told to come back the following day. The net result of this attempt to do just a little work for dependents was inadequate treatment for a very few, and widespread ill will for the Medical Department and the Dental Corps. It appears that a complete suspension of treatment for dependents during the emergency would have been fairest to all concerned and would have created less bad feeling than the temporizing policy actually in effect. The Navy has successfully enforced such a policy for many years, in peace as well as in war.[42]

Civilian Employees and Associated Personnel

Dental care for civilian employees of the War Department in the continental United States was limited to emergency treatment for the relief of pain until definitive care could be provided by a civilian dentist.[43] Overseas, however, where satisfactory dental attention could not be obtained from nonmilitary agencies, the Army had to assume responsibility for the dental care of its civilian specialists. Under these conditions, civilian employees were authorized the same treatment as soldiers, without cost.[44] Red Cross personnel in the United States, where civilian facilities were available, were authorized dental care only when hospitalized and when such dental treatment was an essential part of therapy.[45] In no case was replacement of

---

[42] Statements concerning defects in the policy regarding dental treatment for dependents are very hard to document. Those who received no treatment had no legal basis for complaint, and those who received more than emergency care did not court publicity, for obvious reasons. The author gained personal knowledge of this problem while serving as dental surgeon of two large ZI posts. Most of the facts stated were also common knowledge among dental officers.

[43] Policy in respect to dental treatment for civilian employees in the ZI was published by 1st ind, SG on Ltr, CG, 9th SvC, to SG, 5 Mar 43. Both the original letter and indorsement have been lost, but the latter is quoted verbatim in History of the Army Denal Corps, 1941–43, Professional Sec, p. 42. HD: 314.7–2 (Dental).

[44] Ltr, SecWar to SG, 14 Sep 42, sub: Medical attention for civilians on foreign military missions. SG: 703.1.

[45] 1st ind, TAG, 3 Oct 42, on Ltr, TAG from CO, Sta Hosp, Ft. Lewis, Wash. 21 Sep 42, sub: Dental treatment for Red Cross personnel. SG: 703.1 (Ft. Lewis) N.

missing teeth permitted. Overseas, Red Cross personnel were entitled to all types of dental care without cost.[46]

AUTHORIZED DENTAL TREATMENT

Extent of Authorized Treatment

In deciding what care should be provided military personnel, the Dental Division had to compromise between what was theoretically desirable and what was possible with the maximum resources available. Such operations as the replacement of single missing teeth with fixed bridgework, the treatment of pulpless teeth, the restoration of anteriors with porcelain jacket crowns, and the construction of full-cast, precision-attachment partial dentures could of course be defended as good dentistry, but the expenditure of time on such procedures could not be justified while other soldiers suffered from oral sepsis or were threatened with the loss of additional teeth from rapidly progressing caries. It was therefore necessary to limit the care provided by following the principle of "the greatest good for the greatest number," with primary attention to those conditions which affected the health of the individual or which would result in permanent damage if neglected.

In 1940 the United States was not involved in actual hostilities, and it was expected that inductees would return to civilian life after one year of training. Also, these inductees were required to meet minimum standards of dental health before they were called to active duty. The Dental Division therefore felt that it was both unnecessary and unwise to attempt, in a short time, the complete dental rehabilitation of every individual entering the service in a temporary status. In October 1940 the attitude of the Director of the Dental Division was expressed as follows:[47]

> Under no circumstances is it believed desirable to set up a policy requiring that every man drafted into the Army receive complete dental attention to place him in class IV.... It is believed that it is only right that we should adopt a policy that any Reserve Officer or draftee or National Guard personnel in the Army for a period of one year's training is not to receive dental service replacing teeth lost prior to his entrance into the military service, except in the case of dental pathology involving other teeth or oral tissue where the replacement is necessary to maintain health. In other words, a man who has been able to carry on his business or hold a job in civilian life with

---

[46] Authority for the outpatient dental care of Red Cross personnel overseas has proved impossible to document. Such treatment was obviously essential and to the personal knowledge of the author who served in two theaters, it was rendered without question, but files of The Adjutant General or The Surgeon General fail to reveal any clear-cut reference to the subject. In a telephone interview of 21 August 47, Miss Jeanette Ross of the Insular and Foreign Hospital Service, National Headquarters, Red Cross, stated that it was her understanding that Red Cross employees were authorized hospitalization under AR 40–590, that 40–505 approved medical attention for anyone hospitalized under 40–590, and that AR 40–510 in turn provided for dental attendance for anyone hospitalized under AR 40–505. If strictly interpreted, however, even this complicated series of regulations does not specifically authorize outpatient dental care for Red Cross personnel overseas. It appears that this was a situation where no formal objection was ever raised or a specific directive published.

[47] See footnote 38, p. 207.

his mouth in a neglected state cannot and should not anticipate that a complete and perfect dental service will be given him in the Army, placing his mouth in perfect condition when he would not have gone to the expense to secure such service had he remained in civilian life.

On the basis of this opinion, The Surgeon General recommended to The Adjutant General that dental attendance for temporary personnel be limited to the treatment of emergency conditions, the filling of cavities with routine materials, and the replacement of teeth lost in the performance of duty or as a necessary part of treatment.[48] The Adjutant General disapproved this recommendation, however, because it was against War Department policy to distinguish in any way between temporary and permanent personnel.[49] The Surgeon General then agreed to make the proposed restrictions applicable to all Army personnel [50] and the following policy was published by the Office of The Adjutant General (AGO) on 14 January 1941: [51]

 a. Dental attendance for all military personnel will be confined to the treatment of emergency cases, infectious conditions, and the restoration of carious teeth with amalgam, silicate, or cement fillings, except as provided in b below.

 b. Replacement of missing teeth will not be made, except when teeth were damaged or lost in the performance of duty, while engaged in athletic games, or as a necessary part of treatment. Such replacements will be the standard type of partial or full dentures provided for Army personnel.

 c. Dental attendance for dependents will be limited to emergency treatment. Such treatment will interfere in no instance with the routine dental treatment of military personnel.

With the lowering of dental standards in February 1942, large numbers of men entered the service whose teeth did not meet minimum requirements for health, and it became necessary to remove some of the restrictions against the construction of dentures. On 8 April 1942 the Director of the Dental Division recommended that subparagraph (b) of the aforementioned letter be amended to read as follows: [52]

 Replacement of missing teeth for military personnel will be made when in the opinion of the dental surgeon it is necessary from a health or functional standpoint; that is, insufficient natural or artificial teeth to satisfactorily masticate the Army ration. Such replacements will be the standard type of full or partial dentures provided in the Army, except that anterior teeth lost in line of duty may be replaced by fixed bridgework when in the opinion of the dental surgeon it is advisable. This type of replacement is to be kept at a minimum consistent with the best interests of the Government and the individual.

This change was published verbatim in an AGO letter of 25 April 1942.[53]

---
[48] Ltr, Exec Off, SGO, to TAG, 30 Nov 40, sub: Dental service during the national emergency. SG: 703.1.
[49] 1st ind, 26 Dec 40, TAG on ltr cited in footnote 48, p. 211.
[50] 2d ind, 3 Jan 41, SG on ltr cited in footnote 48, p. 211.
[51] See footnote 39, p. 208.
[52] Memo, Brig Gen R. H. Mills for Gen McAfee, 8 Apr 42. SG: 703.-1.
[53] Ltr, TAG to CGs all CAs and Depts, COs of Exempted Stas, 25 Apr 42, sub: Dental service during and for six months after the war. AG: 703.1.

Limitations on the construction of fixed bridges were still further liberalized by a War Department directive of March 1945 providing that "A fixed bridge may be inserted in the anterior segment, in limited cases, as a morale or functional factor in those instances where extraction has caused a disfiguring space." [54]

Under the terms of War Department policy every soldier was authorized all the care necessary to preserve dental health, though the single missing tooth of one patient would not be replaced as long as other men had insufficient teeth for proper mastication, nor would an inlay be supplied at an expenditure of time that might better be used to save several teeth with standard amalgam fillings.

Quality of Treatment Rendered

Though expensive and time-consuming operations were not authorized when simpler procedures would be effective, the Dental Division consistently demanded that treatment rendered in Army dental clinics be of the highest quality. This policy was partly altruistic in that it was felt that the soldier was entitled to care at least as good as he would receive in civilian life; it was partly selfish because it was believed that work of high quality would prove most economical of both time and money. The attitude of the Dental Division was expressed in the Army Medical Bulletin as follows: [55]

> There is no substitute for quality in the service rendered the soldier by the Army Dental Corps. The Dental Division has on many occasions emphasized that, above all, quality and not quantity is the real objective of the dental service in every hospital, camp or post. There are times and situations which demand an extended effort on the part of the dental officer to complete a certain assignment, but regardless of the circumstances, the dental service cannot afford to be jeopardized by permitting inferior work to leave the dental clinic.

Only standard, high-grade materials were furnished dental clinics, and gold was available when the more common items were not satisfactory. Dentures were normally made of acrylic resin, with gold bars and clasps when required. No charge was made for special materials or treatment, and the practice of having military personnel pay civilian laboratory costs, except in extreme emergency, was specifically prohibited.[56] Surgical procedures were carried out by qualified personnel with due attention to asepsis, and the incidence of infections following oral surgery was very small.[57] Officers with special qualifications were also designated as prosthodontists in all the larger installations. Teeth which could be saved in a healthy condition were not extracted, and the

---

[54] TB Med 148, Mar 1945.
[55] Dental service-accepted procedures no experimentation. Bulletin of the U. S. Army Medical Department 82 : 20, Nov 1944 (cited hereafter as Army Medical Bulletin).
[56] Ltr, SG to CGs, SvCs, 26 Nov 42, sub: Prosthetic dental appliances. SG : 703.1.
[57] Control of dental infections. Army Medical Bulletin 69 : 33, Oct 1943.

number of teeth replaced during the war exceeded the number lost.[58] Liberal use of protective bases under deep fillings was encouraged, but very little root-canal treatment was attempted, both because of the time required and because of the risk that a later acute infection might incapacitate the soldier when he could not get dental care. Only a limited amount of porcelain work was done, though anterior jacket crowns were routinely provided after the acrylic resins became available.

With the exception of hygienists and x-ray technicians, only officers of the Dental Corps were permitted to work on patients at the chair. Army regulations provided that in the absence of a dental officer, medical officers might render dental care "to the extent that their training and skill justify," but such treatment was very rarely given.[59] It was specifically directed that "except as otherwise prescribed . . . the selection of professional procedures to be followed in each case, including the use of special dental materials, will be left to the judgement of the dental officer concerned." [60]

It was especially directed that the soldier would not be used as a guinea pig for testing untried procedures.[61]

Of the 15,000 dentists on duty there were inevitably a few who failed to attain expected standards. There were also a few who mistakenly tried to set records for quantities of work completed, without due regard for quality. As these situations came to the attention of higher authority, men of the first type were placed under responsible supervision or relieved from duty; those of the second were informed that high production, without quality, was not the route to advancement in the Dental Corps.

But while the quality of Army dentistry was generally satisfactory, the amount supplied during the first part of the war was the subject of some critical comment. Due to supply difficulties, and to the enormous accumulation of untreated defects in the civilian population, the Dental Service had to defer a considerable amount of elective treatment during the period of rapid mobilization, before dental facilities reached peak strength. The Director of the Dental Division admitted that: [62]

> The Army Dental Corps has accepted the most momentous job in the history of dentistry, since one man in every four, when inducted, is in a dental state which requires emergency treatment. . . . Time is the biggest handicap since men must be ready and trained in a few months. Then, about three out of every four boys had little dental attention prior to entrance into the service, and about one-half rarely went to

---

[58] Exact figures on the number of teeth replaced are not available, but if the reasonable assumption is made that an average of 8 teeth were replaced by each partial denture, a total of 18,000,000 teeth were supplied soldiers from Jan 1942 through Aug 1945. In the same period 15,000,000 teeth were extracted.

[59] See footnote 31, p. 205.

[60] Ibid.

[61] Accepted dental therapeutics and procedures. Army Medical Bulletin 69: 14, Oct 1943.

[62] 1st ind, SG, 10 Oct 43, on Ltr, Mrs. Walter R. Agard to Gen George C. Marshall, 29 Sep 43. SG: 703.1.

the dentist. . . . It is humanly impossible to complete all of the dental work for all of the inductees.

This statement should not be interpreted to mean that the dental health of military personnel suffered because of their induction into the Army. It merely confirms the knowledge acquired during the World War II period that, in the event of any future mobilization, the Dental Service should not promise the complete dental rehabilitation of every soldier until it has adequate information on the dental needs of inductees, and on the factors which may affect its own ability to mobilize a large number of dentists in a limited time.

The Dental Corps was also accused of being more interested in extracting than saving teeth. This impression was probably gained during mobilization when the first objective was to make men fit for military duties, necessitating the extraction of large numbers of septic or nonrestorable teeth. As any dentist or physician knows, the worst dental infections, chronic in nature, are often painless, and it is easy to understand how soldiers might assume that symptomless teeth had needlessly been extracted. One criticism which came to the attention of The Surgeon General was answered as follows: [63]

> It is the opinion of this office that Dr. . . . has not been correctly informed as to the constructive dentistry now being accomplished by the Dental Corps. . . . A ratio of approximately 27 permanent fillings to every tooth extracted was established during the month (May 1942). The dental reports for the armed forces for the month of May show that conservative constructive dentistry is carried out in every Army dental clinic. Since the lowering of dental requirements for inductees has been in effect, an enormous amount of work has devolved upon the Dental Corps, and many of the men now being inducted into the military establishment present oral conditions which require extensive treatment, and the extraction of many badly broken down teeth.

Qualified civilian dental consultants reported that in general the treatment rendered in the Army met the accepted standards of the American dental profession. The editor of the Journal of the American Dental Association stated in April 1944 that: [64]

> . . . a beneficial result from the preventive and corrective dental program now in operation in the Army and Navy will be that an enormous number of men heretofore dentally deficient will be rehabilitated for military service and a large percentage of them will return from war in improved physical condition as a result of improvement in dental health.

The attitude of enlisted men toward the dental service was not as favorable as the quality of the treatment rendered seemed to justify. In October 1942, 5,538 enlisted men in the AGF and AAF answered questions concerning the medical and dental service as follows: [65]

---

[63] Ltr, SG to Hon. Clyde L. Herring, 20 Jul 42. SG: 703.–1.
[64] Is the Dental Corps meeting its obligations to the Armed Forces? J. Am. Dent. A. 31: 537–540, Apr 1944.
[65] Attitude of enlisted men toward medical, dental, and hospital services, among white enlisted men forming a cross section of Ground Forces and Air Forces, 2 Nov 42. Research Div, Office of Armed Forces Information and Education.

OPERATION OF THE DENTAL SERVICE 215

Question: "Do you think good medical (dental) care is provided by the Army?"

	Yes percent	No percent	Can't decide percent	No reply percent
Medical	80	5	14	1
Dental	68	9	19	4

Question: "Do you think Army dentists try as hard as civilian dentists to keep from hurting their patients?"

Yes percent	No percent	Can't decide percent	No reply percent
44	27	24	5

Question: "Do Army dentists prefer to pull teeth rather than fill them?"

Yes percent	No percent	Can't decide percent	No reply percent
22	45	31	2

Later surveys in England and Alaska showed an even smaller percentage completely satisfied with the dental service, though in all of these studies except the one listed previously the dental service was preferred over the medical service.[66][67] Some of this dissatisfaction was based on general discontent and the normal tendency of the soldier to "gripe." Much of it was based on hearsay rather than personal experience for the percentage who thought that the dental service was good was much higher among men who had actually been patients. Nevertheless, too many enlisted patients had grave doubts concerning the Army dentist's use of the forceps and his humanitarian qualities. More detailed analysis of specific complaints showed that most men felt the end results of treatment were excellent, but they apparently believed that the military practitioner lacked a personal interest in his patient, that he tended to be rough, and that it was sometimes hard to get desired care.

The enlisted patient, lacking the professional knowledge on which to base an informed evaluation of his dental treatment, attached an understandable importance to details which the dental officer considered unimportant. The dentist tended to regard the patient as "another Class II," to be rehabilitated as rapidly as possible, with a minimum of nonessential conversation or explanation; the patient, on the other hand, felt that the situation called for a more sympathetic attitude. There is every evidence that conscientious, careful treatment was the rule in Army dental installations, but it also seems certain that the patient was not made to realize this clearly. Since the soldier's whole attitude toward the Army may be colored by his opinion of the medical care

[66] European Survey No. 17, Dec 1943, of a cross section of men in lettered infantry companies in a division in training in England. Research Div, Office of Armed Forces Information and Education.

[67] Report No. 12, Morale Services Division, Research Unit, Headquarters, Alaskan Department, Aug 1944. Research Div, Office of Armed Forces Information and Education.

he receives, it seems that this factor should be given attention in the event of a future mobilization.

THE PROSTHETIC SERVICE IN WORLD WAR II

Period Prior to World War II

Prior to the First World War, military personnel were expected to have sufficient teeth for mastication when they entered the service. If replacements later became necessary they had to be obtained by the individual. Regulations published in 1916 authorized restorations at Government expense. This, however, applied only to those individuals whose teeth had been lost by traumatic injury in line of duty. Prior approval of a department surgeon or of The Surgeon General was required in each instance and materials had to be obtained by special request to a medical supply depot.[68]

With the entry of the United States into the First World War, however, large numbers of men in poor dental condition were drafted into the Army and more adequate provision had to be made for the construction of prosthetic appliances. After May 1917[69] complete laboratory equipment was issued to the larger installations. In October 1917 The Surgeon General authorized dental officers in base hospitals, general hospitals, and certain larger camps, to repair bridges or dentures for men originally accepted with these appliances and to construct new restorations for soldiers for whom such work was considered essential by a regimental surgeon or dental surgeon. In March 1918 this regulation was further liberalized to permit the replacement, in time of war only, of any teeth essential to mastication. In time of peace, restoration was still to be restricted to teeth lost by traumatic injury in line of duty.

After March 1919 teeth lost otherwise than by traumatic injury in line of duty could also be replaced by the Army but no gold or other precious metals could be expended on these appliances.[70] In October 1920 it was provided that gold could be used for:[71]

> Replacements for teeth lost by traumatic injury in line of duty, in peace or war.
> Partial dentures requiring gold clasps for their retention.
> Repair of crowns or bridges which were originally necessary to establish eligibility of an enlisted man for entry into the service.
> Routine inlays, crowns, or bridges for officers and nurses and for enlisted men with at least 5 years service.

Finally, in 1925, the use of any prosthetic material was authorized for any person entitled to receive dental care at Government expense, including the dependents of military personnel.[72]

---

[68] Manual for the Medical Department. Washington, Government Printing Office, 1916, p. 261.
[69] The Medical Department of the United States Army in the World War. Washington, Government Printing Office, 1928, vol III, p. 611 (cited hereafter as The Medical Department . . . in the World War).
[70] SG Ltr 126, 6 Mar 19.
[71] SG Ltr 129, 27 Oct 20.
[72] SG Ltr 9, 6 Feb 25.

Prior to 1927, prosthetic appliances for soldiers were generally completed by small laboratories in the individual station dental clinics. In these a single assistant often worked on cases under construction whenever he could be spared from other duties. The dental officer commonly had to exercise close supervision over all procedures even if he was not required to do the work personally. Very little organization was possible and technicians were expected to perform all operations, yet men sufficiently skilled to pour up impressions, set teeth, fabricate gold skeletons, and polish the completed dentures were seldom attracted by the wages offered in the Army. As a result, dental officers wasted much time and effort in work which the civilian dentist routinely delegated to trained auxiliary personnel.

In 1927 central dental laboratories (CDL) were established at the Army Medical Center, Walter Reed General Hospital; Letterman General Hospital; and the Station Hospital, Fort Sam Houston.[73] During calendar year 1933 another was installed at Corozal in the Panama Canal Zone, but the laboratory at Fort Sam Houston was closed for lack of personnel while the one at Letterman General Hospital produced only 38 cases.[74] At the end of fiscal year 1935 only the Army Medical Center CDL remained in effective operation.[75] At the same time, however, it was announced that a plan for expanding central dental laboratory facilities was under consideration. By the end of fiscal year 1937 the CDL at Fort Sam Houston was again functioning and another had been established at Fort Clayton in the Panama Canal Zone. On 16 March 1938 The Surgeon General announced a general plan for initiating central dental laboratory service on a large scale [76] and a War Department circular of 16 September 1938 stated further that CDL's would be established in Washington, D. C.; Atlanta, Ga.; St. Louis, Mo.; San Antonio, Tex.; and San Francisco, Calif.[77] By January 1939 all the new CDL's were in operation except the one at St. Louis, completion of which was delayed until July.[78][79] Two subcentral laboratories were also established—at Beaumont General Hospital in El Paso, Tex., and at Fitzsimons General Hospital in Denver, Colo.[80]

All the CDL's except the one in Washington functioned under the control of the respective corps area commanders, but personnel were assigned by The Surgeon General and it was specifically provided that technicians would not

---

[73] Annual Report of The Surgeon General, U. S. Army, 1927. Washington, Government Printing Office, 1927, p. 241 (cited hereafter as Annual Report . . . Surgeon General).

[74] Annual Report . . . Surgeon General, 1934. Washington, Government Printing Office, 1934, p. 163.

[75] Annual Report . . . Surgeon General, 1935. Washington, Government Printing Office, 1935, p. 156.

[76] SG Ltr 9, 16 Mar 38.

[77] WD Cir 53, 16 Sep 38.

[78] Central dental laboratories. The Dental Bulletin, supp. to The Army Medical Bulletin 10: 30, Jan 1939.

[79] Ibid.

[80] Annual Report . . . Surgeon General, 1939. Washington, Government Printing Office, 1939, p. 200.

be used for other duties except in case of urgent emergency. The standard allotment of personnel was set at 2 officers, 1 staff sergeant, 1 sergeant, 2 privates first class, and 2 privates. Extra men and higher ratings were authorized for the CDL at the Army Medical Center, where vitallium cases were constructed.[81]

By the beginning of World War II a central dental laboratory system had thus become well established.

Policies Concerning the Provision of Prosthetic Treatment, World War II

Another major problem which confronted the Dental Service in World War II was the determination of the extent to which it should attempt to provide prosthetic appliances for inductees. Previously this question had been left to the judgment of individual officers, but with the enormous increase in requirements incident to mobilization a more definite policy was necessary. The first directive on this subject was issued by the AGO in January 1941. At that time inductees were expected to be in the Army for only one year, and they were required to meet at least minimum dental standards at the time they entered training. The Dental Division, SGO, felt that it was neither feasible nor necessary to undertake the complete rehabilitation of almost a million men a year when it was expected that most of them would revert to civilian status almost as soon as treatment could be completed. Therefore, the amount of prosthetic treatment to be rendered was limited by the order of 14 January 1941 (see page 211, subparagraph b).

By April 1942 the situation had changed radically. The United States was in the war, inductees were in the Army for the "duration," and dental standards for induction had been lowered to admit men who would require extensive replacements before they could perform their military duties. To meet these new conditions a more liberal dental care policy was established by AGO directive of 25 April 1942 (see page 211) and a subsequent War Department directive of March 1945 (see page 212).[82][83]

For all practical purposes, the interpretation of these directives was again left to the individual dentist. An attempt was generally made to apply the peacetime standard for enlistment which provided that a man with less than 3 posterior teeth above and below in occlusion, and 3 anteriors above and below in occlusion, was not fitted for service. However, one meeting these minimum requirements might actually be a dental cripple. Also the decision in any doubtful case might depend to a considerable degree upon intangible personal factors. One man would wear a denture which was necessary only to preserve the health of the remaining teeth; another would not. One would feel the need of a replacement when only a few teeth were missing; another would wear an

---
[81] SG Ltr 1, 2 Jan 40.
[82] See footnote 53, p. 211.
[83] See footnote 54, p. 212.

appliance only after all his posterior teeth and most of his anteriors had been lost. An SGO circular letter of 22 June 1943 attempted to clarify the situation, but after calling attention to certain fundamental considerations it left the principal responsibility just where it had been before, on the individual dental officer.[84] No rigid formula was found to be universally applicable in World War II and it is doubtful if any fixed standard could ever prove entirely satisfactory.

In view of the difficulty in determining which cases should receive dental replacements it is not surprising that military personnel were sometimes furnished dentures which subsequently rested in a barracks bag or footlocker. One separation center reported that about 1 percent of the men discharged after less than 6 months' service were classified "I–D" (needing prosthetic appliances) but were found, on investigation, to have been provided replacements which they were not wearing. Of the men discharged after more than 6 months' service approximately 4½ percent neglected to wear the dentures which had been supplied them.[85] If we accept the estimate that 10 percent of all military personnel had been provided with dentures, the findings of this separation center indicate that some 40 percent of those for whom appliances had been constructed did not wear them. This figure is admittedly based on a small sample and must be considered highly tenuous; the actual proportion may have been much smaller. But is cannot be said that the dentures which were not worn were "unnecessary" since in most cases their use would have prevented further damage to mouths already partly crippled.

Experience has shown, however, that the policy of relative liberality in authorizing dental replacements, applied reasonably, was in the best interest of all concerned even though some men undoubtedly failed to wear the dentures provided them. The great benefit to the large number who did, justified the extra effort involved. Further, the knowledge that teeth lost would subsequently be replaced, instilled in the soldier a greater confidence in the efforts of the Dental Service.

Requirements for Prosthetic Service as Revealed by Wartime Experience

During the period of hostilities (1942–1945 inclusive) 109 dentures, 32 denture repairs, and 8 bridges were completed *each year* for each 1,000 men. This average rate was far from constant, however, and actual yearly output from 1938 through 1945 varied as follows: [86] [87] [88]

---

[84] SG Ltr 114, 22 Jun 43.

[85] Information on 7,469 men separated at an unspecified separation center from Nov 1944 through 16 Mar 45. Given to Lt Col John C. Brauer by Maj Gen Robert H. Mills, 27 Mar 45. SG : 703.

[86] Figures from 1938–40 taken from annual reports of The Surgeon General for those years.

[87] Data for 1941–43 taken from: A history of The Army Dental Corps, 1941–1943, Professional Service Section. HD: 314.7–2 (Dental).

[88] Figures for 1944–45 calculated by author from data in the files of the Dental Division, SGO.

Prosthetic Operations per 1,000 Men Per Year

Year	Dentures	Dentures repaired	Bridges
1938	36.6	12.1	7.2
1939	41.9	13.8	6.7
1940	26.1	9.1	4.8
1941	14.1	5.1	2.2
1942	45.4	12.6	3.6
1943	125.0	23.8	5.8
1944	129.6	40.0	11.3
1945	96.1	40.0	13.1

The cited figures cannot be interpreted to mean that the need for prosthetic appliances was low in 1940, 1941, and 1942, and high in 1943, 1944, and 1945. The small output of 1941–1942 represented inadequate capacity, which in turn was due mainly to lack of equipment and trained technicians. With the start of mobilization in 1940 the laboratories were unable to increase their facilities to keep pace with the increase in the strength of the Army, and production did not again reach even the per capita rates of 1938–1939 until 1942. In this same period very few bridges were constructed since only the more urgent cases could be handled and the proportion of full dentures to partial dentures was much higher than in the later years of the war.

Improvements in the supply and personnel situation in 1943 made it possible for the prosthetic service to meet current needs and also to start reduction of the accumulated backlog of prosthetic treatment, so that the per capita output of dental appliances reached a figure many times that of the prewar average. At the same time, the number of bridges constructed increased rapidly and the proportion of partial dentures to full dentures approximately doubled, showing that less urgent cases were receiving attention. By 1945, the backlog of treatment accumulated earlier in the war had been substantially depleted and the demand for new dentures began to fall off. Requirements for denture repairs remained high, however, due to the large number of appliances in use, and the high proportion of bridges constructed showed that more optional treatment was being provided as the need for urgent replacements diminished. Unfortunately, pending a detailed study of individual medical records there is no way to break down the preceding figures into requirements for initial rehabilitation and requirements for annual maintenance care.

During the war about 2,566,000 dentures were constructed for military personnel.[89] Since 38 percent of all patients received 2 appliances, about 1,860,000 patients were given dentures. If there had been no replacement of broken, lost, or unsatisfactory prostheses, this would have meant that 19 percent of all soldiers wore artificial replacements. The Dental Division ac-

---

[89] Information compiled by author from monthly reports of dental service on file in the Dental Division, SGO.

tually estimated that 15 percent of all military personnel wore prosthetic devices,[90] but since loss and breakage were inevitably high under wartime conditions, it seems probable that the proportion of men wearing dentures at any one time was somewhat less than that estimated. If 50 percent of all dentures were replaced during the war, the proportion of soldiers wearing these would have been closer to 10 percent, a figure which corresponds more closely with the few available reports from tactical units.

Of the appliances constructed for one group of 107,542 patients in 1943, 17.0 percent were full uppers, 7.4 percent full lowers, 37.5 percent partial uppers, and 38.1 percent partial lowers.[91] Thirty-eight percent of all patients required more than one appliance. These figures were accumulated early in the war, however, and the later trend was toward fewer full dentures and more partial dentures. During 1942, the proportion of partial dentures to full dentures was 2.1;[92] later a more liberal attitude was adopted and in January 1944, 4.4 partial dentures were being supplied for each full denture.[93] The average ratio over the 4 years 1942–1945 was 3.5 partial replacements for each full denture.[94]

The evidence of World War II experience was clear on one point: During a mobilization the need for prosthetic service may be expected to increase out of all proportion to the increase in the strength of the Army. From the end of 1940 to the end of 1943 the strength of the Army increased by about 1,105 percent;[95] during the same period the number of prosthetic cases completed per month increased nearly 5,600 percent, or 5.1 times the increase in the strength of the Army. The number of dentures supplied each 1,000 men in 1944 was 3.5 times the number supplied in 1938.[96] Though some increase had been expected because of lowered dental standards, it certainly was not foreseen that a thousand inductees would require approximately four times as many prosthetic appliances as an equal number of men in the peacetime establishment.

Professional Standards of the Prosthetic Service

Certain "luxury" types of denture service, such as full-cast gold appliances, cast-base full dentures, and those involving the use of special attachments were obviously out of place in the wartime prosthetic service. However, every effort was made to provide soldiers with replacements which met the standards of ethical civilian practice. Materials employed were of the highest quality and included all of the commonly accepted types. The usual partial denture was constructed on an acrylic resin base, with assembled gold clasps and a gold

---

[90] Final Rpt for ASF, Logistics in World War II. HD: 319.1–2 (Dental).
[91] See footnote 87, p. 219.
[92] Army reveals data on denture construction. J. Am. Dent. A. 15 Aug 45, p. 1080.
[93] Ibid.
[94] Calculation by author from monthly reports in the files of the Dental Division, SGO.
[95] Strength of the Army, 1 Mar 46.
[96] Calculation by author from monthly reports in the files of the Dental Division, SGO.

lingual bar. Cast gold and vitallium dentures were available when no other materials would be satisfactory, though their use was kept to a minimum. Little ceramic work was done in Army laboratories but acrylic resin was used in the construction of crowns and bridges when indicated. Whenever possible, specially skilled dentists were put in charge of the prosthetic service, and laboratories operated under the close supervision of full-time dental officers. Each model sent to a laboratory was surveyed and the necessary replacement designed by a dentist before being turned over to a technician.

No attempt was made to prescribe any uniform technique for taking impressions or constructing dentures. So long as acceptable standards were maintained each dental officer was free to use the methods with which he was familiar. However, inferior models and registrations were sometimes received in the laboratories, and certain generally recognized requirements were therefore established by directives published in July 1943 and March 1945.[97] [98] These did not state *how* results were to be attained, but did prescribe certain essential objectives (e. g. all full denture impressions to be muscle-trimmed, relations to be taken with well-fitted bite rims, etc.).

Prosthetic consultants reported that in general the dentures constructed by the Army met all requirements for health, comfort, function, and appearance. In isolated instances, however, the overwhelming demand for prosthetic service and the need for completing cases in a limited period resulted in the adoption of methods which left much to be desired. Such practices as the use of acrylic resin in place of gold lingual bars, the use of one-armed clasps, and soldering clasps on the same model which was later to be used for vulcanization were rare, but sufficiently frequent to warrant some criticism.[99] Dentures were occasionally inserted before the ridges had become reasonably stabilized after extractions, though the dental surgeon usually had no choice but to supply a replacement to a soldier who would soon leave for an active theater, even when he was certain that the appliance would have a short useful life.[100] Since these difficulties were due in large part to such factors as inadequate dental care for the civilian population and inability to obtain equipment during the early part of the war, it is surprising that they were not more common. On the other hand, the fact that they existed, even temporarily, emphasized the importance of planning for an extensive prosthetic service from the start of any future mobilization.

From 1 January 1942 until the end of August 1945, the prosthetic service completed the following operations for military personnel:[101]

---

[97] SG Ltr 128, 17 Jul 43.
[98] See footnote 54, p. 212.
[99] Personal knowledge of the author who was successively the dental surgeon of a replacement training center, an overseas theater, and a large permanent post in the ZI.
[100] Memo, Col Rex McK. McDowell for Exec Off, SGO, 18 Jan 44. SG: 703.–1.
[101] Information assembled by the author from monthly reports in the files of the Dental Division, SGO.

Dentures _____ 2,566,000
Denture repairs _____ 743,000
Bridges _____ 206,500

About 800,000 of the above operations were carried out overseas. An additional 10,300 full dentures, 35,500 partial dentures, and 16,600 denture repairs, were completed for prisoners and nonmilitary personnel.

REFUSAL OF DENTAL TREATMENT

No soldier could refuse dental treatment if failure to correct the dental defect could normally be expected to interfere with the efficient performance of his military duties. A War Department General Order of 31 January 1942 provided that:[102]

> In time of war if a person in the military service refuses to submit to dental or surgical operations or dental, surgical or medical diagnostic procedures or dental or medical treatment, such person will be examined by a board of three medical officers convened by a corps area or department commander or a commander of a base or general hospital, or a commanding officer of any post, camp, or station where there are four or more officers of the Medical Department on duty. If, in the opinion of the board, the operation or diagnostic procedure or medical or dental treatment advised is necessary to enable such person to perform properly his military duties and will normally have such effect, and he persists in his refusal after being notified of the findings of the board, he may be tried by court martial.

In practice, it was seldom necessary to apply the provisions of this order, but it recognized that a soldier had no right to maintain a condition which might damage his health or make him unavailable in some future emergency.

"QUOTA" DENTISTRY

A persistent problem of the Dental Service during the first part of the war was the tendency of dental surgeons to prescribe daily quotas of operations to be performed by their subordinates. The plans proposed ranged from a simple requirement that each dental officer complete from 10 to 30 fillings a day, to ingenious schemes under which the dentist received "points" of credit for each different operation, with a minimum total established for the day's work. The pressure on the dental clinics, especially in the camps which were preparing men for duty overseas, was so formidable that it is not surprising that heads of clinics sometimes fell back on desperate measures to speed treatment. The Dental Division did not minimize the need for maximum output of all clinics, but the defects of any quota system were so serious that all such plans were disapproved individually and in principle. Among these defects the following were most important:

---

[102] WD GO 8, 31 Jan 42.

1. The dentist who produced superior work was made to appear inferior to the careless operator.

2. Dentists varied greatly in the speed with which they normally operated. If a moderate quota was set the fast operator might reduce his output, feeling that he was expected to accomplish no more than the prescribed average. The slow operator could increase his speed only at the expense of quality.

3. When too high quotas were established the conscientious dental officer, who required no spur, became discouraged and apathetic. The lazy operator could easily take refuge in such practices as falsifying records, selecting only the smallest cavities for attention, polishing old fillings to make them appear new, and generally doing slipshod work.

The Dental Division wanted to handle the question of quota dentistry with as little publicity as possible and no specific prohibition against it was ever published, but repeated statements of policy in respect to "quality versus quantity" could have left no doubt of its official position. The War Service Committee of the American Dental Association reported in November 1944 that: [103]

> It was called to the attention of the committee that, in some Army (and Navy) installations, certain dental officers were required to perform services under a "speed-up" system. These complaints were presented to officials of the armed services in Washington, who stated that they would be thoroughly investigated and, if such practices did exist, they would be discontinued. The officials further stated that this was not the policy of the Corps, which was to encourage quality and not quantity dentistry, and that they would cooperate in every way possible.

The Dental Division went further to condemn even the appearance of quota-setting by registering its disapproval of such schemes as that established by the Control Division, Seventh Service Command, under which the "efficiency" of various hospitals was reported, even though no minimum output was prescribed. This Service Command had determined that a dentist should see 1.58 patients an hour. Using this figure as a norm, it rated the relative production of the various hospitals on the basis of the number of patients actually seen. The response of the Dental Division to this plan was clear and to the point. In a memorandum to the Control Division, SGO, on 12 March 1945, it stated that: [104]

> The principal criterion used in making such an analysis is sittings. A sitting is recorded for every visit to the dental clinic, and with a large turn-over of patients in a hospital it is possible to show a large number of examinations recorded as sittings. Likewise, a post-operative treatment is recorded as a sitting, and an inefficient oral surgeon might have ten (10) post-operative treatments (sittings) when a very competent surgeon could accomplish the same with one POT (sitting). Furthermore, an inefficient dental officer or one who wants to see the total number of sittings high can insert one small filling per appointment (15–20 minutes), when the more efficient operator, who is vitally interested in the patient and the service, would place several fillings which would require an hour or more. Then too, the operator who places a

---

[103] Report of the War Service Committee. J. Am. Dent. A. 15 Nov 44, p. 1551.

[104] Memo, Maj Gen Robert H. Mills for Control Div, SGO, 12 Mar 45, sub: Efficiency of work measurement reports of dental service, general hospitals. SG: 703.–1.

superior filling, produces a superior denture, or who is more considerate of his patient in oral surgery, will require more time with resultant less fillings than the careless, fast, inconsiderate operator.

A method which attempts to evaluate the efficiency of a dental service on sittings is decidedly unfair and impractical. Such a method places a premium on poor work, injudicious consideration of the patient and the service, and will terminate in an inferior quality of dental service. This method, or any method where mathematical figures are employed, leads to false impressions, and the true values cannot be analyzed. Anyone can pile up an impressive figure in sittings, but it is an inaccurate, incomplete, and dangerous criterion to use in determining the efficiency of work measurement. . . .

The Army Dental Corps has been stigmatized wrongly and criticized editorially as being interested only in, and sponsoring, quantity. This office has continually emphasized quality with a full measure of service and duty hours, but never quantity at the expense of quality. Efficiency reports such as those instituted by the Seventh Service Command . . . can only lead to an inferior service and an inadequate evaluation of the dental service.

Recommend that suitable steps be taken to eliminate such unwarranted ratings which deal with mathematical evaluation of the dental service.

Whenever the quota system was reported in operation at any installation, the Dental Division took prompt and vigorous action, usually in the form of a personal letter from the Director, so that the practice was gradually and quietly, but effectively, eliminated.[105]

DENTAL REHABILITATION OF SELECTIVE SERVICE REGISTRANTS BEFORE INDUCTION

World War I

In the First World War, the Preparedness League of American Dentists, operating under the auspices of the National Dental Association, proposed a plan for completing as much dental work as possible for draftees before they were called for active duty. Members of the League pledged themselves to assist in the program on a voluntary basis, without cost to the Government or to the individual, and The Surgeon General and The Provost Marshal General authorized the local boards to refer registrants needing care to the cooperating dentists. By 30 June 1918, 375,000 operations had been carried out by league members [106] and a total of nearly 1,000,000 operations were performed by 1,700 civilian dentists during the entire war.[107]

World War II

During World War II no plan similar to that of the Preparedness League of American Dentists was attempted. In the first place, the Army Dental Corps

---
[105] Statement of Maj Gen Robert H. Mills (Ret) to author, 8 Sep 47.
[106] Annual Report . . . Surgeon General, 1918. Washington, Government Printing Office, 1918, p. 413.
[107] The Medical Department . . . in the World War. Washington, Government Printing Office, 1923, vol I, p. 193.

was much better prepared to assume the burden in 1941. Also, it seems to have been the general opinion of all concerned that the dental rehabilitation of military personnel was a responsibility of the entire nation and was too big a problem to be delegated to any limited group. From the start of the war, however, the American Dental Association offered to cooperate in any matter affecting the dental health of inductees.

In February 1941 Selective Service announced that a Dental Advisory Committee of prominent members of the profession had been appointed "to guide us in all matters pertaining to dentistry." [108] With the assistance of this Committee a tentative plan for the "prehabilitation" of registrants was proposed in July 1941.[109] Initially this plan was very limited in scope, and was designed to accomplish little more than to acquaint dentists with the requirements for military service and encourage them to give special attention to the care of men of military age. Responsibility for obtaining and paying for dental treatment remained with the Selective Service registrant.

On 2 July 1941 a more elaborate program was proposed by the Commission on Physical Rehabilitation, a subcommittee of the Health and Medical Committee of the Federal Security Agency. The principal provisions of this plan were as follows: [110]

1. Congress to appropriate sufficient funds to defray the cost of treatment for men not able or willing to obtain care at their own expense.

2. State and local rehabilitation committees to be formed under the joint auspices of the Federal Security Agency and the Selective Service System. These committees would administer the program in their areas, determine how payment for treatment would be made, and designate the facilities which would render dental care. Private dentists, semipublic clinics or hospitals, or any combination of dental facilities might be utilized.

3. Local Selective Service boards to indicate on examination records whether or not disqualifying defects found were correctible, the registrant to be directed to his own dentist or to a designated agency for treatment. The board would also set a time-limit within which treatment would have to be completed.

The Commission on Physical Rehabilitation recognized that:

> Only a small percentage of the population can afford to pay or will be willing to pay for corrective measures which may make them available for military or industrial service, but which do not as yet interfere with their present civilian occupations. . . . Because of widespread shifting of population during and after the National Emergency, the responsibility is national as well as local. In order to meet the situation realistically it is recommended that Congress enact legislation to defray the cost. . . . Without federal legislation of this nature, it can be predicted that little progress in voluntary rehabilitation is to be expected.

---

[108] Rowntree, L. G.: Dentistry and Selective Service. J. Am. Dent. A. 28: 636–638, Apr 1941.
[109] Plan for the prehabilitation of registrants. J. Am. Dent. A. 28: 1161, Jul 1941.
[110] Report of the Commission on Physical Rehabilitation. J. Am. Dent. A. 28: 1362–1364, Aug 1941.

The Commission stated that:

> ... the alternative to such a program is lower physical standards of eligibility for selective service and compulsory physical rehabilitation after induction into the Army. Action is required along the lines of one or the other of these alternatives, for the present standards of physical eligibility have reduced the nation's reservoir of eligible registrants to a number far lower than had been expected.

In August 1941 the President of the American Dental Association urged consideration of the problem of dental rehabilitation in the following discussion: [111]

> It is well-known, of course, that many registrants under the Selective Service and Training Act of 1940 have been rejected for active military service because of dental defects. The large number of such rejections has been a matter of grave concern to officials of the American Dental Association as well as to our military authorities. A good deal of study has been devoted to the development of a practicable plan through which the correction of dental defects, either before or after the registrant has been examined by his local draft board, can be promoted.
>
> The problem of rehabilitation, in its initial stage, proposed certain questions of a jurisdictional nature in addition to many others. Was a program of rehabilitation to be set up by the Selective Service System or was such a program to be developed by the American Dental Association in consultation with the proper governmental agencies? What types of dental care would be made available under such a program?
>
> By whom and under what conditions was dental care to be provided for a deficient registrant? Was the financial burden of such a rehabilitation program to be borne by the dentist, the registrant himself, the government or the organized profession?

The President of the American Dental Association went on to state that the National Health Program Committee of that organization had been directed to cooperate with the governmental agencies and that the American Dental Association had officially offered its services to the Coordinator of Health, Welfare, and Related Activities in the National Defense Program, to The Surgeon General of the United States Public Health Service, and to the Director of the Selective Service System.

On 3 August 1941 the President of the American Dental Association called a joint meeting of the board of trustees and members of the committees on Dental Preparedness, Legislation, and the National Health Program. After an all-day session this group made the following recommendations: [112]

1. It was believed that dental rehabilitation would be most effectively accomplished by inducting deficient registrants into the Armed Forces under lowered physical standards, necessary treatment to be rendered subsequent to induction by dental officers of the respective services.

2. If a "prehabilitation" program was considered necessary by Selective Service, consideration should be given to a plan similar to that proposed by the Commission on Physical Rehabilitation. If the latter program were

---

[111] Robinson, W. H.: President's Page. J. Am. Dent. A. 28: 1332–1333, Aug 1941.
[112] Program for rehabilitation of registrants rejected for dental defects under the Selective Service Act. J. Am. Dent. A. 28: 1518–1519, Sep 1941.

adopted, however, it was recommended that the state rehabilitation committees contemplated in the proposed plan should be headed by the ranking dental officer in the state government as executive officer and that they should include representatives of the appropriate state agencies, the organized dental profession, and such other groups and agencies as were deemed necessary. The American Dental Association also recommended that the majority of the members of these committees should be dentists nominated by the organized dental profession. Local committees would be organized along similar lines under the jurisdiction of the state committees. Standards of fees, methods of payment, and the designation of the agencies to render treatment would be largely the responsibility of the local committees.

On 9 October 1941, the President told a conference of the Secretary of War, the Chief of Staff, and Selective Service officials, that he desired action to effect the rehabilitation of an estimated 100,000 men with correctible dental defects out of a total of 188,000 rejected.[113] The following day the President announced a program to "salvage" 200,000 men out of 1,000,000 rejected for all causes. He stated that treatment would be made available by the registrant's own dentist or physician, with the cost borne by the Government through funds made available to Selective Service.[114] The President also stated that it was believed that care could be provided by local medical personnel at less cost than by the Armed Forces.

In February 1942 the Selective Service System inaugurated a test rehabilitation program in the states of Maryland and Virginia. From February to September about 300 men received medical care, but reports from the pilot test headquarters did not distinguish between medical and dental cases, so the number of inductees who had dental defects corrected is not known.[115] Average time required for dental cases was 38.5 days.[116] Reports on the cost are conflicting; one official placed the average expense at $54.19,[117] another at $78.00.[118]

The reasons why this test was considered a failure are not clear, but as early as June 1942 General Lewis B. Hershey, Director of the Selective Service System, told the annual meeting of the American Medical Association that "results of the pilot test did not justify the current adoption of a rehabilitation program on a nation-wide basis. . . ."[119] In July 1944 a representative of Selective Service told a Senate Subcommittee on Wartime Health and Education that:

> It appears that dental rehabilitation by the armed forces during the basic training period of personnel offered a more logical method than the slower method contemplated

---

[113] Wells, C. R.: Role of dentistry in the war effort. J. Am. Dent. A. 29: 835–841, May 1942.
[114] Plans for rehabilitation of rejected draftees. J. Am. Dent. A. 28: 1884–1885, Nov 1941.
[115] Ltr, Brig Gen Carlton S. Dargusch to Brig Gen Thomas L. Smith, 5 Dec 46. SG: 702.
[116] Hearings before a subcommittee of the Committee on Education and Labor, United States Senate, Seventy-eighth Congress. Washington, Government Printing Office, 1944, pt. 5.
[117] Ibid.
[118] See footnote 115, above.
[119] Ibid.

in the offices of civilian dentists, particularly since the ranks of civilian dentists were becoming rapidly depleted due to the demand for thousands of dentists by the Armed Forces and the lowering of dental standards made more men available for military service without prior dental rehabilitation.[120]

The Senate Subcommittee itself found that:

> Early in the war, test rehabilitation programs were undertaken by the Selective Service System, but yielded meager results and were abandoned. In sharp contrast to the results of the Selective Service efforts are those of the Army rehabilitation program. Here remarkable success has been achieved. Approximately one and one-half million men with major defects have been inducted and rendered fit for duty, including 1,000,000 men with major dental defects.[121]

It has been hinted, but not specifically stated, that the civilian prehabilitation program was unsatisfactory because:

1. Selective Service was too deeply involved in other matters to be able to devote the time and effort necessary.[122]

2. The time required for treatment in busy civilian offices was too long.[123]

3. Civilian dentists were already working at top capacity and could not accept new patients without neglecting essential civilian needs.[124]

In any event, it seems clear that if the Armed Forces take approximately one-third of the dentists in the country, the remaining dentists will be too busy to assume responsibility for preinduction care of Selective Service registrants.

The poor results attained in the Selective Service test program discouraged further efforts to promote large-scale dental rehabilitation by civilian agencies. The American Dental Association, which had from the first favored rehabilitation by the Army, continued to sponsor a "Victory" program to encourage high school students to maintain dental health on a voluntary basis, but the care of inductees became the sole responsibility of the Armed Forces.

DENTAL CRITERIA FOR OVERSEAS SERVICE

The Dental Service of World War II was organized to provide approximately twice as many dental officers per capita in the United States as were alloted to overseas theaters. This ratio was justified by the obvious fact that it would be more satisfactory to carry on dental rehabilitation during training rather than after the soldier had assumed his military duties in the field. The basic authorization of 1 dentist for each 1,200 men in tactical units was expected to provide only routine maintenance care of troops who were in good dental condition when received into the organization. Un-

---

[120] See footnote 116, p. 228.
[121] 'Report of Senate Committee on Wartime Health and Education. J. Am. Dent. A. 32: 270–284, 1 Mar 45.
[122] See footnote 116, p. 228.
[123] See footnote 116, p. 228.
[124] Ibid.

fortunately, shortages of personnel, equipment, and lack of a definite dental standard for foreign service led to the shipment overseas during 1942 and 1943 of large numbers of men with serious dental defects. The reports of almost all theaters during this period note that their dental facilities were unable to cope with the unexpected demand. The Southwest Pacific Area, for instance, found that up to 80 percent of the men arriving in Australia early in the war needed some form of dental treatment.[125] The Director of Training, ASF, stated as late as May 1943 that ". . . men were still leaving replacement training centers and replacement depots for subsequent shipment overseas prior to the completion of apparently necessary dental work." [126]

On 20 June 1942 the War Department directed that all enlisted men designated for combat units overseas must meet physical standards prescribed in MR 1–9, though limited service categories could be sent to overseas hospitals and other Zone of Interior-type installations.[127] However, this publication was rescinded in November of the same year.[128] In October of 1942 it was provided that nonprogressive dental defects would not bar shipment of officers overseas, implying, though not stating specifically, that other serious dental defects would prevent transfer to a foreign theater.[129] Neither of these directives was sufficiently explicit in respect to dental deficiencies.

On 26 March 1943 War Department Circular No. 85 provided that "all replacements so ordered [overseas] will be mentally and physically qualified for service in an overseas combat theater"; limited service categories were not to be shipped outside the continental United States.[130] A subsequent War Department circular stated that officers were still arriving for overseas shipment with Class I dental conditions and that the provisions of the previous circular were not being complied with, so it would appear that Circular No. 85 was intended to prevent shipment of Class I dental cases overseas. Its very general terms were not always so interpreted, however, and about a month after it was published the Commanding General, AGF, notified the Assistant Chief of Staff G-1 that great difficulty was being experienced because of differences of opinion as to what constituted "dental fitness." He recommended that "definite standards of dental requirements relative to overseas eligibility be established." [131] This recommendation was forwarded to The Surgeon General for comment, and on advice of the Dental Division, The Surgeon General suggested that:

---

[125] See footnote 34, p. 206.
[126] Memo, Brig Gen Walter L. Weible for Brig Gen Robert H. Mills, 13 May 43. SG: 703.
[127] WD Cir 198, 20 Jun 42.
[128] WD Cir 363, 4 Nov 42.
[129] WD Cir 349, 19 Oct 42.
[130] WD Cir 85, 26 Mar 43.
[131] Memo, Maj Theodore R. Pitts, Asst Ground Adj Gen, AGF, for ACofS, G-1, 24 Apr 43, sub: Eligibility of enlisted men as overseas replacements. SG: 702.-1.

OPERATION OF THE DENTAL SERVICE

> ... the following should be accomplished for military personnel prior to departure for staging areas and ports of embarkation for service overseas: "Dental correction of all Class I cases to include those with 'insufficient teeth to masticate the Army ration' as outlined in Change 1, dated September 10, 1942, of AR 40–510 and so far as practical correction of Class II cases." [132]

On 13 May 1943 the Director of Military Personnel, ASF, recommended to the Assistant Chief of Staff G–1 that approximately the same provisions be published as a change to War Department Circular No. 85.[133] This request was disapproved on technical grounds as it was desired to keep War Department Circular No. 85 couched in general terms, with specific requirements on any individual point to be published separately.[134] Definite requirements for dental health of personnel ordered overseas were finally established in "Preparations for Overseas Movement," in August 1943, as follows: [135]

> All necessary dental treatment, from a health and functional standpoint, will be provided troops *prior to their departure from home station.* The following policy will govern dental qualifications for overseas service: dental correction of all Class I cases as outlined in AR 40–510, including Change 1 and, as far as practicable, correction of Class II cases.

The same provisions were essentially repeated in War Department Circular No. 189, published 21 August 1943.[136] These directives remained in effect during the remainder of the war, though a slight modification was made in June 1945 when the suspicion that some men were intentionally destroying their dental appliances to delay shipment caused the War Department to direct that soldiers requiring dentures were not to be withheld from shipments if they had been able to perform their military duties previously and if their history indicated that replacement was not absolutely essential.[137]

It will be noted that the published standard did not make mandatory the completion of all dental treatment. In fact, the Director of the Dental Division stated in September 1943 that it was physically impossible to complete all work prior to shipment.[138] Routine care of nonemergency conditions was to be rendered whenever possible, but a man was not to be kept from shipment overseas for such treatment.

The order directing that essential dental care would be rendered before departure for a combat area was aimed more directly at commanding officers than at dentists. Prior to its publication, unit commanders had been extremely reluctant to release men from training schedules for dental appointments; now

---

[132] 1st ind, SG, 5 May 43, on memo cited in footnote 131.
[133] Memo, Brig Gen Russel B. Reynolds, Dir, Mil Pers Div, SOS, for ACofS, G–1, 13 May 43, sub: Eligibility of enlisted men as overseas replacements. SG: 702.–1.
[134] Memo, R. W. Berry, Exec Off, ACofS, G–1, for TAG, 17 May 43, sub: Eligibility of enlisted men for overseas service. SG: 702.–1.
[135] See footnote 33, p. 206.
[136] WD Cir 189, 21 Aug 43.
[137] WD Cir 196, 30 Jun 45.
[138] Memo, Maj Gen Robert H. Mills for Brig Gen W. L. Weible, 8 Sep 43. [D]

they knew that they would lose the men anyway if the latter did not meet required standards when the unit went overseas, and they vigorously supported the dental surgeon's efforts to provide urgent treatment.

As a result of improvements in dental facilities, and the establishment of definite standards for foreign service, men received as replacements overseas after 1943 were in much better dental condition than those who preceded them. The change was so marked, in fact, that the Southwest Pacific Area, which had claimed that 80 percent of new troops needed dental care, now reported that 85 percent were in Class IV on arrival.[139] In general the shipment of men in poor dental condition ceased to be a serious problem in the latter part of 1943.

USE OF CIVILIAN DENTISTS

The amount of dental care rendered military personnel by civilian dentists during World War II was not important in spite of the fact that such attendance had been authorized, in an emergency, for many years. In October 1925, AR 40-510 provided that when no dental officer was available, emergency civilian dental treatment could be obtained by military personnel on a duty status at Government expense and without prior authority. Routine dental care could be provided with the prior authorization of The Surgeon General.[140] Military personnel on duty overseas without troops could procure civilian dental attendance without prior authority, subject to later approval by The Surgeon General. In July 1942, it was further authorized that personnel on leave or furlough could procure emergency dental care at Government expense.[141]

The cited regulations were not interpreted to authorize civilian dental treatment as a routine procedure when Army facilities were inadequate due to shortages of equipment or personnel, though such an interpretation was possible and it was actually the basis for the use of civilian dental laboratories on a large scale at one stage of the war.

EXCESSIVE LOSS OR DESTRUCTION OF DENTURES

The careless loss or intentional destruction of dentures was an annoying problem throughout the war. Varying circumstances led to this waste of effort and materials. In many cases dentures were lost through simple failure to observe normal precautions in caring for a fragile and expensive appliance. The soldier who daily saw millions of dollars worth of property destroyed was not likely to be impressed with his responsibility for such a small item as a denture. In time of stress the denture often went into a hip pocket, where it suffered irreparable damage when its owner rode in a truck or hit a fox-

---

[139] See footnote 34, p. 206.
[140] AR 40-510, 10 Oct 25.
[141] See footnote 31, p. 205.

hole. Some were lost because soldiers neglected to remove them when they became nauseated on a sea-crossing. Also, since the appliance cost the soldier nothing, he was likely to be very impatient of defects. It was reported that in some cases men discarded dentures if a single tooth was broken because they knew that a new one would be forthcoming without delay.[142] It has also been stated that partial dentures containing gold were occasionally sold in France, where they brought a good price.[143]

Even more serious in its effect on morale was the intentional destruction of dental appliances to avoid dangerous duty or to delay departure for an overseas theater. The Commanding General of the Army Ground Forces stated in April 1943:

> Although it is not possible to obtain positive evidence in any considerable number of cases, this headquarters has observed indications that individual enlisted men in proper dental condition upon departure from Replacement Training Centers have destroyed their dental fittings and rendered themselves unsuitable for overseas shipment, with a view to shirking hazardous duty.[144]

The North African theater reported in January 1944:

> It is impossible to say that men break or lose their dentures intentionally, but the incidence of this type of accident is so high that the suspicion seems warranted.[145]

The Seventh Army, in the Mediterranean area, noted that:

> Accurate figures were not available as to the deliberate loss or breakage of dentures in order to be evacuated from combat, but it was believed that the rate was highest just before and during amphibious operations.[146]

One step recommended to give dental surgeons information on past prosthetic treatment was to record dental appliances in individual service records.[147] The Dental Division did not concur in this plan since it was believed that even with a clear record that a denture had existed, it would be impossible to prove intent in case of loss or destruction.[148] The further course of this recommendation is not certain, but a War Department directive of 1 August 1943 provided that dentures would be listed in the service records of enlisted men going overseas.[149] In October 1943 it was further provided that prosthetic appliances of officers be listed in the Immunization Register.[150] In January 1945 the War

---

[142] The fact that soldiers discarded dentures on slight provocation was reported by the 5th Auxiliary Surgical Group in Europe. This report was seen by the author in 1946 but it was subsequently lost or misplaced. The situation noted has since been confirmed, however, in conversations between the author and numerous senior dental surgeons.

[143] Information from Maj Gen Thomas L. Smith who was dental surgeon in Europe during the war.

[144] See footnote 142, above.

[145] Essential Technical Medical Data Report, Headquarters, North African Theater, 27 Jan 1944. HD: 350.05.

[146] Seventh Army Section, supp. to the Dental History, MTO. HD: 314.7-2.

[147] Ltr, Dental Surg, Sta Hosp, Ft. McDowell, Calif, to TAG, 19 Mar 43, sub: Entry in service record. SG: 703.

[148] 1st ind, Col McDowell, 14 Apr 43, on footnote 147.

[149] See footnote 33, p. 206.

[150] Preparation for overseas movement, 1 Oct 43.

Department finally directed that a record of all prosthetic appliances be entered in the individual's Immunization Register.[151]

Late in 1943 the question of charging military personnel for dental appliances lost through carelessness or intent was brought up by the Army Ground Forces Replacement Depot No. 1, at Fort George G. Meade, Md. This station reported that men who had been given replacements were arriving without them and stated its intention to enter a statement of charges in such cases.[152] At about the same time the Army Service Forces Replacement Depot at Camp Reynolds, Pa., reported that in a recent shipment to that station 18 men were found not to meet dental requirements for overseas duty. Investigation showed that 9 of these men had been supplied dentures within the past 3 months. One had been given his replacement only a few days before. None had any reasonable excuse for the shortage. This station therefore recommended that dentures be entered on the individual soldier's record of personal equipment and that a charge be made in case of negligent loss.[153] On the basis of these recommendations the Commanding General, Army Ground Forces, asked The Adjutant General for an opinion as to the legality of making a charge for dentures and spectacles lost through carelessness. Noting that "There have been cases where it is apparent that enlisted men have wilfully destroyed or wrongfully disposed of dentures and spectacles in order to forestall their shipment overseas" and that "such acts are highly prejudicial to good order and military discipline" AGF recommended that "in the event that soldiers cannot be penalized under present regulations for loss or destruction of the subject items . . . regulations be changed so that punitive action may be sustained, at least to the extent of requiring enlisted men to pay for such losses."[154] The Adjutant General referred the matter to The Surgeon General for comment and the latter stated that in the opinion of his Legal Division dentures and spectacles became the personal property of the soldier and that there was no basis for a charge even if the man deliberately destroyed the appliances. He stated further that his Office would be opposed to establishing property accountability for dentures since it was believed that the procedures involved would be too cumbersome to justify the effort. The Surgeon General recommended, as an alternative, that court martial action be taken to punish offenders.[155] The Adjutant General concurred in the recommendations of The Surgeon General and notified the Commanding General, AGF, that men could not be charged for destroyed dental appliances.[156] In March 1944 a Bulletin

---

[151] WD Cir 32, 27 Jan 45.

[152] Ltr, CG, AGF Replacement Depot No 1, Ft. George G. Meade, Md, to CG, AGF, 5 Nov 43, sub: Replacement of dentures and spectacles. SG: 413.75–2 (Ft. George G. Meade).

[153] Ltr, Hq, ASF Replacement Depot, Camp Reynolds, Pa, to TAG, 12 Nov 43, sub: Issue of dentures and corrective appliances to replacements. SG: 220.31–1 (Camp Reynolds).

[154] 1st ind. CG, AGF, 2 Dec 43, on ltr cited in footnote 152, above.

[155] Ltr, Chief, Oprs Br, SGO, to Enlisted Br, AGO, 15 Jan 44, sub: Replacement of dentures and spectacles. SG: 413.75–2 (Ft. George G. Meade).

[156] 2d ind, TAG, 22 Feb 44, on ltr cited in footnote 152, above.

of The Judge Advocate General's Office confirmed the opinion of the Legal Division, SGO, that military personnel could not be charged for dental appliances under existing regulations.[157]

As a result of the above opinions no further attempt was made to penalize soldiers for the loss or destruction of dental appliances. It was true that a man could be tried for such action, but the burden of proof was on the prosecution and the very nature of the offense was such that no matter how strong the presumptive evidence it was practically impossible to prove intent to the degree required for conviction before a court martial.

The chief of the Operations Service, SGO, suggested in 1944 that port medical officers should hold as few men as possible for the replacement of dentures;[158] and a War Department circular of June 1945 provided that Class I dental patients who needed only replacement of missing teeth would not be held back when they had previously performed their military duties satisfactorily and if their history indicated that restoration was not necessary.[159] In May 1944 it was directed that all dentures would carry the names and serial numbers of their owners, partly to assist in the return of lost appliances and partly to aid in identification of the patient in case of accident.[160] All of these measures did not greatly deter the few men who were inclined to use any means to avoid shipment overseas, or any other dangerous assignment, from "losing" or destroying their dentures.

It would appear that a practical solution to this problem would be to enter dental appliances on the list of articles for which the soldier is responsible, to be paid for if lost through negligence. Under such circumstances, a commanding officer could collect the cost of a denture through a simple administrative action. No charge would have to be made if negligence were not involved, but the soldier would have the same responsibility for a dental appliance as for any other valuable piece of equipment issued for his use.[161]

ROLE OF THE DENTAL SERVICE IN THE DEVELOPMENT OF THE ACRYLIC RESIN ARTIFICIAL EYE

In the latter part of 1943 the Army was faced with a critical shortage of satisfactory artificial eyes. Replacements were needed for the casualties which were arriving from the battle zones and physical requirements had been lowered to permit the induction of men with only one eye. At the same time, the normal supply of glass eyes from Europe had been cut off. Ordinary glass eyes had many disadvantages for military use. They were extremely fragile and even

---

[157] Bulletin of the Judge Advocate General of the Army, 1944–45. Washington, Government Printing Office, 1944, vol. 3–4, p. 126.
[158] See footnote 155, p. 234.
[159] See footnote 137, p. 231.
[160] TB Med 44, May 1944.
[161] Brig Gen Thomas L. Smith, Chief of the Dental Consultants Division, in 1947, in a statement to the author said that he favored some system for property accountability for dental appliances.

small factors like sudden changes in temperature might result in breakage; they became etched in the fluids of the socket so that they required frequent replacement; custom-fitted eyes for difficult conditions required as much as 2 months for construction and some men lost up to 8 months' duty in a single year while getting successive eye replacements; stocks of as many as a hundred thousand eyes were required for the proper fitting of only a thousand patients.[162] As a result of this situation which was almost as serious for the civilian population as for the military, several agencies undertook investigations to develop an artificial eye which would readily be available and which would be superior to the glass eye in common use.

A clear synthetic resin (methyl methacrylate) had been in use for some years for the construction of artificial dentures. It was strong, well tolerated by human tissues, and easy to form into irregular shapes. It is not surprising, therefore, that the idea of using this material for ocular prostheses suggested itself to several persons at approximately the same time.[163] As early as 1941 the pink acrylic resin used in denture work was made up into temporary eyes to maintain socket form until a permanent appliance could be placed.[164]

Captain Stanley F. Erpf, DC, on duty with the 30th General Hospital in England, was probably the first Army officer to produce a satisfactory acrylic eye; Captain Erpf's own statement of his work is as follows:[165]

> *May 1943 to December 1943.* Initial research begun. Forty prostheses constructed for patients of the 30th General Hospital.
>
> *December 1943.* Research report and training manual written and submitted to the Office of the Chief Surgeon, ETOUSA.
>
> *January 1944 to May 1944.* Training program conducted at the 30th General Hospital for 40 U.S. Army and 10 British Army dental officers.
>
> *June 1944.* Training center at 30th General Hospital terminated and Capt. Erpf en route to the United States to aid in setting up center at Valley Forge General Hospital in the United States.
>
> *July 1944 to December 1944.* Research and training program conducted at Valley Forge General Hospital in collaboration with Major Victor Dietz and Major Milton Wirtz, who had also been working independently on development of the acrylic prosthesis.

At approximately the same time that Captain Erpf was doing his work in England, Major Victor H. Dietz and Major Milton S. Wirtz were experimenting along similar lines at Thomas M. England General Hospital, Atlantic City, N.J., and at Camp Crowder, Mo.[166] It appears that these two officers of the Dental Corps produced acrylic eyes for patients somewhat later than Captain

---

[162] Randolph, M. E.: History of the artificial eye program (glass and plastic), 2 Jan 46. HD: 314.7-2.

[163] At least three Army Dental Corps officers and an unknown number of Naval officers and civilian investigators apparently worked independently along similar lines.

[164] Holmes, A. G.: Use of acrylic resins in the construction of temporary artificial eyes. Dental Bulletin, supp. to Army Medical Bulletin 12: 265-266, Oct 1941.

[165] Personal letter from Dr. Stanley F. Erpf to the author, 9 Oct 46. HD: 422.2.

[166] Erpf, S. F., et al.: Prosthesis of the eye in acrylic resin. Army Medical Bulletin 4: 76-86, Jul 1945.

Erpf, but determination of this point must await decision by the United States Patent Office. In any event, each worked on his own initiative and each was awarded the Legion of Merit for his contribution. In July 1944 both officers joined Captain Erpf in developing a standard technique.

The acrylic eye proved so superior in every respect that it was eventually adopted as the exclusive type of replacement by the Army. In October 1944 it was announced that 12 Eye Centers would accept patients for acrylic eyes, though glass eyes were still furnished on request.[167] By August 1945, 29 general hospitals and 1 regional hospital were rendering this service.[168] The exact number of acrylic eyes constructed is not known, though 7,500 appliances had been made in the United States alone by October 1945.[169][170] Captain Erpf estimated that about 10,000 eyes were made in the first 18 months of the program.[171] The Army technique was adopted by the Veterans Administration when it took over responsibility for the continued care of former soldiers. The part played by dental officers in developing and staffing the artificial eye program reflected great credit on the Dental Corps and the Medical Department.[172]

ROLE OF THE DENTAL SERVICE IN THE DEVELOPMENT OF THE ACRYLIC HEARING-AID ADAPTER

For a decade or more before the war it had been known that the efficiency of hearing-aids depended to an important extent on the accuracy with which the receiver was adapted to the external auditory canal. An ear mold custom-fitted to the individual case eliminated outside noise, prevented "feedback" to the receiver, and channeled sound waves directly to the tympanum without loss of intensity. At the start of the war, ear molds were being constructed by civilian laboratories from individual impressions of the canal, but this system was not altogether satisfactory for the following reasons:[173]

1. Patients had to be held in the hospital while time was lost in mailing work to commercial laboratories.

2. Impressions were subject to distortion or breakage in the mail.

3. Commercial laboratories could not take chances on their ear molds impinging on the tympanum so they habitually shortened the mold to a degree which sometimes resulted in loss of efficiency.

---

[167] WD Cir 398, 11 Oct 44.
[168] SG News Notes 26, 15 Aug 45.
[169] Erpf, S. F., et al.: Plastic-artificial-eye-program, U. S. Army. Am. J. Ophth. 29: 984–992, Aug 1946.
[170] The Army technique was adopted by the Veterans Administration when it took over responsibility for the continued care of former soldiers. SG News Notes, 15 Jan 47. HD: 000.71.
[171] See footnote 165, p. 236.
[172] The subject of the chronological development of the acrylic eye is not considered in detail in this discussion because it is believed that only the U.S. Patent Office can evaluate claims of the military and civilian personnel involved.
[173] McCracken, G. A.: Construction of ear molds for hearing-aid appliances. HD: 314.7–2.

Late in 1943 the Chief of the Aural Rehabilitation Service and Col. Gerald A. McCracken, Chief of the Dental Service at Deshon General Hospital, Butler, Pa., consulted on the possibility of constructing ear molds in a laboratory established in the hospital itself. The project appeared practical and it was presented to the Dental Division and The Surgeon General for approval. The Surgeon General not only concurred in the plan but also directed that laboratories be established at Borden General Hospital (Chickasha, Okla.) and Hoff General Hospital (Santa Barbara, Calif.).[174] The laboratories were supervised and operated by dental personnel because of their experience in taking impressions and handling plastics. Improvements were made in the techniques commonly used by the commercial laboratories and the work produced was eminently satisfactory. While it is not yet known how many ear molds were fabricated, it was reported that Deshon General Hospital alone employed 6 technicians on 2 shifts to turn out from 250 to 350 cases a month while the plan was at peak operation.[175]

ROLE OF THE DENTAL SERVICE IN THE FABRICATION OF TANTALUM PLATES FOR THE REPAIR OF SKULL DEFECTS

Tantalum plates for the repair of skull defects were first used in the Army in September 1942. They were found to be strong and well-tolerated, but the fabrication of a plate with irregular outline and contour offered considerable difficulty. Lt. Col. Arthur J. Hemberger, of the Dental Service at Walter Reed General Hospital, suggested that dental procedures might be applicable to the problem and thereafter dental officers were given the responsibility for taking impressions of cases before operation and forming appliances which could be adapted with a minimum of alteration at the time of repair. Impressions were first made of the area involved. A model was then poured and built up to the desired contour. From this model dies were formed which were used to mold the sheet of tantalum under high pressure. The plate was then trimmed to the desired outline on the model and was ready for insertion after cleaning and sterilization.

This technique was described to Army neurosurgeons at the annual meeting at Walter Reed General Hospital in 1943. Motion pictures of the process were distributed throughout the Army and Navy and the method was reported in the Journal of Neurosurgery in 1945.[176] [177]

---

[174] Ibid.
[175] Ibid.
[176] Hemberger, A. J.: The fabrication of tantalum plates for the repair of skull defects. HD: 314.7-2.
[177] Hemberger, A. J.; Whitcomb, B. B.; and Woodhall, B.: The technique of tantalum plating of skull defects. J. Neurosurg. 2: 21-25, Jan 1945.

INCIDENCE OF THE PRINCIPAL DENTAL DISEASES AND THE AMOUNT OF TREATMENT RENDERED

Tables 4 through 6 show the incidence of some of the more important dental diseases during the period 1 January 1942 through 31 August 1945. Tables 7 through 14 show the more significant treatments rendered in the same period. (In some instances, reports on the incidence of dental diseases, and the amount of treatment rendered, contained no breakdown for military and "other" personnel; however, the number of "others" treated was generally so small that the rates for military personnel were not greatly affected.) The incidence of five important dental diagnoses are shown graphically in Charts 2 through 6. Considerable confusion has existed in the dental profession concerning the diagnosis of Vincent's infection. It is probable that the rates reported for this disease were excessive and included many cases which should properly have been listed as "gingivitis." The statistics shown for Vincent's stomatitis are probably no more nor less accurate than those which would have been obtained from a similar group of civilian dentists.

CHART 2. INCIDENCE* OF CELLULITIS OF DENTAL ORIGIN IN THE UNITED STATES ARMY, 1938–1945.

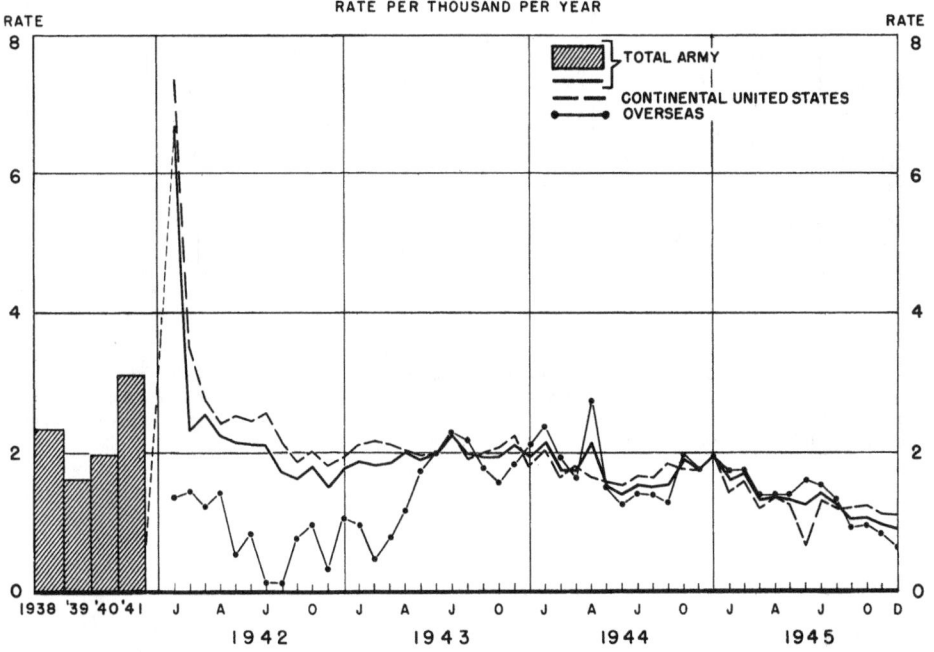

*Includes new cases, readmissions, and both in- and out-patients.
Source: Bar graphs (1938–40), prepared from statistical data obtained from Annual Reports of The Surgeon General, U. S. Army, 1938–41. Washington, Government Printing Office, 1938–41. Other graphic presentation, including bar graph for 1941, prepared by the author from reports received in the Dental Division, SGO.

CHART 3. INCIDENCE* OF FRACTURED MANDIBLES IN THE UNITED STATES ARMY, 1938–1945.

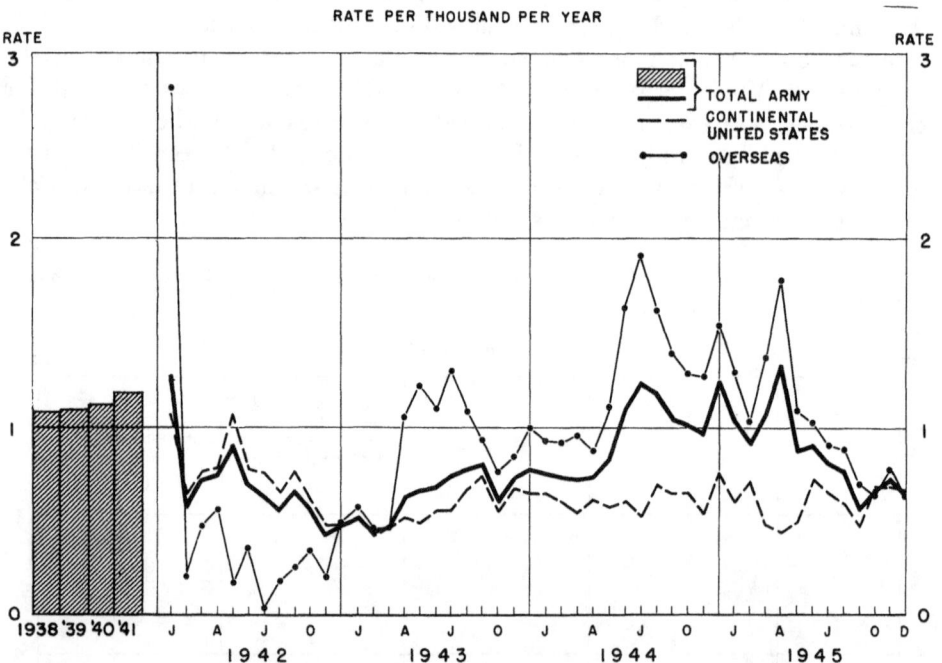

*Includes new cases, readmissions, and both in- and out-patients.
Source: Bar graphs (1938–40), prepared from statistical data obtained from Annual Reports of The Surgeon General, U. S. Army, 1938–41. Washington, Government Printing Office, 1938–41. Other graphic presentation, including bar graph for 1941, prepared by the author from reports received in the Dental Division, SGO.

CHART 4. INCIDENCE* OF FRACTURED MAXILLAE IN THE UNITED STATES ARMY, 1938–1945.

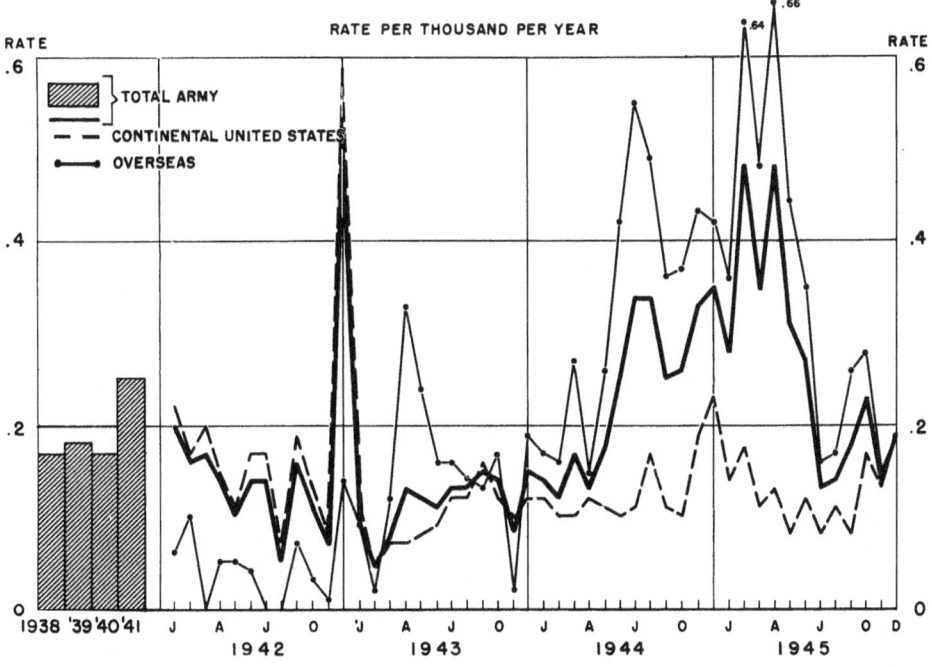

*Includes new cases, readmissions, and both in- and out-patients.
Source: Bar graphs (1938–40), prepared from statistical data obtained from Annual Reports of The Surgeon General, U. S. Army, 1938–41. Washington, Government Printing Office, 1938–41. Other graphic presentation, including bar graph for 1941, prepared by the author from reports received in the Dental Division, SGO.

CHART 5. INCIDENCE* OF OSTEOMYELITIS OF ORAL STRUCTURES IN THE UNITED STATES ARMY, 1938–1945.

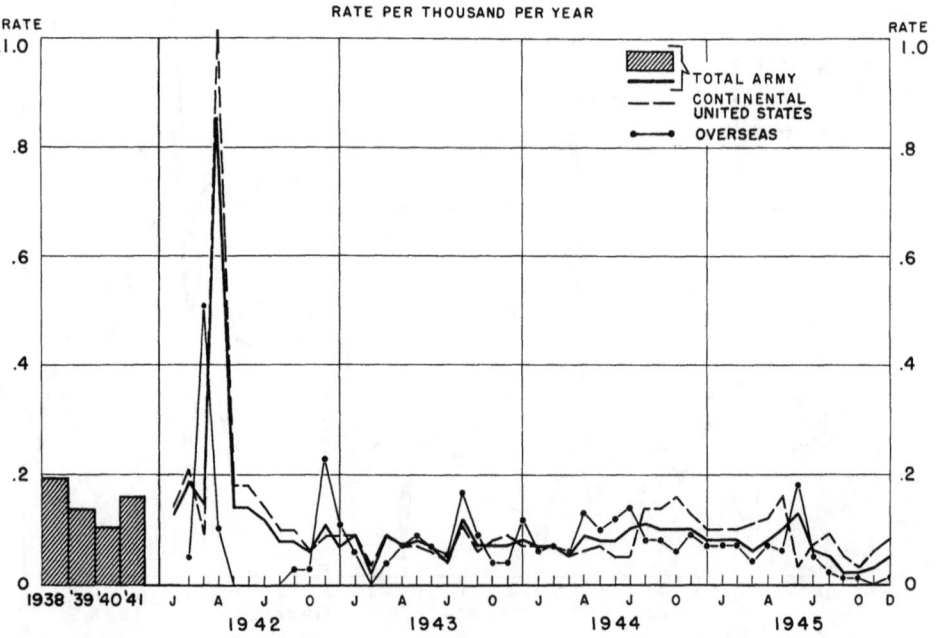

*Includes new cases, readmissions, and both in- and out-patients.
Source: Bar graphs (1938–40), prepared from statistical data obtained from Annual Reports of The Surgeon General, U. S. Army, 1938–41. Washington, Government Printing Office, 1938–41. Other graphic presentation, including bar graph for 1941, prepared by the author from reports received in the Dental Division, SGO.

CHART 6. INCIDENCE* OF VINCENT'S STOMATITIS IN THE UNITED STATES ARMY, 1938–1945.

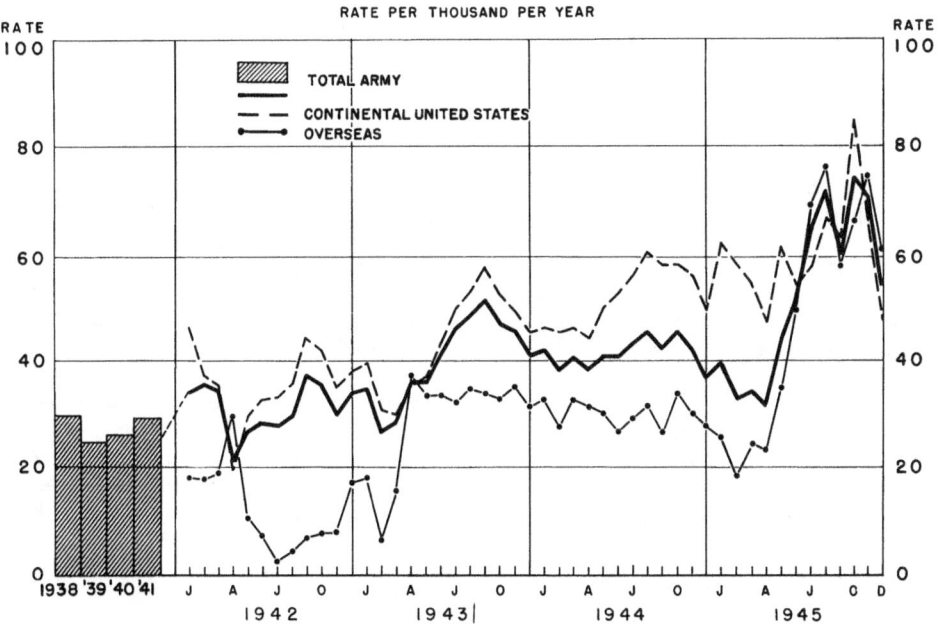

*Includes new cases, readmissions, and both in- and out-patients.
Source: Bar graphs (1938–40), prepared from statistical data obtained from Annual Reports of The Surgeon General, U. S. Army, 1938–41. Washington, Government Printing Office, 1938–41. Other graphic presentation, including bar graph for 1941, prepared by the author from reports received in the Dental Division, SGO.

TABLE 4. INCIDENCE [1] OF CELLULITIS OF DENTAL ORIGIN, UNITED STATES ARMY, AND OTHER PERSONNEL, 1 JANUARY 1942–31 AUGUST 1945

Area	Army [2]		Others [3]
	Number	Number per 1,000 mean strength per year	Number
1942–45			
Total	[4] 41,320	1.7	[4] 3,643
United States	[4] 26,080	1.9	[4] 1,865
Overseas	[4] 15,240	1.6	[4] 1,778
1942			
Total	7,416	2.1	147
United States	6,949	2.5	147
Overseas	467	0.7	
1943			
Total	[4] 13,647	2.0	([4])
United States	[4] 10,595	2.1	([4])
Overseas	[4] 3,052	1.8	([4])
1944			
Total	12,561	1.6	1,236
United States	6,061	1.5	866
Overseas	6,500	1.6	370
1945 [5]			
Total	7,696	1.4	2,260
United States	2,475	1.2	852
Overseas	5,221	1.4	1,408

[1] Includes new cases, readmissions, and both inpatients and outpatients.

[2] Except where otherwise indicated, consists of Army personnel and a negligible number of Navy and Allied military personnel.

[3] Consists of dependents, civilian employees, prisoners of war, and all other personnel not part of the Allied Armed Forces.

[4] During 1943, data for "Other" personnel were not reported separately from "Army" personnel. The statistics shown for "Army" for this year include therefore, data for both "Army" and "Other" personnel.

[5] Data are for 1 January–31 August only.

Source: Compiled by the author from reports received in the Dental Division, SGO.

TABLE 5. INCIDENCE [1] OF VINCENT'S STOMATITIS, UNITED STATES ARMY, AND OTHER PERSONNEL, 1 JANUARY 1942–31 AUGUST 1945

Area	Army [2]		Others [3]
	Number	Number per 1,000 mean strength per year	Number
1942–45			
Total	[4] 958,940	40	[4] 18,203
United States	[4] 657,482	47	[4] 6,993
Overseas	[4] 301,458	31	[4] 11,210
1942			
Total	102,133	30	957
United States	96,519	35	957
Overseas	5,614	9	
1943			
Total	[4] 277,174	40	([4])
United States	[4] 228,932	45	([4])
Overseas	[4] 48,242	28	([4])
1944			
Total	327,116	41	3,106
United States	215,183	54	1,813
Overseas	111,933	28	1,293
1945 [5]			
Total	252,517	46	14,140
United States	116,848	59	4,223
Overseas	135,669	39	9,917

[1] Includes new cases, readmissions, and both inpatients and outpatients.

[2] Except where otherwise indicated, consists of Army personnel and a negligible number of Navy and Allied military personnel.

[3] Consists of dependents, civilian employees, prisoners of war, and all other personnel not part of the Allied Armed Forces.

[4] During 1943, data for "Other" personnel were not reported separately from "Army" personnel. The statistics shown for "Army" for this year include therefore, data for both "Army" and "Other" personnel.

[5] Data are for 1 January–31 August only.

Source: Compiled by the author from reports received in the Dental Division, SGO.

TABLE 6. INCIDENCE [1] OF OSTEOMYELITIS OF ORAL STRUCTURES, UNITED STATES ARMY, AND OTHER PERSONNEL, 1 JANUARY 1942–31 AUGUST 1945

Area	Army [2]		Others [3]
	Number	Number per 1,000 mean strength per year	Number
1942–45			
Total	[4] 2,136	0.08	[4] 213
United States	[4] 1,372	0.09	[4] 121
Overseas	[4] 764	0.08	[4] 92
1942			
Total	507	0.15	19
United States	458	0.17	19
Overseas	49	0.08	
1943			
Total	[4] 500	0.07	([4])
United States	[4] 376	0.07	([4])
Overseas	[4] 124	0.08	([4])
1944			
Total	689	0.08	113
United States	344	0.08	83
Overseas	345	0.09	30
1945 [5]			
Total	440	0.08	81
United States	194	0.10	19
Overseas	246	0.07	62

[1] Includes new cases, readmissions, and both inpatients and outpatients.

[2] Except where otherwise indicated, consists of Army personnel and a negligible number of Navy and Allied military personnel.

[3] Consists of dependents, civilian employees, prisoners of war, and all other personnel not part of the Allied Armed Forces.

[4] During 1943, data for "Other" personnel were not reported separately from "Army" personnel. The statistics shown for "Army" for this year include therefore, data for both "Army" and "Other" personnel.

[5] Data are for 1 January–31 August only.

Source: Compiled by the author from reports received in the Dental Division, SGO.

TABLE 7.—PERMANENT FILLINGS PLACED BY THE UNITED STATES ARMY DENTAL SERVICE, 1 JANUARY 1942—31 AUGUST 1945

Area	Army [1]		Others [2]
	Number	Number per 1,000 mean strength per year	Number
1942-45			
Total	68,092,479	2,880	1,454,081
United States	55,393,744	4,000	1,266,310
Overseas	12,698,735	1,290	187,771
1942			
Total	7,768,357	2,300	91,851
United States	7,122,475	2,580	68,808
Overseas	645,882	1,030	23,043
1943			
Total	23,643,902	3,420	176,962
United States	20,898,379	4,060	149,352
Overseas	2,745,523	1,560	27,610
1944			
Total	24,426,685	3,080	594,258
United States	19,306,933	4,860	540,333
Overseas	5,119,752	1,290	53,925
1945 [3]			
Total	12,253,535	2,250	591,010
United States	8,065,957	4,050	507,817
Overseas	4,187,578	1,210	83,193

[1] Except where otherwise indicated, consists of Army personnel and a negligible number of Navy and Allied military personnel.
[2] Consists of dependents, civilian employees, prisoners of war, and all personnel not part of the Allied Armed Forces. The great increase in treatment after 1943 largely represents care given prisoners of war.
[3] Data are for 1 January–31 August only.

Source: Compiled by the author from reports received in the Dental Division, SGO.

TABLE 8.—EXTRACTIONS PERFORMED BY THE UNITED STATES ARMY DENTAL SERVICE, 1 JANUARY 1942–31 AUGUST 1945

Area	Army [1]		Others [2]
	Number	Number per 1,000 mean strength per year	Number
1942–45			
Total	15,189,936	643	1,041,328
United States	12,627,293	912	705,900
Overseas	2,562,643	262	335,428
1942			
Total	3,246,910	960	53,940
United States	3,030,146	1,099	40,945
Overseas	216,764	347	12,995
1943			
Total	6,007,658	870	164,005
United States	5,316,079	1,032	118,612
Overseas	691,579	393	45,393
1944			
Total	3,842,788	484	395,105
United States	2,919,953	735	282,813
Overseas	922,835	233	112,292
1945 [3]			
Total	2,092,580	384	428,278
United States	1,361,115	684	263,530
Overseas	731,465	212	164,748

[1] Except where otherwise indicated, consists of Army personnel and a negligible number of Navy and Allied military personnel.

[2] Consists of dependents, civilian employees, prisoners of war, and all other personnel not part of the Allied Armed Forces.

[3] Data are for 1 January–31 August only.

Source: Compiled by the author from reports received in the Dental Division, SGO.

TABLE 9. FULL DENTURES CONSTRUCTED BY THE UNITED STATES ARMY DENTAL SERVICE, 1 JANUARY 1942–31 AUGUST 1945

Area	Army [1]		Prisoners of war
	Number	Number per 1,000 mean strength per year	Number
1942–45			
Total	568,669	24	10,359
United States	467,108	34	9,103
Overseas	101,561	10	1,256
1942			
Total	41,208	12	
United States	39,530	14	
Overseas	1,678	3	
1943			
Total	214,368	31	
United States	196,708	38	
Overseas	17,660	10	
1944			
Total	208,263	26	3,023
United States	159,594	40	2,939
Overseas	48,669	12	84
1945 [2]			
Total	104,830	19	7,336
United States	71,276	36	6,164
Overseas	33,554	10	1,172

[1] In addition to Army personnel, consists of dependents, civilian employees, and a negligible number of Navy and Allied military personnel.

[2] Data are for 1 January–31 August only.

Source: Compiled by the author from reports received in the Dental Division, SGO.

TABLE 10. PARTIAL DENTURES CONSTRUCTED BY THE UNITED STATES ARMY DENTAL SERVICE, 1 JANUARY 1942–31 AUGUST 1945

Area	Army [1]		Others [2]
	Number	Number per 1,000 mean strength per year	Number
1942–45			
Total	1,997,162	85	35,522
United States	1,636,757	118	25,247
Overseas	360,405	36	10,275
1942			
Total	115,648	34	1,860
United States	108,072	39	1,691
Overseas	7,576	12	169
1943			
Total	638,435	92	1,598
United States	588,951	114	1,137
Overseas	49,484	28	461
1944			
Total	819,921	103	18,226
United States	669,750	169	9,985
Overseas	150,171	38	8,241
1945 [3]			
Total	423,158	78	13,838
United States	269,984	136	12,434
Overseas	153,174	44	1,404

[1] Except where otherwise indicated, consists of Army personnel and a negligible number of Navy and Allied military personnel.

[2] Consists of dependents, civilian employees, prisoners of war, and all personnel not part of the Allied Armed Forces.

[3] Data are for 1 January–31 August only.

Source: Compiled by the author from reports received in the Dental Division, SGO.

TABLE 11. DENTURES REPAIRED BY THE UNITED STATES ARMY DENTAL SERVICE, 1 JANUARY 1942–31 AUGUST 1945

Area	Army [1]		Others [2]
	Number	Number per 1,000 mean strength per year	Number
1942–45			
Total	743, 261	31	16, 596
United States	464, 699	34	10, 841
Overseas	278, 562	28	5, 755
1942			
Total	39, 507	12	1, 020
United States	35, 858	13	874
Overseas	3, 649	6	146
1943			
Total	160, 978	23	1, 495
United States	125, 972	24	750
Overseas	35, 006	20	745
1944			
Total	316, 711	40	4, 787
United States	200, 058	50	3, 255
Overseas	116, 653	29	1, 532
1945 [3]			
Total	226, 065	41	9, 294
United States	102, 811	52	5, 962
Overseas	123, 254	36	3, 332

[1] Except where otherwise indicated, consists of Army personnel and a negligible number of Navy and Allied military personnel.

[2] Consists of dependents, civilian employees, prisoners of war, and all personnel not part of the Allied Armed Forces.

[3] Data are for 1 January–31 August only.

Source: Compiled by the author from reports received in the Dental Division, SGO.

TABLE 12.— FIXED BRIDGES CONSTRUCTED BY THE UNITED STATES ARMY DENTAL SERVICE, 1 JANUARY 1942–31 AUGUST 1945

Area	Army [1]		Others [2]
	Number	Number per 1,000 mean strength per year	Number
1942–45			
Total	206,484	8.7	1,584
United States	169,980	12.3	1,178
Overseas	36,504	3.7	406
1942			
Total	11,110	3.3	175
United States	10,038	3.6	148
Overseas	1,072	1.7	27
1943			
Total	39,235	5.7	192
United States	34,549	6.7	139
Overseas	4,686	2.7	53
1944			
Total	89,488	11.3	600
United States	74,057	18.7	426
Overseas	15,431	3.9	174
1945 [3]			
Total	66,651	12.2	617
United States	51,336	25.8	465
Overseas	15,315	4.4	152

[1] Except where otherwise indicated, consists of Army personnel and a negligible number of Navy and Allied military personnel.

[2] Consists of dependents, civilian employees, prisoners of war, and all personnel not part of the Allied Armed Forces.

[3] Data are for 1 January–31 August only.

Source: Compiled by the author from reports received in the Dental Division, SGO.

TABLE 13.—TEETH REPLACED BY THE UNITED STATES ARMY DENTAL SERVICE, 1 JANUARY 1942–31 AUGUST 1945

(Based on an estimated 8 teeth replaced per partial denture)

Area	Army [1]		Prisoners of war	Teeth replaced for Army personnel and others [2] per 100 extractions
	Number	Number per 1,000 mean strength per year	Number	
1942–45				
Total	18,306,800	775	309,305	115
United States	15,060,978	1,086	284,195	115
Overseas	3,245,822	332	25,110	113
1942				
Total	980,769	290	----------	30
United States	931,293	338	----------	30
Overseas	49,476	79	----------	22
1943				
Total	6,466,248	936	----------	105
United States	5,953,376	1,156	----------	110
Overseas	512,872	292	----------	70
1944				
Total	7,067,700	891	103,697	169
United States	5,721,652	1,441	101,847	182
Overseas	1,346,048	339	1,850	130
1945 [3]				
Total	3,792,083	696	205,608	159
United States	2,454,657	1,232	182,348	162
Overseas	1,337,426	387	23,260	152

[1] In addition to Army personnel, consists of dependents, civilian employees, and a negligible number of Navy and Allied military personnel.
[2] "Others" include prisoners of war, in addition to those listed in footnote 1.
[3] Data are for 1 January–31 August only.
Source: Compiled by the author from reports received in the Dental Division, SGO.

TABLE 14.—DENTAL PROPHYLAXES PERFORMED BY THE UNITED STATES ARMY DENTAL SERVICE, 1 JANUARY 1942–31 AUGUST 1945

Area	Army [1]		Others [2]
	Number	Number per 1,000 mean strength per year	Number
1942–45			
Total	8,187,932	346	271,347
United States	5,999,091	433	229,653
Overseas	2,188,841	224	41,694
1942			
Total	978,769	290	19,089
United States	880,458	319	14,050
Overseas	98,311	157	5,039
1943			
Total	2,301,367	333	31,123
United States	1,865,542	362	24,356
Overseas	435,825	248	6,767
1944			
Total	2,995,851	377	88,824
United States	2,109,597	531	77,876
Overseas	886,254	223	10,948
1945 [3]			
Total	1,911,945	351	132,311
United States	1,143,494	574	113,371
Overseas	768,451	222	18,940

[1] Except where otherwise indicated, consists of Army personnel and a negligible number of Navy and Allied military personnel.

[2] Consists of dependents, civilian employees, prisoners of war, and all personnel not part of the Allied Armed Forces.

[3] Data are for 1 January–31 August only.

Source: Compiled by the author from reports received in the Dental Division, SGO.

DISCHARGES FOR DENTAL DEFECTS

Discharges for physical disability due to dental defects were negligible during the war. Of 956,232 enlisted men separated from the Army for disability from January 1942 through December 1945, only 312 were separated due to pathology of the teeth.[178] This figure, however, does not cover other possible losses due to dental or oral defects since oral structures may have been involved for some of the men reported as separated for other diseases or traumatic injuries.

CASH VALUE OF TREATMENT RENDERED BY DENTAL OFFICERS

Table 15 gives the average number of five of the more important operations completed per dental officer per year in the continental United States, overseas, and in the Army as a whole, for the period 1 January 1942 through 31 August 1945. Under Veterans Administration fee-schedules published in May 1946 the average yearly work of each dentist, for these five items only, would be valued at over $16,000 a year. The value of the other miscellaneous care given cannot be determined with accuracy, but since it constituted numerically more than half of all treatments rendered, an estimate of $4,000 a year would seem conservative, bringing the gross value of the dental officer's yearly work to about $20,000.

---

[178] Separations from the Army for Physical and Mental Reasons, Health of the Army, Vol 1, No. 2, Aug 1946, pp. 20–23.

TABLE 15. AVERAGE NUMBER OF FIVE PRINCIPAL OPERATIONS COMPLETED PER DENTAL OFFICER PER YEAR, 1 JANUARY 1942–31 AUGUST 1945

Operation	1942 [1]	1943	1944	1945 [2]	Total [3]
Permanent fillings:					
Total Army	1,307	1,950	1,678	1,315	1,630
United States		2,058	1,944	1,630	1,898
Overseas		1,392	1,099	948	1,067
Extractions:					
Total Army	549	505	284	258	340
United States		531	314	309	391
Overseas		370	220	199	232
Dentures:					
Total Army	26	70	70	56	65
United States		77	83	68	77
Overseas		34	44	42	42
Dentures repaired:					
Total Army	7	13	22	24	20
United States		12	20	21	17
Overseas		18	25	28	26
Fixed bridges:					
Total Army	2	3	6	7	6
United States		3	7	10	7
Overseas		2	3	3	3

[1] Accurate statistics are not available on the number of dental officers overseas and in the continental United States.
[2] Average based on figures for the period 1 January–31 August 1945.
[3] Average based on figures for the period 1 January 1943–31 August 1945.

CHAPTER VII

Dental Service in Zone of Interior

FACILITIES PROVIDED, ZONE OF INTERIOR

General Considerations

From the start of mobilization the Dental Division recommended that wherever possible dental facilities should be centralized into large, efficient, clinics which would permit specialization and skilled supervision. In July 1940 the Director of the Dental Division proposed:[1]

> 1. That the plan for the professional service of divisional camps and other new stations include a central dental clinic.
> 2. That the War Department be asked to include in its building program suitable housing for such a clinic.
> 3. That central clinics be located in, or suitably near, the station hospitals.

Preliminary plans called for 2 types of dental clinics, of 25 and 15 chairs, respectively. It was later found necessary to provide smaller units for certain exceptional situations, and by the end of the war the following types had been authorized:

DC-1	25 chairs	DC-4	3 chairs
DC-2	15 chairs	DC-5	1 chair
DC-3	8 chairs	DC-6	1 chair

DC-1 Clinic

The DC-1 clinic of 25 chairs was authorized for divisional camps or other stations with a strength of approximately 15,000 men.[2] It was housed in a separate, 2-story, frame building 110 feet long and 30 feet wide. The floor plans of the DC-1 are shown in figure 17. This clinic (figs. 18 and 19) was furnished with the most modern base equipment, including laboratory (fig. 20), x-ray, prosthetic, and oral surgical facilities. Each operator was supplied a standard chair, unit, cabinet, and operating light.

DC-2 Clinic

The DC-2 clinic consisted of a separate, single-story building with space for 15 chairs. It was a smaller edition of the DC-1, designed to meet the needs of camps of about 10,000 men.[3] It was also used as a dental clinic in all station hospitals of 250 beds or more.[4] In camps of less than 10,000 men, but large enough to have a 250-bed hospital, the hospital DC-2 supplied all dental care

---

[1] Memo, Brig Gen Leigh C. Fairbank for SG, 17 Jul 40, sub: Definitive dental service in divisional camps and other large installations. AG: 632.

[2] Dental expansion program. The Dental Bulletin, supp. to the Bulletin of the U. S. Army Medical Department (cited hereafter as Army Medical Bulletin) 11:177, Oct 1940.

[3] Ibid.

[4] 3d ind, TAG to SG, 20 Nov 40, on ltr, SG to TAG, 2 Nov 40, sub: Dental service in cantonment hospitals—dental laboratory service, divisional areas. AG: 632.

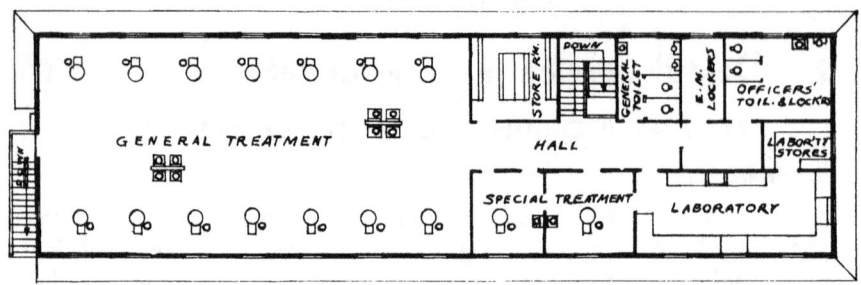

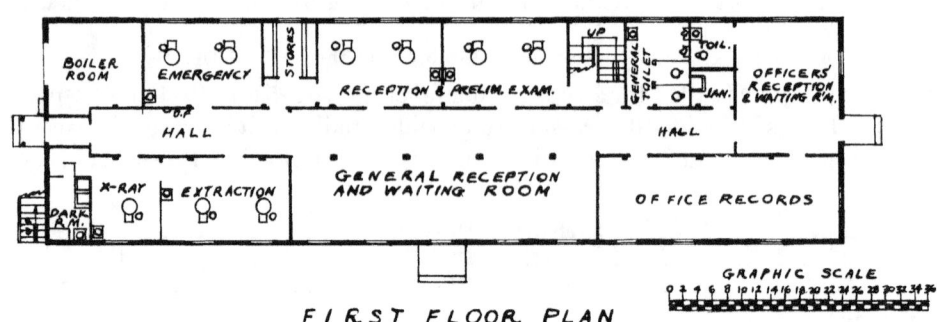

Figure 17. Floor plan, dental clinic type DC-1.

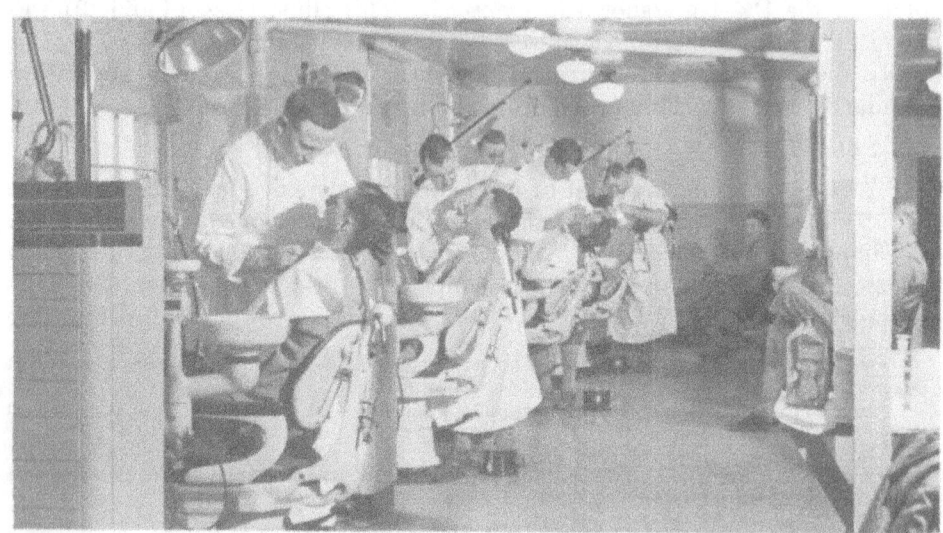

Figure 18. Part of general operating room, DC-1.

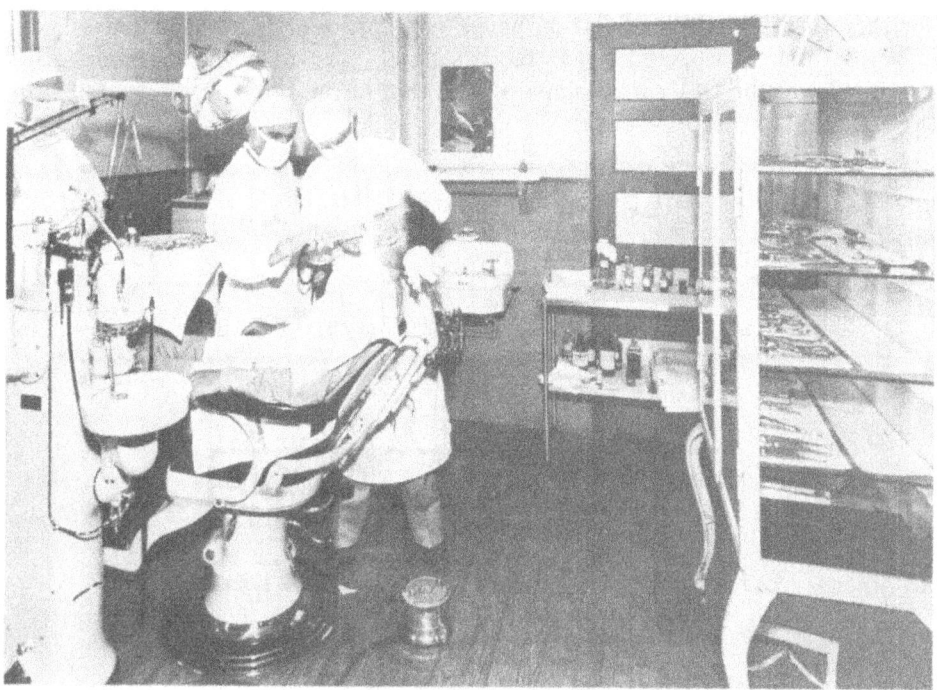

Figure 19. Oral surgical operating room, DC-1.

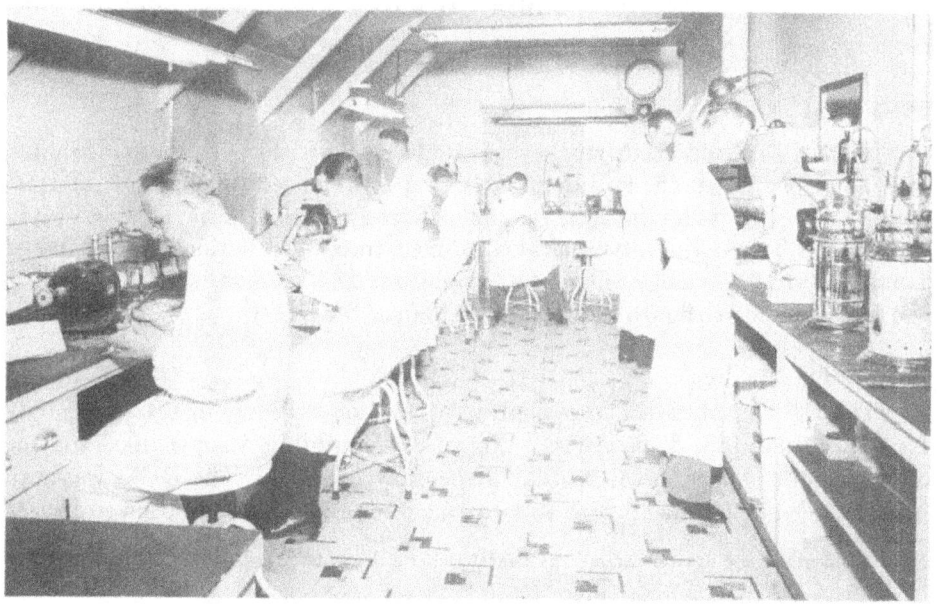

Figure 20. Dental laboratory, DC-1.

for the camp. If the installation had a population of more than 10,000 men, but less than 15,000, additional facilities were provided in the troop area. Equipment of the DC-2 was comparable to that of the DC-1. See figure 21 for the floor plan of the DC-2 clinic.

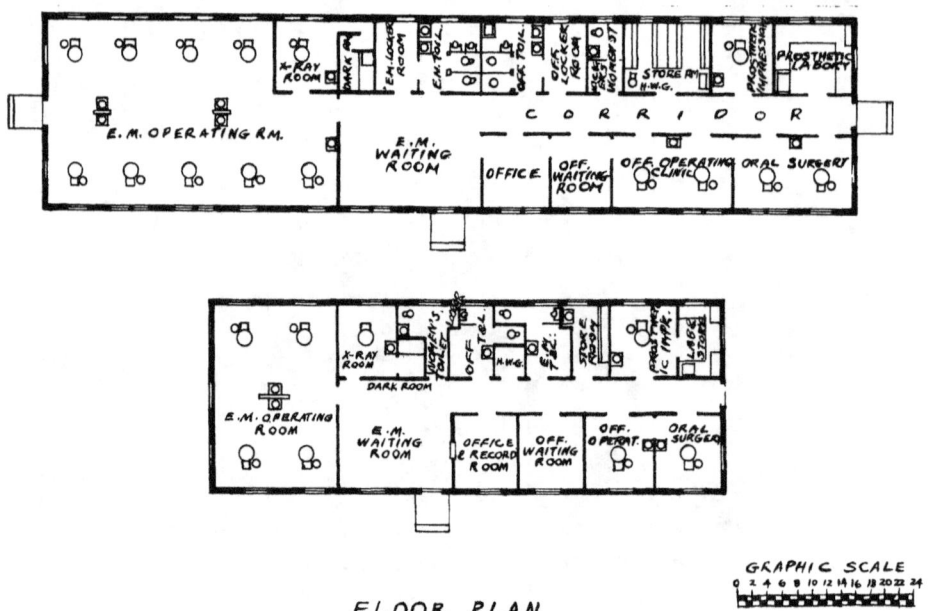

Figure 21. Floor plans of DC-2 and DC-3 clinics.

DC-3 Clinic

The DC-3 clinic, occupying a separate building with space for eight chairs, was developed about the middle of 1941 to meet the needs of posts of intermediate size.[5] Policy for its use was not definitely stated, however, until early 1942, when The Adjutant General approved these installations for camps of from 3,000 to 6,000 men. The DC-3 clinic was also used in hospitals of from 100 to 200 beds. See figure 21 for the floor plan of the DC-3.

DC-4 Clinic

The DC-4 clinic, with three chairs, was authorized early in 1943, primarily for use in small unit dispensaries. No separate building was provided and the clinic occupied space in the regular dispensary quarters. The DC-4 was supplied base-type equipment, with an x-ray machine and some laboratory supplies.[6]

---

[5] The dental clinic number three. The Dental Bulletin, supp. to Army Medical Bulletin 12: 249, Jul 1941.

[6] MD Equipment List No. 95058, 6 Dec 44.

DC-5 Clinic

The DC-5 clinic, with 1 chair, was also authorized in 1943 for use in the smaller dispensaries where the 3 chairs of the DC-4 were not needed. It had no x-ray machine and only the most essential laboratory equipment was provided.[7] Like the DC-4, it occupied space in a regular dispensary building.

DC-6 Clinic

The DC-6 clinic, which was a simplified version of the DC-5, was intended for use in prisoner of war camps. It was authorized a base-type chair but no cabinet. A mobile dental engine was substituted for the operating unit.[8]

Cost of the Various Clinics

The cost of the aforementioned installations was approximately as follows:[9]

Type	Equipment	Building approximate	Total
DC-1	$33,684	$25,000	$58,684
DC-2	20,535	15,000	35,535
DC-3	11,356	10,000	21,356
DC-4	5,717	(1)	5,717
DC-5	2,425	(1)	2,425
DC-6	1,192	(1)	1,192

[1] None provided.

By September 1942, 100 DC-1, 150 DC-2, and 138 DC-3 clinics were in operation or nearing completion.[10][11]

THE DENTAL SERVICE IN A REPLACEMENT TRAINING CENTER

General Considerations

Major dental rehabilitation for the inductee was not initiated until arrival at a replacement training center, which was recognized to be the most favorable place in which to concentrate dental facilities. It was the first installation in which an inductee spent enough time to permit the completion of extensive treatment.

The replacement training center was a large, fairly stable establishment where the dental service could be organized for maximum efficiency. Specially qualified dental officers could be assigned to the more critical positions

---

[7] MD Equipment List No. 95059, 6 Dec 44.

[8] MD Equipment List No. 95054, 6 Dec 44.

[9] Cost of equipment listed is taken from the ASF Medical Supply Catalog of 1 Mar 44, on file in HD. The cost of buildings of course varied greatly in different locations and at different times. The figures quoted are approximate, obtained from the Fiscal Div, CE, Mr. Jonas Stein. They were given the author in a telephone conversation, 7 Mar 47.

[10] Mills, R. H.: Dentistry in the war. J. Am. Dent. A. 15 Sep 42, p. 1754.

[11] At the time this history was prepared (1947) information was not available on the clinics constructed subsequent to 1942.

and trained auxiliary personnel and clerical assistants were available to take over many time-consuming, nonprofessional duties.

Soldiers usually went directly from a replacement training center to duty with operational units and a high percentage were sent overseas within a short time. It was therefore desirable that all possible treatment be completed during the training period, and absolutely essential that men leaving the center should at least meet minimum dental standards for foreign service.[12] From the start of the war the Director of the Dental Division, SGO, recommended that replacement training center dental clinics meet the main burden of dental rehabilitation.

Operation of the Dental Service in a Replacement Training Center

Time for the treatment of inductees in a replacement training center was limited; it was also necessary to avoid as far as possible interruption of normal activities. The dental service in a replacement training center was therefore organized to attain three primary objectives:

1. To examine every man with the least possible delay and start his treatment immediately.

2. To check the progress of his work and make such additional examinations as were necessary to insure completion of all required treatment before his departure from the center.

3. To provide dental treatment at times which would interfere least with scheduled training.

No uniform system was prescribed, and each dental surgeon used the methods which best conformed to his own ideas and to conditions encountered in his particular camp. The operation of a typical training center dental service (Fort Knox, Kentucky) has been described as follows:[13]

> Dental surveys were conducted 3 times during each training cycle of 17 weeks. The first was made within 48 hours after the arrival of the trainees from the induction centers. A second was made at the completion of the basic training period, before the start of specialist training. The third or final dental check was conducted during the final week of the training cycle, just prior to shipment.
>
> All dental surveys were scheduled by the S-3 officer of the center as a part of training and the company commander was responsible for the presence of all trainees at every dental check within his unit. Surveys were conducted in the unit area by the dental surgeon and one assistant. Clerks for the examination were supplied by the unit.
>
> The company was requested to furnish duplicate copies of a current roster for every survey. At the time of examination an individual survey form was given to each trainee, who filled in all data on the form except the dental classification and information concerning his dental condition. This form was collected by the clerk at the time of examination and entry made of the dental classification and pertinent information regarding prosthetic appliances. Forms and rosters were then taken to the office

---

[12] Memo, Brig Gen R. H. Mills for Exec Off SGO, 27 Apr 42. SG: 322.0531.
[13] Incl to Personal Ltr, Dr. H. L. Davidson to Col Walter Love, 2 Dec 46. SG: 703.

of the dental surgeon where individual classifications were entered on both copies of the roster and a record of prosthetic appliances made on the original copy. This copy was retained by the dental surgeon and the duplicate sent to the company commander for use in filling appointments allotted his organization.

From the data on the individual survey forms an MD Form 79 [now AG Form 8–116, Register of Dental Patients] was made out for each trainee in need of dental care and held in the files of the dental surgeon for use at such time as the man was ordered in for treatment.

Patients were treated at four widely scattered clinics but all orders for trainees to appear for treatment were issued from the office of the dental surgeon as an official memorandum over the signature of the commanding general. The dental surgeon consulted flow charts and training schedules so that patients might be called for treatment during the least important parts of their training cycle, though dental care held preference over all training. A carbon copy of the memorandum directing men to report for treatment, a list of the trainees requiring care, and the previously prepared MD Forms 79 were forwarded to the clinic named in the memorandum.

Patients were ordered for treatment by classification only, and the unit commander was charged with the responsibility for selecting men of the indicated classification from his dental roster, detailing them to the specified clinic. Changes in classification were reported directly from the clinic to the unit of the patient receiving care and to the office of the dental surgeon. All completed MD Forms 79 were returned daily to the files of the dental surgeon.

Should the individual clinic chief find it necessary to make changes in the flow of patients, or should he be confronted by any delinquency in keeping appointments, he discussed the matter with the dental surgeon, who took the necessary steps to correct the situation.

The midtraining survey was necessary because a considerable number of trainees were transferred to new companies due to sickness, emergency furloughs, etc. These men did not appear on the dental survey rosters of their new organizations and were easily lost to the dental service. It was therefore deemed advisable to conduct a new survey at the end of basic training and carry through a second time as the original had been handled, except that new MD Forms 79 were made for new patients only.

The dental check made a few days before completion of training gave the dental surgeon a final chance to correct any defects still existing among the men about to be shipped out. These patients were given the highest priority.

The aim of the dental service of this replacement training center was to put every man in Class III or IV prior to completion of his training. This policy was rigidly followed, especially in respect to men being sent to Army Ground Forces replacement depots. The dental surgeon had the authority to request the removal of specific persons from shipping orders for dental reasons.

A check of original dental survey rosters over a period of 42 months revealed the following average classification of men arriving in the replacement training center from civilian life:

Class	Percentage
Class I	22.5% (35% of these would require prosthetic replacements before completion of treatment.)
Class I–D	5.0%
Class II	22.5%
Class III	1.5%
Class IV	48.5%

Treatment Rendered

The personnel of the larger camp dental clinics included specialists in oral surgery and prosthetics, and the station hospital was able to give institutional care when it was required. As a result, very few dental patients had to be sent off the post for other than highly specialized treatment. However, when such treatment was necessary for conditions which involved badly comminuted or displaced fractures, severe infections, the removal of tumors, or plastic reconstruction, the patient was usually transferred to a general hospital. Dental hygienists provided many soldiers with their first instruction in the individual care of the teeth and the supporting structures. In general, the centralized clinics of the replacement training centers and other major installations were well designed to provide rapid, efficient treatment of routine conditions and at the same time to give the more complex defects the extra attention they required.

The "production line" organization of the larger clinics, with all surgical and prosthetic care given by specialists, undoubtedly increased output and improved the quality of the treatment rendered. It was not without disadvantages, however. In particular, the strain on men in the general operative section was severe. The placing of even routine fillings is meticulous work, hard on the eyes and nervous system, and requiring a tiring posture. In his civilian office the dentist is able to get a "change of pace" by doing surgical, prosthetic, or laboratory work, but in a large Army clinic, the officer works continuously at the chair "plugging amalgams," with another patient always waiting to take the place of the one just completed. The monotony and physical strain of performing one task over and over for months at a time was a constant cause of complaint. Further, the dentist had no chance to maintain his skill in other branches of dentistry. The bitterness of young officers toward the "amalgam line" was certainly a factor in their lack of interest in a career in the Army Dental Corps after the war.

Personnel Problems

In determining the number of dental officers to be assigned replacement training centers it was necessary to compromise between what was theoretically desirable and what was practical with available resources. The Dental Division, SGO, recommended a ratio of 1 officer for each 300 men in training and this figure probably represented both the largest number which could be spared and the smallest number which could provide effective treatment.[14] However, the number of dentists actually provided varied greatly and cannot accurately be determined, but figures on the overall assignment of dental officers in the Zone of Interior give some indication of the working ratio.

On 30 November 1942 there was 1 dentist for each 473 soldiers in the United States. This ratio decreased steadily until April 1943 when each dental officer

---

[14] Memo, Chief, Oprs Serv SGO, for CG ASF, 5 Jun 44, sub: Requirements for Dental Corps officers. HD: 314.

was responsible for 586 men. Thereafter the proportion of dentists again increased until in November 1944 [15] it reached a fairly stable level of 1 officer for each 350 men. Some Zone of Interior installations (e. g. hospitals) had more than the average ratio; others had less (e. g. air fields); the proportion of 1 dentist for each 350 men is probably not far from the ratio actually provided replacement training centers in 1944.

THE DENTAL SERVICE IN A ZONE OF INTERIOR REPLACEMENT DEPOT

The function of the dental service in Zone of Interior replacement depots was to detect and provide treatment,[16] within a maximum of 15 days, for men who, when reporting for shipment overseas, still failed to meet minimum dental standards.

The details of operating the dental service in a replacement depot varied in different installations, but two fundamental requirements had to be kept in mind: (1) early detection of the men needing treatment, and (2) a system for insuring that patients were called to the dental clinic without delay and with minimum chance that they would be "lost" administratively. At one replacement depot, Camp Reynolds, Pa., new arrivals were first assigned to a casual battalion where processing was completed. Men reporting to this battalion were marched directly to the dental survey office where 2 dental officers and 3 clerks were constantly on duty. Those in Class I were placed in a separate company and carried as "unavailable for shipment" until their essential treatment had been completed. The dental service notified the Classification and Assignment Section whenever a man was ready for shipment and he was then taken out of the "dental" company and returned to his unit, or to the regular processing line if he was a casual.[17]

Personnel were allotted in about the same proportion as for replacement training centers, for though the men were passing through the replacement depot in a much faster flow they had generally received more or less complete dental care at previous stations, so that the average amount of work per individual was much less than in a replacement training center.

Since only the most essential treatment was rendered at replacement depots it might have been expected that extractions and dentures would have constituted a high proportion of all operations performed. Apparently, how-

---

[15] The proportion of dental officers to total strength of the Army was calculated by author from data in Strength of the Army, 1 Mar 46.

[16] This service was also to be rendered at ports of embarkation, redistribution and redeployment stations, but in actual practice these played a minor role in the process; ports of embarkation were primarily concerned with the supervision of embarkation, and with the sudden end of the war in Asia the activities of the redistribution and redeployment stations were curtailed almost before they could reach stable operation.

[17] Annual Rpt, Surg Cp Reynolds, 1944. HD.

ever, these major dental deficiencies had usually been corrected at home stations, and work completed at replacement depots consisted of a higher proportion of permanent fillings. The following tabulation compares the treatment rendered in a replacement depot (Camp Reynolds) in 1944 with the treatment rendered in the total Army in the same period: [18] [19]

Operation	Percentage of five principal operations in a replacement depot	Percentage of five principal operations in the Army as a whole
Permanent fillings	87.6	78.1
Extractions	6.3	18.0
Dentures	3.8	2.8
Denture repairs	2.2	0.9
Bridges	0.1	0.2

THE DENTAL SERVICE IN A SEPARATION CENTER

Prior to 1944 the problem of providing dental treatment for men being discharged from the Army was overshadowed by requirements for the rehabilitation of inductees. A circular letter of 2 September 1943 prohibited the practice of informing separatees that they could have their dental work completed in Veterans Administration facilities after discharge and also stated that "The status of the soldier with reference to his retention in the service should be clearly understood before any extensive dental treatment is started. Every effort will be extended to complete all essential dental treatment for a soldier, once begun, prior to his discharge." [20] While this letter encouraged the completion of work which had already been initiated, it also had the probable unintentional effect of discouraging extensive treatment for men due for early discharge. It was not the desire of the Dental Division or The Surgeon General to limit treatment for men leaving the service and on 7 March 1944 the Dental Division recommended that care be made available for all Class I patients prior to relief from active duty.[21] On 31 March 1944 this recommendation was substantially repeated in a memorandum to the Medical Practices Division, SGO, but no formal action resulted. In a Physical Standards Division conference on 27 December 1944 the following points were agreed upon with the concurrence of the Dental Division: [22]

1. Soldiers with Class I defects to be offered treatment prior to discharge.
2. Treatment to be optional with the man concerned.
3. Priority for treatment of separatees over other personnel to be given only at separation centers.

---

[18] See footnote 17, p. 265.
[19] Data on the Army as a whole taken from Army Medical Bulletin 4: 632, Dec 1945.
[20] ASF Ltr 156, 2 Sep 43.
[21] Memo, Act Dir Dental Div for Oprs Serv SGO, 7 Mar 44, sub: Dental treatment for personnel during demobilization. SG: 703.
[22] Memo for Record, 27 Dec 44, sub: Office policy regarding dental treatment at separation centers. HD: 314.

In spite of informal agreement on general policies for the operation of separation centers no official directive was issued until 10 September 1945. Technical Manual (TM) 8–255, published on that date, provided that:[23]

> Individuals having Class I dental defects which are incapacitating or likely to interfere with performance of duties in military or civilian life, or individuals who have lost anterior teeth in line of duty, will be provided with appropriate treatment and/or prosthetic appliances prior to separation if the individual so desires. Routine dental treatment, such as for Class II's, etc., may be provided for individuals, providing time, facilities and dental personnel are available, and providing the individual elects to have such treatment.

It was further directed that dental officers would be provided on examining teams, in accordance with the number of separatees processed daily, as follows:

Number of daily examinations	Number of dental officers on teams
75–150	1
200–300	2
400	3
500–600	4
800	6
1,000	7
1,800	12

These dental officers were concerned only with examinations; treatment was given in established clinics. In a memorandum of June 1944 it had already been recommended that dentists be provided separation centers in the ratio of 1 officer for each 300 separatees,[24] though the number actually assigned to each center was determined by the respective service command.

A letter to the service commands, dated 6 September 1945, quoted the tentative provisions of TM 8–255 and elaborated on them as follows:[25]

> Every effort should be made to use existing dental facilities to the fullest capacity, and when such facilities are inadequate, additional dental equipment should be installed in other available quarters to meet the local demands.
>
> Dental personnel, officers and enlisted men, should be shifted within the Service Command to permit the greatest service.
>
> Under the provisions of AR 40–510, C 1, paragraph 5b (3), 10 September 1942, the procurement of civilian dental laboratory service may be authorized by the Commanding Generals of Service Commands where adequate dental laboratory facilities are not available and when there is insufficient time to have the cases completed at Central Dental Laboratories. . . .

At many stations the Dental Service operated a double shift.

The Dental Division was not in a position to predict how much work would have to be accomplished at separation centers. The dental classification of the Army was known, but this classification was based on the urgency of the treatment required rather than upon its amount. A man in Class II, for instance,

---

[23] TM 8–255, Terminal physical examination on separation from military service, 10 Sep 45.
[24] See footnote 14, p. 264.
[25] Ltr, SG to CG 1st SvC, 6 Sep 45, sub: Dental treatment prior to separation from the Army. HD: 314.

might have 1 cavity or 10, so that information on total classifications was of little value in estimating future needs. Above all, it was impossible to predict what percentage of men needing treatment would ask for it. Previous experience had indicated that only a small proportion of separatees would risk delaying their discharge even a few hours, but many factors influenced their decisions. It was found, for instance, that more men applied for dental care during the period when 45-day furloughs for recuperation and recreation were being granted than after that privilege was discontinued.[26]

Since the requirements for separatee dental service might change from day to day faster than personnel could be shifted, the service command dental surgeons could only establish the separation center clinics to meet average expected demands, thereafter maintaining an even flow of patients by varying the types of service rendered. When the flow of separations was slow, all kinds of treatment were offered and every effort made to complete routine fillings without delaying the departure of patients from the center. When the flow of separations was rapid, treatment had to be limited to the urgent cases specified in TM 8-255.

The organization of the dental service of a separation center offered peculiar problems which were solved in different ways on different posts. Separatees were understandably impatient to be released from the Army, even when they had asked to be held for dental care. They wanted furloughs and passes and often failed to return in time for appointments. Keeping in touch with the men under treatment was in itself a major problem, and constant supervision was needed to insure that service was rendered as speedily as possible and that patients were released for discharge as soon as their dental work was completed. Men requiring prolonged treatment were withdrawn from processing, but every effort was made to complete minor care without delaying departure of the patient, although in many cases only a few nighttime hours were available for such treatment out of the 48 which the separatee spent in the center.

The system in operation at Fort Monmouth was typical of the elaborate methods used to control the dental patient in a separation center.[27] The salient points of the Fort Monmouth plan were as follows:

1. Patients were classified into three broad groups according to the type and amount of treatment needed:

   a. Men for whom treatment was urgent, including those requiring replacement of missing teeth, received first priority and at their own request were withdrawn from processing until treatment was completed. No man in this group was refused care regardless of the backlog of patients.

---

[26] Incl to ltr, Col Arne P. Sorum to Dental Div SGO, 30 Oct 46, sub: Dental treatment at a separation center. HD: 314.

[27] Memo, Maj Joseph G. Rosen for CG 1260th SCU, 16 Nov 45, sub: Plan of dental treatment at separation center, Fort Monmouth, N. J. SG: 703 (Ft. Monmouth) N. J.

b. Men needing extensive but routine dental care were also withdrawn from processing at their own request if the backlog of patients was sufficiently small to permit starting their work within a reasonable time. But these were not accepted unless they could be given appointments within 36 hours.

c. Men needing routine care which could be completed at one sitting were given appointments during free periods of their processing schedule if such were available. Because these men were often fully occupied during the few daylight hours they passed in the installation, their work was frequently done at night. If no free time was available for completing their work during the normal processing period they could be voluntarily withdrawn from the schedule under the same provisions as men in group *b.*

2. A dental officer was on duty at the Initial Receiving Point (IRP) at all times when separatees were being processed. This officer was notified in advance as to how many appointments of each type he might give out during the day. The IRP dental officer explained to each group the possibilities of getting dental treatment. If ample appointments of all types were available he notified the separatees that those requiring extensive care could be withdrawn from processing for such treatment and that those with minor defects could have their work completed without delaying their departure from the separation center. If appointments could not be given during the normal period of processing, but would be available within 36 hours, it was explained that all men needing treatment could be given appointments but that it would be necessary to withdraw them from processing until such treatment was completed. If the accumulated backlog of patients was such that no appointments could be given within 36 hours it was explained that only urgent cases would be accepted and that it would be necessary to hold these from processing. The IRP dentist then examined those separatees who felt that they qualified for treatment and who volunteered to delay their departure if that was necessary. Those in the first two groups were immediately suspended from processing by notification to the IRP officer and given colored cards which they took to the dental clinic as authority for starting treatment (blue cards for Class I's, pink cards for Class II's). Men in the third group were given white appointment cards to the dental clinic for a period when they were not required for processing.

3. All separatees were given a chance to request dental care at the IRP, as explained above. Those in Class I were given another opportunity to request treatment when they were given the dental examination during processing. To avoid withdrawing partially-processed men from the line, those who did not require urgent care were not accepted later unless they had asked for treatment when given the opportunity at the IRP.

4. On arrival at the dental clinic men in the first two groups were given appointments and their names entered on "suspense logs." The IRP dentist also sent in a list of those placed on suspense during the day and this was

checked against the clinic suspense log to insure that all men withheld had actually reported to the dental clinic. This log was checked periodically to detect for investigation any patient who had been on suspense for an unusually long period. Any Class II patient who failed to keep an appointment was automatically released from suspense. The colored cards which patients brought to the dental clinic were clipped to their dental records and, when treatment was completed, were filled in on the reverse side and placed in a box which was emptied every hour. Separation center headquarters was in turn given, by telephone, an hourly list of men whose cases had been closed, and this list was verified in writing at the end of the day. A patient was thus released to continue his processing within an hour after his treatment had been completed. No special check was needed for men given white cards for minor care since they were not withdrawn from the processing schedule.

The proportion of separatees needing treatment was only a fraction of the number who had needed care when they entered the service. Of 278,309 separatees processed at Fort Dix between 1 March and 30 September 1946 only 0.86 percent needed extractions or other urgent treatment, only 1.75 percent, replacement of missing teeth, and 10.15 percent, fillings or other routine care.[28] Of those requiring treatment only a small percentage were willing to delay their discharge even a few days.

The total number of separatees who received dental treatment *at the time of separation* is not known since a report was made only of those suspended from processing, and many thousands had minor work completed while on the normal separation center schedule. During the demobilization period, from May 1945 through October 1946, about 111,800 persons were withdrawn from the examining line because they needed urgent oral treatment requiring a delay in their separation. Of these, about 104,900 were for dental defects, and about 6,900 for mouth and gum defects. These withdrawals constituted 1.6 percent of all personnel processed for separation during this period: 1.5 percent for teeth, and 0.1 percent for mouth and gum defects. While the proportion of men withdrawn from the line for dental reasons may seem to be relatively small, the number of persons who received such care is obviously quite important. In fact, the withdrawals for dental reasons made up about 36 percent of the withdrawals for all physical reasons. About 2.6 percent of the persons withdrawn for dental reasons required inpatient treatment.[29]

Among the soldiers willing to wait for dental treatment, a high proportion needed extensive prosthetic replacements. Over 65 percent of the men held for treatment at Fort Dix required replacement of missing teeth. Special prosthetic sections had to be set up in many clinics and civilian laboratories called

---
[28] See footnote 26, p. 268.
[29] Unpublished data from Medical Statistics Div SGO, based on special reports dealing with the processing of military personnel at separation centers, points, and bases.

upon to carry some of the unusual load. At Fort Dix, when 4,500 men were being discharged daily, 1 officer with a staff car was kept busy delivering and picking up cases from civilian laboratories.[30]

As a means of saving money the program for dental treatment of separatees was not too successful. The Veterans Administration soon provided dental care for "service connected" defects of former military personnel and the many men who had refused such treatment at a separation center were able to have their work completed later at Government expense. The program did give the soldier a last chance to have essential work completed before he returned to civilian life, however, and those who took advantage of the offer were generally the most urgently in need of care and the most deserving of consideration by the Army.

Summary, Dental Service in Separation Centers

1. After extensive service in the Army the average separatee needed relatively little dental care.

2. The majority of the men willing to delay their discharge to receive dental treatment required extensive replacements, necessitating special prosthetic facilities and the use of civilian laboratories.

3. To be effective, the dental service of a separation center must have the facilities and organization adequate to handle as many patients as possible during the normal separation period. Very few men will take advantage of the proffered treatment if they must be suspended from processing to receive it. To reach as many of these as possible it becomes necessary to operate extensive facilities outside of regular duty hours.

THE DENTAL SERVICE IN ZONE OF INTERIOR STATION HOSPITALS

Each Zone of Interior post of any importance had its own station hospital for the institutional medical care of local personnel. These hospitals were not expected to render highly specialized treatment but were equipped and staffed to handle all routine medical and surgical conditions. They varied in size from 25 to 1,000 beds or more. In small hospitals of less than 100 beds the dental clinic normally occupied a part of the administration building. Intermediate hospitals of from 100 to 200 beds were authorized a separate dental clinic of 8 chairs (DC–3), while hospitals of 250 beds or larger were provided a separate clinic building of 15-chair capacity.[31] The hospital clinics were

---

[30] See footnote 26, p. 268.

[31] Data on the dental clinics provided the smaller station hospitals obtained by the author from Mr. James J. Souder, Act Chief Hospital Construction Br Hospital Div SGO, on 14 Apr 47. Hospitals of 250 beds or larger were authorized DC–2's by 3d ind, TAG, 20 Nov 40, on Ltr, SG to TAG, 2 Nov 40, sub: Dental service in cantonment hospitals—dental laboratory service, divisional areas. AG: 632.

authorized base-type chairs, units, cabinets, x-ray machines, and laboratories. Equipment and instruments were adequate for all routine operations.

Unlike overseas station hospitals, the Zone of Interior station hospitals had no prescribed allotments of personnel. The number of officers and enlisted men required in each situation was determined within the service command on the basis of relative strength, the primary activity of the post, and individual ideas of the staff officers concerned. Late in the war (October 1945), ASF published a "guide" for the allotment of officers and men to station hospitals. It suggested that 1 dental officer and 1½ enlisted men be provided for each 200 hospital beds. Since the hospital dental clinics on the smaller posts had to furnish all dental care for the troop areas as well as for hospital patents, it was recommended that they be allowed 2 additional dental officers and 3 enlisted men for each 1,000 troops.[32] This directive was only advisory, however, and not binding on local commanders.

The station hospital dental clinics fulfilled different functions on posts of different sizes, as follows:

1. On posts of less than 10,000 men the hospital dental clinic normally furnished all definitive dental treatment for the command, including routine care for outpatients, laboratory service, and any treatment of hospital patients which was not of a highly specialized nature. If tactical units were present on the post their own dental officers conducted surveys, held sick call, and rendered emergency care to their men, but all other treatment was carried out in the hospital clinic, sometimes with the aid of the tactical dentists on temporary duty. The hospital clinic constructed prosthetic appliances, placed permanent restorations, treated infections about the mouth, extracted diseased or impacted teeth, and rendered emergency treatment to serious facial injuries pending their transfer to a hospital where specialized care would be given.

2. On posts of more than 10,000 men the hospital dental clinic provided routine care only for hospital patients. In addition it undertook the more difficult types of treatment such as the construction of complicated prosthetic replacements or the extraction of impacted teeth. It provided care for infections or other conditions which could not be treated on a duty status and rendered emergency treatment for serious facial injuries. Simple fractures might be handled in the hospital dental clinic but more difficult surgical cases were normally transferred to a general hospital. Routine fillings, prosthetic restorations, and extractions for nonhospitalized personnel were taken care of in the troop-area clinics.

The maximum number of station hospitals in the United States was reached at the end of 1943 when 611 hospitals provided bed space for 270,499 patients.[33]

---

[32] ASF Ltr 389, 16 Oct 45.
[33] Info from files of Medical Statistics Div SGO.

THE DENTAL SERVICE IN ZONE OF INTERIOR GENERAL HOSPITALS

Zone of Interior general hospitals were strategically located to provide highly specialized medical and surgical care which could not be furnished in the station hospitals. A circular letter of 1 January 1943, stated that:[34]

> General hospitals are established and maintained to afford better facilities than ordinarily can be provided in station hospitals for the observation, treatment, and disposition of complicated or obscure cases; for the performance of the more formidable surgical operations; and to provide beds for the evacuation of station hospitals. . . .
>
> No hard and fast rules can be laid down, but in general it will be the policy of the Medical Department to treat as general hospital cases all patients who require more than 90 days' hospitalization, as well as all cases requiring specialized treatment which is not available at station hospitals. . . .
>
> Complicated or severe fractures of the long bones, facial bones, and fractures of the vertebrae should be transferred to a general hospital as early as possible. . . .

It was soon apparent, however, that not even all of the general hospitals could provide certain types of treatment. The Adjutant General therefore directed, in March 1943, that maxillofacial cases would be sent to one of the following general hospitals:[35]

Bushnell General Hospital, Brigham, Utah.
O'Reilly General Hospital, Springfield, Mo.
Valley Forge General Hospital, Phoenixville, Pa.
Walter Reed General Hospital, Washington, D. C.

The number of hospitals offering maxillofacial care increased gradually until the following eight installations were designated as maxillofacial hospitals in August 1944:[36]

Baker General Hospital, Martinsburg, W. Va.
Beaumont General Hospital, El Paso, Tex.
Cushing General Hospital, Framingham, Mass.
Dibble General Hospital, Menlo Park, Calif.
Northington General Hospital, Tuscaloosa, Ala.
O'Reilly General Hospital, Springfield, Mo.
Valley Forge General Hospital, Phoenixville, Pa.
Wakeman General Hospital, Camp Atterbury, Ind.

These installations were given specially trained personnel and every item of equipment needed for performing the most exacting operations on the oral and facial structures. The other general hospitals had qualified oral surgeons, prosthodontists and operative personnel, and laboratory and x-ray equipment, for the treatment of any but the most unusual cases.

As in the case of the station hospitals, allotments of personnel for general hospital dental clinics were determined within the service commands. Pro-

---
[34] SG Ltr 1, 1 Jan 43.
[35] WD AG Memo W40-9-43, 6 Mar 43, sub: General hospitals designated for special surgical treatment. AG: 705.
[36] WD Cir 347, 25 Aug 44.

curement was based on the following hypothetical authorization of dental officers, but the hospitals concerned were not necessarily provided the numbers listed: [37]

Number of beds	Number of dental officers
1,000	7
1,500	8
1,750	9
2,000	12
2,500	14
3,000	16
3,500	19
4,000	21

The maximum number of general hospitals in the United States was reached in 1945 when 65 installations provided bed space for 153,595 patients.[38]

DENTAL SERVICE ON HOSPITAL SHIPS

Since the primary purpose of hospital ships was transportation rather than definitive treatment, the Dental Service operated on a slightly smaller scale than in a hospital of corresponding size. Ships of 400-bed capacity or less had a single exodontist in the grade of captain or lieutenant; with 500 beds an oral surgeon in the grade of major was authorized; with 600 to 800 beds 2 officers were allotted, with the senior in the grade of major; ships with 900 or 1,000 beds had a lieutenant colonel, a major, and a captain or lieutenant; vessels carrying 1,500 beds had a lieutenant colonel, a major, and 2 captains or lieutenants.[39]

Hospital ships carried full base dental equipment, including prosthetic and x-ray facilities. As mentioned, the smaller vessels were authorized an exodontist, larger craft an oral surgeon. All types of work were possible and needs of seriously wounded or ill patients could be met en route.

The Dental Service of hospital ship platoons proved less satisfactory. These auxiliary units were used to provide medical care for patients returning to the Zone of Interior on ordinary transports. Each platoon with a capacity of 100 or more patients was authorized a dental officer.[40] A large proportion of all patients with maxillofacial injuries were transported by air, however, and these small contingents had little need for a dentist. Also, much valuable time was wasted in long "layovers" between trips. Since specially qualified exodontists or oral surgeons could not be spared for such minor organizations it was found that the men assigned were often young and inexperienced.[41] In view of these considerations the Dental Division decided that it would be in

---

[37] WD Cir 209, 26 May 44.
[38] See footnote 33, p. 272.
[39] T/O&E 8-537T, 7 Dec 43; T/O&E 8-537, 3 Mar 45.
[40] T/O&E 8-534, 21 Oct 43.
[41] History of the Dental Division, Hq ETOUSA, 1 Sep-31 Dec 1944. HD.

the best interests of all concerned if the dental officers and their equipment were removed from hospital ship platoons.

A recommendation to this effect was made to the Operations Service, SGO, 7 March 1944.[42] No action being taken, it was repeated 7 December 1944.[43] The new recommendation was approved by the Technical Division, to which it was first sent, and forwarded on 20 December 1944 to the Hospital Division for comment. The Hospital Division disapproved the proposed action because (1) it was felt that the dental officer would be of some use treating patients, (2) dentists were filling administrative positions which would have to be filled by Medical Administrative Corps officers if the dental officers were removed, and (3) it was believed that the dentists with the hospital ship platoons would serve as a useful pool of officers from which to draw in case of special need.[44] Faced with this nonconcurrence the Dental Division dropped the matter, though it still held that the use of dentists in hospital ship platoons was wasting manpower needed elsewhere.

DENTAL SERVICE ON ARMY TRANSPORTS

In World War I regular dental service on Army transports, as distinguished from incidental treatment rendered by transient dental officers, was not inaugurated until the latter part of 1919, when most ships on the Atlantic run were provided dental personnel and equipment. The Surgeon General's annual report for that year stated that experimental installations had proved so successful that new transports were being built with space for a dental clinic especially provided.[45] In the period of retrenchment following World War I, however, and with the withdrawal of most troops from overseas areas, this project was neglected. In the period preceding World War II the transport surgeon was normally equipped with a few essential dental instruments, and if no dental officer was on board as a passenger he took what measures he could to relieve pain until the ship docked. Army regulations authorized the assignment of dentists "if required," but did not specify definite conditions under which such assignment would be made.[46] So long as transports were small the absence of a dental officer was not serious, but when ships capable of carrying 10,000 men were taken over at the start of the war adequate dental facilities became a necessity.

On 26 January 1942 the Dental Division recommended to the Finance and Supply Division, SGO, that a dental field chest be placed on every transport

---
[42] Biweekly Dental Service Reports, 1 Jan 1944–30 Oct 1945. HD: 024.
[43] Memo, Dir Dental Div for Dir Technical Div SGO, 7 Dec 44. HD: 314.
[44] Memo, Col A. H. Schwichtenberg, Dep Chief Hosp Div for Chief Technical Div SGO, 23 Jan 45, sub: Dental officers in medical hospital ship platoons. HD: 314.
[45] Annual Report of The Surgeon General, U. S. Army, 1920, Washington, Government Printing Office, 1920, p. 303.
[46] AR 30–1150, 16 Sep 42.

so that emergency treatment could be rendered, presumably by personnel travelling on the ship.[47] No specific action was taken, and in August 1942 the Dental Division resubmitted the recommendation, accompanied by the following extract from a letter received from the European theater:[48]

> One of my greatest headaches, and the source of my greatest complaints, is the dental service on board transports en route to this theater of operations. As previously stated, in many cases there is little or no dental equipment on board these transports to relieve the urgent dental emergencies. Reports come to me of acute conditions going untreated during the entire voyage.

The Chief of the Finance and Supply Division answered that he knew of no convoys which had not had an adequate number of field chests assigned and suggested that the trouble lay in coordination at the ports.[49] On 16 September 1942 The Surgeon General directed all port surgeons to make maximum use of the available dental equipment and officers to insure that each transport complement was afforded at least emergency dental care.[50] On 23 November 1942 Col. Thomas C. Daniels, DC, was assigned to the New York Port of Embarkation to supervise the transport dental service under the port surgeon, and to take any action required to provide dental officers and equipment on transports leaving the harbor. These steps were apparently effective, at least so far as the eastern seaboard was concerned, for the dental surgeon of the European theater reported in October 1943 that he had had no further trouble due to inadequate dental treatment on transports bound for England.[51] Dental field chests were still not standard components of the medical equipment of transports, however, and on 7 March 1944 the Dental Division again recommended to the Operations Division of the SGO that M. D. Chest No. 60 be routinely authorized for all ships carrying Army personnel.[52] An equipment list published about a month later listed the dental field chest as a regular item for troop ships.[53]

When used on the larger transports field equipment left much to be desired. The amount of treatment to be rendered might equal that of a small post, and one ship reported that the dental clinic was in constant use from 8 a. m. to 9 p. m.[54] In addition, the light wooden chair of the field set proved very unstable at sea and the foot engine was difficult to operate on an undulating platform. On 20 June 1944, after a conference with the Director of the Dental Division, the surgeon of the San Francisco Port of Embarkation

---

[47] Memo, Col Don G. Moore for Finance and Supply Div SGO, 28 Jan 42. SG: 444.4–1 (BB).
[48] Memo, Col Rex McDowell for SG, 26 Aug 42. SG: 703.1 (BB).
[49] Memo, Col F. C. Tyng, Finance and Supply Div SGO, for Gen J. C. Magee, 28 Aug 42. SG: 703.1 (BB).
[50] Ltr, SG to CGs of all ports of embarkation, 16 Sep 42, sub: Dental attendance of troop transports. SG: 703.–1.
[51] Ltr, Col William D. White to Maj Gen Robert H. Mills, 22 Oct 43. HD: 703 (ETO).
[52] See footnote 42, p. 275.
[53] Incl 4, Equipment List No. 9N809, to Ltr, Chief Oprs Serv to CofT, 3 Jul 44, sub: Dental equipment for transports. SG: 444.4 (BB).
[54] Rpt, dental surg of an unnamed transport, 21 Jul 44. HD: 460 (Army Transport).

asked that permanent outfits be authorized for troop transports operating out of that base [55] and 4 days later his medical supply officer submitted a requisition for 50 units, chairs, cabinets, air compressors, and operating lights.[56] On the recommendation of the Dental Division this requisition was approved.

On 28 June 1944 the Dental Division recommended to the Technical Division, SGO, that current equipment lists be amended to authorize base-type dental outfits for Army transports.[57] For reasons which remained obscure, this recommendation was neither adopted nor disapproved. Its status on 14 December 1944 was described in a letter from the Chief of the Technical Division to the Chief of Operations Service, in which it was stated, in effect, that all efforts to get a decision from the Chief of Transportation had failed but that under existing instructions port surgeons could get the necessary equipment when they wished. It was further stated that "It is informally understood that the Chief of Transportation prefers this arrangement to any set requirement which would necessitate the automatic installation of dental equipment on all transports regardless of the circumstances under which they operate or the availability of permanent dental personnel." [58] By 6 February 1945 the Dental Division had apparently given up any hope of having permanent dental outfits authorized as standard equipment and asked the Technical Division to distribute a list of recommended items to assist port surgeons in ordering supplies on their own responsibility.[59] The Technical Division concurred in this request since it also had many inquiries from port surgeons concerning appropriate outfits.[60] The Supply Service, SGO, disapproved, however, for the reason that it would be tantamount to authorizing the issue of items for which no formal procurement authority existed.[61] Meanwhile, port surgeons had been able to have the desired equipment installed in many transports without the formal approval of either the Chief of Transportation or The Surgeon General. By the end of November 1944, 35 ships had been so equipped [62] and by March 1945, 63 transports had permanent chairs and units. Since the most important needs had been met by these conversions the Dental Division notified the Technical Division on 7 March 1945 that no further efforts would be made to have the base outfits placed on the standard equipment list.[63]

---

[55] Ltr, Brig Gen Wallace DeWitt to Col Rex McDowell, 20 Jun 44. SG : 444.4–1 (BB).

[56] Incl 3, ltr, Col F. C. Tyng to Chief of Supply Div SGO, 24 Jun 44, sub : Requisition No. D 4424–44, to ltr, Chief Oprs Serv to CofT, 3 Jul 44, sub : Dental equipment for transports. SG : 444.4 (BB).

[57] Incl 1, Memo, Col Rex McDowell for Technical Div SGO, 28 Jun 44, to ltr, Chief Oprs Serv to CofT, 3 Jul 44, sub : Dental equipment for transports. (SG : 444.4 (BB).

[58] Ltr, Chief Technical Div to Chief Oprs Serv SGO, 14 Dec 44, sub : Dental equipment for Army transports. HD : 314.

[59] Memo, Dental Div for Chief Technical Div SGO, 6 Feb 45. HD : 314.

[60] Memo, Chief Technical Div for Chief Supply Serv SGO, 21 Feb 45, sub : Dental equipment for Army transports. HD : 314.

[61] 1st ind, Chief Supply Serv, 26 Feb 45, to memo cited in footnote 60 above. HD : 314.

[62] Memo, Col Rex McDowell for Chief Technical Div SGO, 30 Nov 44. HD : 314.

[63] Ibid.

PROSTHETIC FACILITIES IN THE ZONE OF INTERIOR

Prior to World War II, prosthetic facilities were concentrated in central dental laboratories (figs. 22, 23, and 24). For a peacetime Army, or for small stations scattered over a corps area, these well-equipped laboratories, staffed with skilled technicians, could complete dentures or appliances with enough efficiency and economy to outweigh the disadvantages of transporting these cases considerable distances. However, with a fully mobilized Army, it was recognized that the facilities of the existing central dental laboratories were inadequate to meet the demands of the increased prosthetic needs [64] and plans were made to inaugurate laboratory facilities in the larger camps.

From the outset some laboratory space and equipment was provided in all the larger dental clinics. To reinforce these facilities The Surgeon General recommended to The Adjutant General on 2 November 1940 [65] that a DC-2 clinic be established in each station or general hospital of 250 beds or more. On 20 November 1940 The Adjutant General approved this action with additional comment as follows: [66] [67]

> In camps of less than 10,000 strength the building will provide dental chairs for all camp personnel, including hospital patients, and laboratory space for necessary making of prosthetic appliances. In camps of over 10,000 strength the building will provide dental chairs for hospital patients only, and laboratory space for making prosthetic appliances. The division of floor space between chairs and laboratory will be made locally.

Four months later, in March 1941, the Dental Division found it necessary to ask that laboratory equipment for these station hospitals be increased slightly, though it was still expected that the hospital laboratories would sufficiently reinforce the small prosthetic facilities in the camp dental clinics.[68]

By May 1941 the Director of the Dental Division foresaw that larger laboratories would be required in training camps and other strategic locations and announced a plan for their construction.[69] Responsibility for obtaining these installations, however, was left largely to local dental surgeons. In fact, Maj. Gen. Robert H. Mills, who became Director of the Dental Division early in 1942, subsequently stated that he had at first attempted to have additional CDL's authorized, and only after this recommendation had been rejected by The Surgeon General did he definitely decide to establish laboratories in each

---

[64] Final Report for ASF, Logistics in World War II. HD: 319.1-2 (Dental Div).
[65] Ltr, SG to TAG, 2 Nov 40, sub: Dental service in cantonment hospitals—dental laboratory service, divisional areas. AG: 632.
[66] 3d ind, TAG, 20 Nov 40, to ltr cited in footnote 65.
[67] The footnote referred to here is found only on a single copy of the basic communication. AG: 632.
[68] Memo, Brig Gen Leigh C. Fairbank for Finance and Supply Div SGO, 13 Mar 41. SG: 444.4-1.
[69] Fairbank, L. C.: Prosthetic dental service for the Army in peace and war. J. Am. Dent. A. 28: 798-802, May 1941.

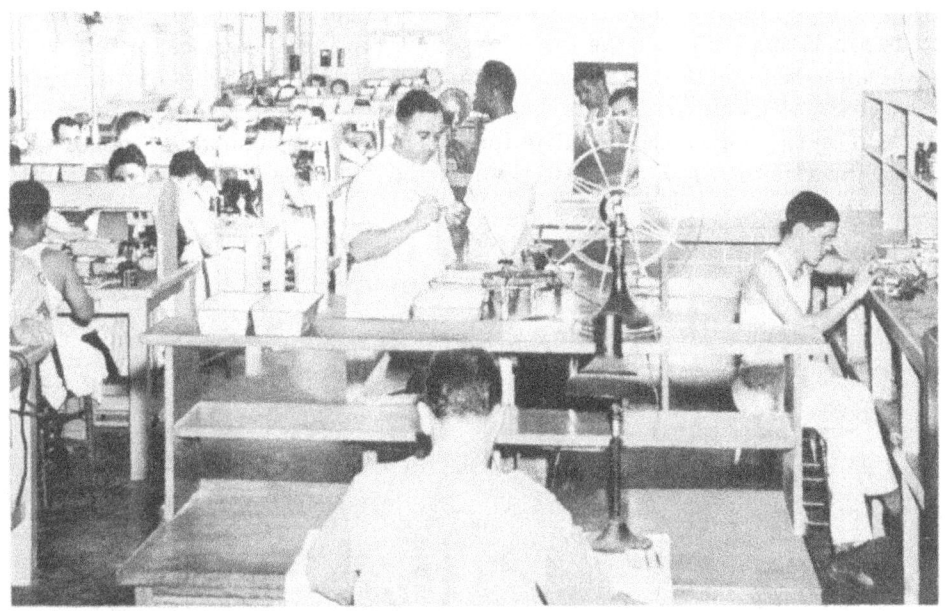

Figure 22. Surveying and designing unit, Central Dental Laboratory.

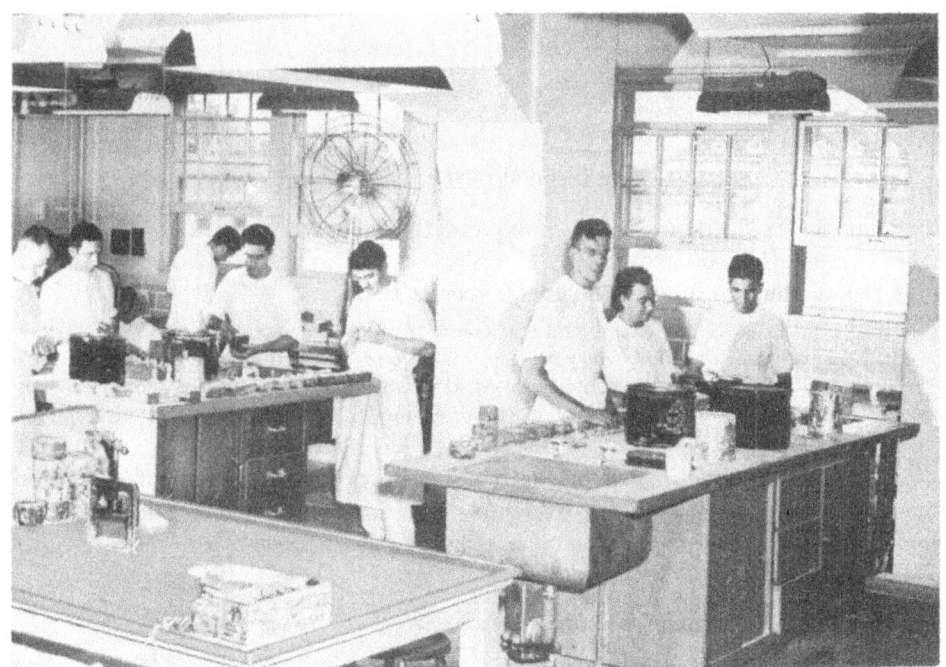

Figure 23. Flasking and deflasking unit, Central Dental Laboratory.

camp of 10,000 men or more.[70] Standard camp laboratory equipment was prescribed in March 1943. In the annual report of the Dental Service for the fiscal year ending 30 June 1943, it was noted that "An increasing number of the larger camps have been able to institute their own laboratory service, thereby reducing the load on the central dental laboratories." [71] From the annual report of the Dental Service for fiscal year 1944 it was noted "The tremendous requirements

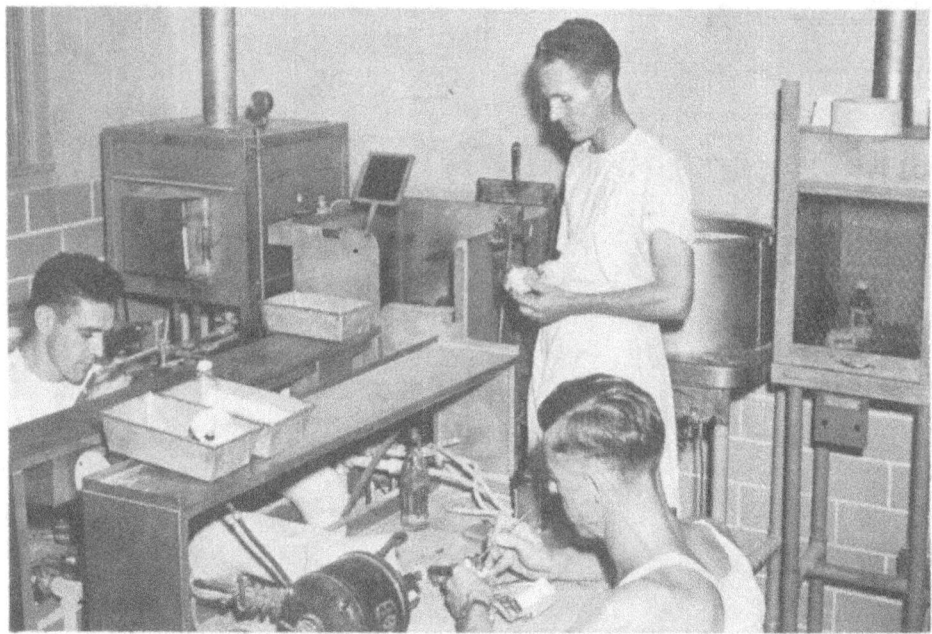

Figure 24. Vitallium unit, Central Dental Laboratory.

for dentures made it necessary to expand the laboratory facilities to include those camps of 10,000 or over. . . ." [72] It was not until 1946, however, that a War Department circular stated unequivocally that:

> All general hospitals, camps and stations with a military strength of 10,000 or over will furnish their own laboratory service, with the provision that each of those stations is authorized to forward cases to the central dental laboratory serving its service command when local facilities cannot meet the demands, and cases which require special fabrication methods available only at central dental laboratories.[73]

Laboratories established in the more important camps were often larger than the peacetime CDL's. Fort Knox, Ky., for instance, had 2 laboratories employing a total of about 25 men to provide prosthetic service for a strength of from 15,000 to 20,000 trainees.[74]

---

[70] Memo, Brig Gen R. H. Mills for Supply Serv SGO, 15 Feb 43. SG : 322.15–16.
[71] Annual Rpt, Dental Serv, 1943. HD.
[72] Annual Rpt, Dental Serv, 1944. HD.
[73] WD Cir 21, 22 Jan 46.
[74] Info given to author by Col Walter D. Love, former dental surg at Ft. Knox.

General approval by the War Department did not in itself insure that adequate facilities would be provided these camp installations, however. Under the usual system of assigning enlisted men, camp dental surgeons still had to obtain allotments of personnel in competition with all other branches. Moreover, there was no backlog of trained laboratory men in replacement centers in 1942 and 1943. Often a large proportion of all enlisted men allotted to the dental clinic had to be put on duty in the laboratory, leaving few assistants for the operating sections. Later, civilian assistants were hired to replace the technicians so lost, but at first, when demands were greatest, the activities of many dental clinics were hampered by the necessity of assigning half or more of their men to the construction of prosthetic appliances.

The camp laboratories reduced the strain on the CDL's, but prosthetic service still had to be provided for a large number of stations too small to operate their own establishments. It was therefore necessary to multiply the facilities of the five existing CDL's, and their increasing output from 1940 through 1944 is shown in the following tabulation: [75] [76] [77]

Year	Total cases completed
1940	10,658
1941	10,658
1942	48,012
1943	216,358
1944	178,034
1945	153,908

But while the total output of the CDL's expanded about 2,000 percent between 1940 and 1943, they completed in 1943 only 22 percent of all prostheses constructed in the United States, as compared with over 50 percent in 1940.

Operation of the Laboratory Service

There can be no doubt that the prosthetic service was severely hampered by shortages of personnel and equipment at a period when the demand for dental appliances was increasing many times as rapidly as the strength of the Army.[78] In spite of these difficulties there was surprisingly little delay in the processing of cases. In July 1943 the Director of the Dental Division stated that the current time interval from impression to insertion of the finished appliance was as follows: [79]

---

[75] Data on the annual output of the CDL's in 1940 are taken from Annual Report . . . Surgeon General, 1941.

[76] Figures for 1941–43 are found in Annual Rpt, Dental Serv, 1944. HD.

[77] Figures for 1944 are found in Annual Rpt, Dental Serv, 1945. HD.

[78] For discussion of personnel and supply difficulties see chapters on "Personnel and Training" and "Equipment and Supply."

[79] Memo, Brig Gen R. H. Mills for Chief Prof Serv SGO, 19 Jul 43, sub: Construction of dentures. SG: 444.4–1.

Elapsed time	Percentage of appliances completed
1–7 days	33
8–10 days	21
11–14 days	18
15–21 days	17
22–28 days	6
over 28 days	5

Actual laboratory time (CDL's and station laboratories combined) was:

Elapsed time	Percentage of appliances completed
1–7 days	54
8–10 days	18
11–14 days	11
15–21 days	10
22–28 days	5
over 28 days	2

A comparison of the time required for the completion of cases in CDL's and station laboratories is given in the following tabulation, based on 21,156 appliances processed in CDL's and 73,416 in station laboratories between 1 June and 31 August 1943:[80]

Elapsed time	Percentage completed in camp laboratories	Percentage completed in CDL's
0–6 days	39.9	67.3
7–10 days	23.8	17.7
11–14 days	14.8	7.2
15–21 days	12.4	4.8
22–28 days	4.0	1.6
over 28 days	5.1	1.4

It is evident that CDL's were able to process cases in considerably less time than the camp laboratories. This advantage was somewhat reduced, of course, by loss of time in the mails for cases sent to the CDL's, and 21.8 percent of all cases completed in camp laboratories were actually inserted within 6 days after the impression was taken, compared with only 15.3 percent of the cases completed in CDL's. But for any laboratory time over 6 days the greater speed of the CDL more than offset the time required for mailing, so that except for the 21.8 percent of the camp laboratory cases completed in less than 6 days the actual elapsed time between taking of impressions and insertion of the finished denture was less for appliances made by the CDL's than for appliances completed at the patient's home station. Actual elapsed time from impressions to insertion of the finished dentures for cases completed in CDL's and camp laboratories is shown in the following tabulation:[81]

---

[80] History of the Army Dental Corps, 1941–43, Table 16. HD.
[81] Ibid.

Elapsed time	Percentage completed in camp laboratories	Percentage completed in CDL's
0–6 days	21.8	15.3
7–10 days	24.8	35.8
11–14 days	17.6	22.8
15–21 days	17.8	15.6
22–28 days	8.6	5.7
over 28 days	9.4	4.8

Data on the output per technician are limited to the larger laboratories because of obvious difficulties in determining how much time was actually devoted to technical procedures in the smaller units. Figures given for the large laboratories include all dentures, repairs and bridges, though the latter item constituted a negligible part of the total. On this basis each technician completed 58.6 cases per month in 1943 and 51.0 cases per month in 1944.[82][83] The decrease in output per technician in 1944 was probably due to a slackening in the demand for dental appliances, which had made it necessary to operate with considerable overtime in 1943.

Use of Civilian Laboratories

In some individual centers the situation was more critical than indicated by the aforementioned figures. In July 1943 Fort Bragg reported that minimum time required for completion of a prosthetic case was 35 days; average time 56 days, while some patients had had to wait 120 days for their appliances. Fort Riley reported an *average* period of 91 days between impression and completion of dentures.[84] To meet these emergency situations the Dental Division was forced to make temporary use of civilian laboratories. In a letter of 26 November 1942 The Surgeon General called the attention of local commanders to their authority to send cases to civilian installations and requested that they take necessary action when military facilities were inadequate.[85][86] The following day a second letter placed some restrictions on the amounts and types of service to be obtained from the civilian laboratories, as follows:[87]

> a. This is an emergency measure to relieve the present critical situation in construction of needed prosthetic appliances only until our dental laboratories are established and equipped to take care of our needs. It is in no manner to be construed as a reason for any delay of effort to establish and place in full operation laboratories adequate to care for all local needs in all large camps. The Central Dental Laboratories will then be able to meet the demands made upon them by smaller stations.

---

[82] Data for 1943 computed from History of the Army Dental Corps, 1941–43. HD.

[83] Data for 1944 computed from Annual Report of the Dental Service, Jan–Dec 1944. HD.

[84] Memo, Lt Col R. S. Nourse, AG Replacement and School Command AGF for CG AGF, 13 Jul 43, sub: Eye correction and dental restorations. SG: 444.4–1.

[85] AR 40–510, C 1, 10 Sep 42.

[86] Ltr, SG to CG 1st SvC, 26 Nov 42, sub: Prosthetic dental appliances. SG: 703.

[87] Ltr, SG to CG 1st SvC, 27 Nov 42, sub: Dental appliances constructed by civilian laboratories. SG: 703.

b. When laboratories are established as above, except in isolated cases, there will be no need for further employment of civilian laboratories for the construction of dentures.

c. No special appliances, such as all-cast dentures of gold, ticonium, vitallium, or similar materials, are to be authorized under provisions of this letter.

d. In approving vouchers for payment care will be taken to assure that the prices charged are reasonable and not above those charged civilian dentists for similar work in the locality.

After March 1944 payment for civilian laboratory service was made by the service commands and it is therefore not known how many cases were completed under this plan. In 5 months, from March through July 1943, 16,607 dentures were constructed by civilian laboratories,[88] amounting to 5 percent of the total of 327,838 appliances constructed for Army personnel in the United States in the same period. From April 1943 through January 1944 a single medical depot at Los Angeles paid vouchers for dentures constructed for 8,643 patients, costing $276,271.35, or an average of $31.96 per patient.[89] At this installation the cost of dentures increased gradually from $23.09 per patient at the start of the program to well over $30.00 at the end of the period reported upon. (About 40 percent of these patients received 2 appliances.)

Important as the civilian laboratory service was in an emergency, it did not supply a significant proportion of the total cases completed. By September 1944 the central laboratories were able to handle all cases not completed in their home stations and a circular letter announced that a station unable to complete any appliance within 1 week would forward such appliance to a CDL. It also directed that station laboratories would be discontinued where diminishing activities warranted this step.[90]

Coordination of the Activities of Camp and Unit Dental Officers

Tactical units in training in the United States or awaiting shipment overseas were concerned primarily with the instruction of their personnel in the duties they would have to perform in action. They were unable and unwilling to assume responsibility for the routine operation of the permanent stations on which they were temporarily quartered. Nevertheless, many post functions had to go on whether the units housed there were in barracks or absent on maneuvers or field exercises. A camp where tactical units were quartered was therefore authorized a permanent service detachment which provided the necessary utilities and such special facilities as medical and dental service. Since it was undesirable to change the camp administrative staff with each successive tactical organization, this service detachment was put under a post commander and its activities were independent of those of the tactical units.

---

[88] Memo, Voucher Audit Br AGO, for Col Rex McDowell, 18 May, 3 Jun, 22 Jul, and 11 Aug 43. SG : 703.

[89] Weekly Civ Lab Rpts, LA Med Depot, 24 Apr 43–8 Feb 44. SG : 703.

[90] SG Ltr 295, 8 Sep 44.

During the early period of mobilization the fact that tactical unit dentists were administratively independent of the post dental surgeons led to some confusion. Unit dental officers had to devote much of their time to training activities, and were equipped with field dental chests only. They were therefore not expected to meet the routine needs of their organizations. However, though post dental officers were expected to assist the unit dentists, they were not authorized in sufficient numbers to enable them to provide full dental care for both permanent and temporary personnel. Adequate treatment could be rendered only by using both groups of dentists to the limit of their availability. Post clinics were planned to provide extra working space for as many tactical unit dentists as could be spared from their units, but some difficulty was encountered in obtaining their services when needed. Organization commanders disliked to release their dental officers for duty in the camp clinic and often gave them nonprofessional duties to occupy their time when not engaged in training. Unit dental surgeons also felt that they should have control of any installation where their men were receiving dental treatment and sometimes refused to cooperate when told that the camp dental clinic would remain under the direction of the camp dental surgeon.

To clear up any misunderstanding concerning respective responsibilities for dental care on posts having both types of dental personnel, The Adjutant General directed in January 1941 that:[91]

1. Camp dental clinics would operate under the camp commander.

2. Camp dental facilities would be operated and maintained so that the using troops would derive the utmost benefits therefrom.

3. Tactical unit dentists would be used in the camp dental clinic whenever they were not required for essential duties in their own organizations.

4. The use of tactical unit dentists in camp clinics would be arranged by mutual agreement between the commanding officers concerned. In case of failure to come to an agreement the matter would be forwarded to the War Department for decision.

At the same time it was explained in the Dental Bulletin that:[92]

> . . . under its provisions [the directive mentioned above] the dental clinics will be activities operated by the personnel assigned or attached to the post, camp, or station complements *and not by field force personnel*, although the dental clinics may be operated in areas occupied by the field force. Under this same authority, the permanent personnel of the dental clinics (i. e. those assigned to post, camp, or station complements) has been limited to that necessary for the operation and maintenance of the post when all units of the field forces are absent therefrom. This personnel will be augmented by members of units of the field forces only when the field forces are present. When the field forces leave the post for maneuvers or for any other reason, these men will be relieved from duty with the dental clinic and will rejoin their units. . . .

---

[91] Ltr, TAG to CGs of Armies and Corps Areas, 11 Jan 41, sub: Station complement activities and agencies. SG: 320.3-1.

[92] The control and operation of central dental clinics. The Dental Bulletin, supp. to the Army Medical Bulletin 12: 118, Apr 1941.

A second directive of 11 April 1941 provided that:[93]

a. Dental service at regimental and separate battalion dispensaries and aid stations will consist of emergency service and dental surveys in the tactical units to which the dispensaries are attached and will be provided by dental officers attached to the regiment or separate battalion.

b. Definitive dental treatment, serious extractions, and treatment which demands more extensive dental equipment will be provided in camp or hospital dental clinics and will be under the control of the Corps Area Service Command.

c. Dental officers of the tactical units will receive training in medical tactics as auxiliary medical officers and in emergency treatment of jaw casualties in their respective units. Technical instruction in more extensive definitive dental treatment will be provided in the camp or hospital dental clinics. . . .

d. Training activities in medical tactics and functions of the regimental and separate battalions will be under the direction of the division or unit surgeon. Technical training in camp or hospital dental clinics will be under the direction of the camp or station surgeon.

In July 1942 still more specific instructions were issued, as follows:[94]

1. a. The current shortage of Dental Corps officers requires the maximum utilization for professional duties.

b. It is desired that all Dental Corps officers under your jurisdiction who are now engaged in nonprofessional duties be relieved of those duties and returned to professional work with the Dental Corps as soon as practicable, and that in the future no dental officers be assigned to nonprofessional duties. You are authorized to make exceptions to the foregoing policy only when the immediate release of such officers will severely interfere with the functions of the medical service. In these exceptional cases dental officers will be permitted to continue on nonprofessional duties only until they can be replaced by qualified Medical Administrative Corps officers.

2. a. Instructions are being issued to division and other tactical unit commanders that up to 50 percent of the dental officers assigned to and present for duty with such organizations while they are at camps or stations where dental clinics are in operation are to be made available for duty at such clinics at all times.

b. It is desired that in cases of dental officers from tactical units made available for duty in clinics under your jurisdiction, mutual arrangements be effected locally to insure that although the clinics will be fully staffed at all times, no individual dental officer from a tactical unit will spend more than 50 percent of his time on such duty and that during the remainder of the time, each officer be returned to his organization for such training as may be directed by the appropriate tactical commander.

The restriction on the nonprofessional use of dental officers curbed the tendency of some commanders to use dentists for purely administrative functions, and at the same time the provision that 50 percent of the dentists with tactical units would be on duty in the camp dental clinics whenever their organizations were on the post helped the service detachments complete essential dental treatment for these units before they were sent overseas.

---

[93] Ltr, TAG to CGs of Armies and Corps Areas, 11 Apr 41, sub: Organization, training, and administration of medical units. SG: 320.2.

[94] Ltr, TAG to CGs all SvCs, 31 Jul 42, sub: Utilization of dental officers for professional duties. HD: 314.

CHAPTER VIII

Administration of the Dental Service in a Theater of Operations

GENERAL CONSIDERATIONS

In the administration of the Dental Service in theaters of operations, it was at first believed that the flexibility needed to meet rapidly changing situations could be attained only by assigning dentists directly to the small organizations which they were expected to serve, together with equipment which could be moved on short notice and set up near the actual combat area. Such assignments were made to small units the size of a battalion or regiment, in each of which 1 or 2 dentists were responsible for the care of from 400 to 3,000 men.

The unit dental officer was normally part of the organization medical detachment, responsible directly to the unit surgeon and through him to the unit commander. He was concerned mainly with the care of the men of his own organization and was involved very little in the problems of the Dental Service as a whole. His relation to the dental surgeon of a higher headquarters was often vague; the latter might offer technical advice, but the unit surgeon actually exercised direct supervision over the dental surgeon's activities. Under such control, the unit dental service had the advantage of flexibility; without waiting for specific orders from higher authority the dental officer and his equipment accompanied the command wherever it might move. Unfortunately, however, there resulted a system of highly dispersed, loosely supervised dental installations with certain very serious weaknesses.

Two of the outstanding defects of the unit dental services, the difficulty of providing uniform dental care in the larger commands and the inefficient utilization of dental personnel, are discussed in connection with the dental service of a division. A third difficulty was the practical impossibility of making an equitable assignment of dental officers to separate small organizations.

In much of the period between World Wars I and II dental officers were provided in an overall ratio of 1 dentist for each 1,000 men. Some officers were required for hospitals and administrative positions, however, and the number available for field units was therefore somewhat less than this figure. In the absence of any formal policy, a ratio of 1 dentist for each 1,200 men in tactical commands seems to have been generally accepted; this ratio was eventually made official in 1943.[1] But since very few units had a strength of exactly 1,200 men, or a multiple of that figure, the application of any fixed ratio was not simple. Even if the doubtful assumption that 1 dental officer could care

---

[1] WD AG Memo W310-9-43, 22 Mar 43, sub: Policies governing tables of organization and tables of equipment. AG: 320.2.

for 1,200 soldiers was accepted, what was to be done about the organization with 600 men, or the one with 1,800 men? In the final analysis each case still had to be decided on its own merits, and many unsatisfactory compromises were necessary. Some commands which would have been entitled to a dentist under the prescribed policy were allowed none if it was felt that they would be able to get attention from nearby units, while smaller commands were sometimes given a dental officer when they were expected to function independently.

The Dental Division recognized the need for a more equitable distribution of dental personnel. In 1944, with the approval of The Surgeon General and the Air Forces, it recommended that 1 dentist be authorized for each 1,000 troops. At that time the proposed increase was disapproved by Ground Forces and Army Service Forces, and even by the end of the war when it was clear that fundamental changes were needed in the tables of organization of tactical units, no further action on this recommendation had been taken.

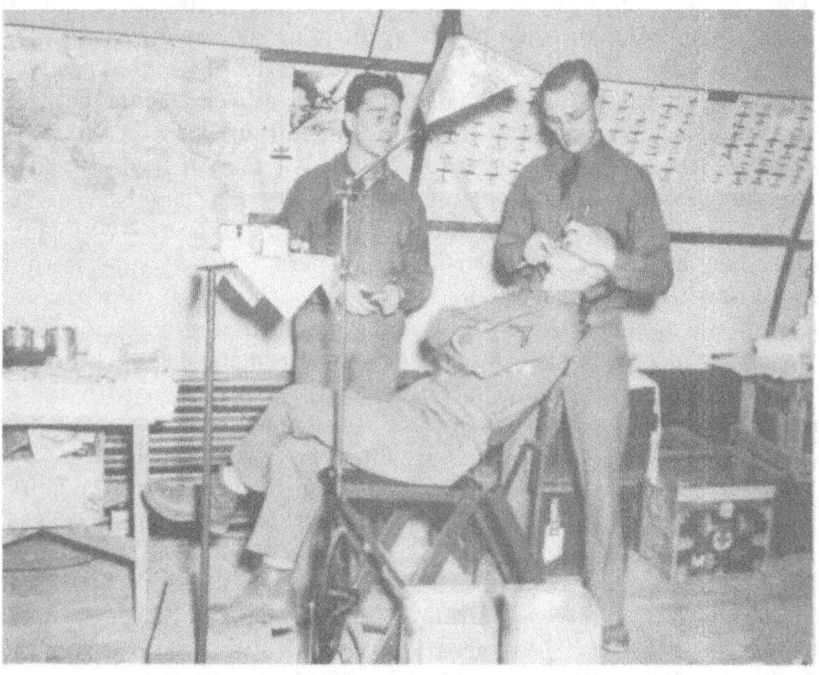

Figure 25. Dental Clinic of the 61st Coast Artillery Battalion (AA). Kaldadarnes, Iceland, 1942.

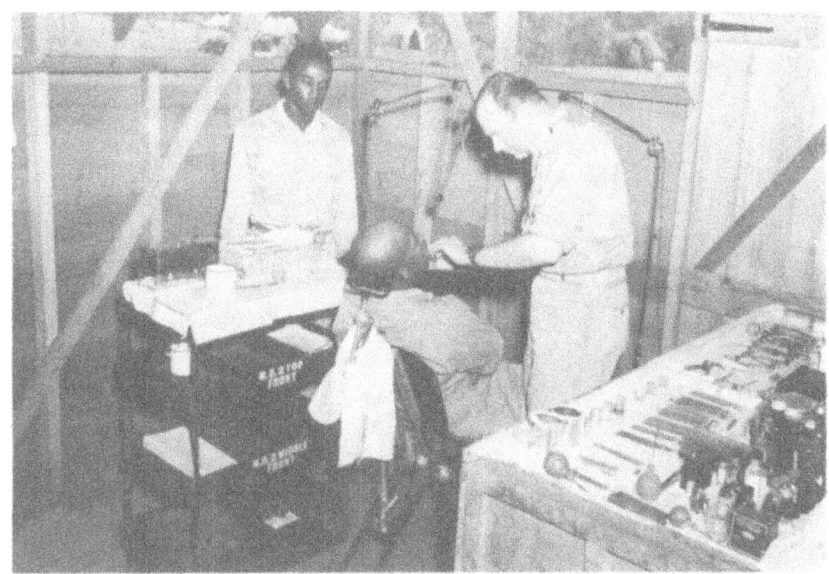

Figure 26. Dental Clinic of the 48th Quartermaster Truck Regiment. Queensland, Australia, 1942.

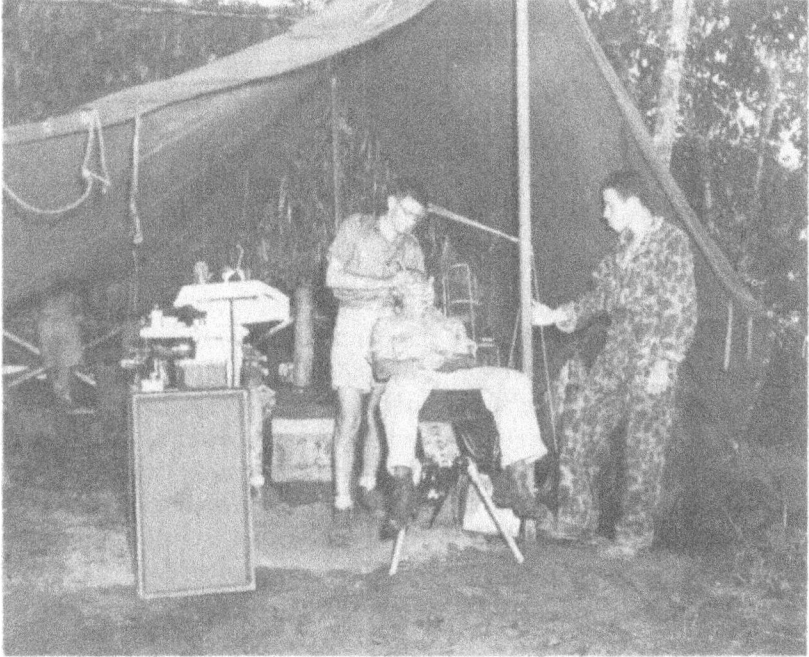

Figure 27. Dental Clinic of Headquarters Company, 41st Infantry Division, New Guinea, 1943.

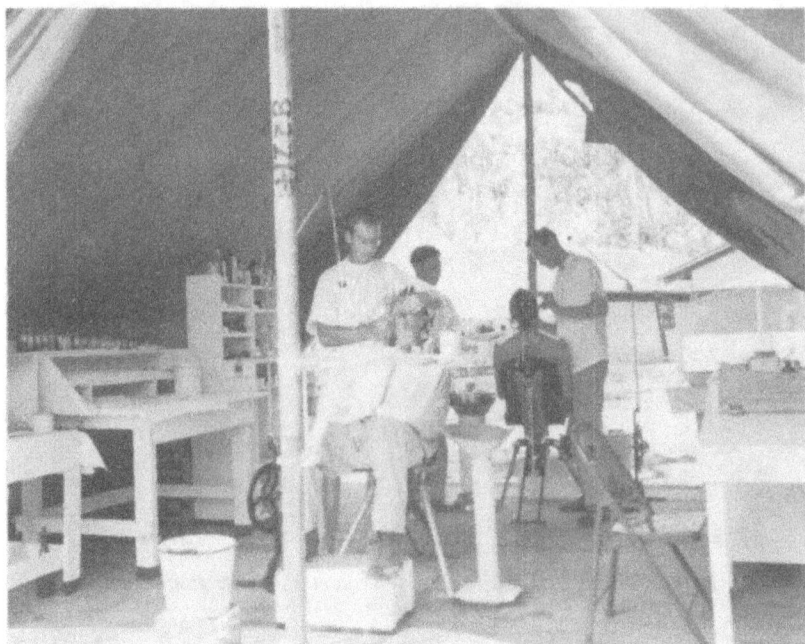

Figure 28. Dental Clinic of the 2d Field Hospital. Woodstock, Australia, 1943.

DENTAL SERVICE OF A DIVISION

In the administration of the dental service the division was an important organization for it was the smallest complete combat team comprised of many arms and services in which coordination of the activities of individual dental officers could be attempted. The division dental service, however, was a very loosely organized activity. It consisted essentially of the separate unit dental services of its component commands, supervised by a division dental surgeon.

At the start of World War II the dental service of a "square" infantry division numbered 30 officers under a division dental surgeon in the grade of colonel. In the "streamlining" of the division to its "triangular" form during the early part of the war this figure was reduced by approximately one-half, otherwise the internal organization of the dental service was changed only in minor details. With something less than 15,000 men the infantry division was authorized 12 dentists. One, in the grade of major, was assigned to the medical section of division headquarters as division dental surgeon. Eleven dentists, captains or lieutenants, were assigned to the larger component tactical units as follows: [2]

---

[2] T/O&E 7, 15 Jul 43.

3 Infantry regiments (3,256 men each)	6
Division artillery (2,219 men)	1
Engineer battalion (664 men)	1
Special troops (943 men)	1
Medical battalion (469 men)	2

One of the first responsibilities of the division dental surgeon was to coordinate the activities of seven or more separate dental services to provide equitable care for the organization as a whole. Under the system officially in effect during most of the war, this task involved formidable difficulties. Many smaller units had no assigned dental officers; moreover, the division was commonly reinforced with a number of auxiliary commands which were also without their own dentists. The total strength of these "orphan" units might reach several thousand men. In theory the personnel of the smaller organizations were expected to receive dental attention from the officers of nearby regiments or battalions, but in practice they were often given treatment under protest, if at all. The dentists of the larger units, who were individually responsible for a thousand or more men, were naturally reluctant to neglect their own troops to care for adjoining commands, and in this attitude they usually had the full support of their commanders and surgeons. The General Board of the European theater found that "personnel of units whose tables of organization did not authorize dental personnel received as a rule only mediocre dental service. These units depended upon dispensaries, hospitals, clinics, and other units in the area for their dental care, and in most instances the emergency cases only received attention." [3] Even among units with assigned dental officers there was no uniformity in the quality of the dental service provided. The dental officer of the engineer battalion, for instance, was able to render adequate treatment for all his 664 men, but the dental officer with the division artillery could meet only a fraction of the needs of his 2,219 soldiers. Even with unlimited authority the solution of this problem would not have been simple, and the practical powers of a division dental surgeon were anything but unlimited.

As previously stated, the dental officer of any individual unit was directly under the surgeon of that unit, who in turn was under the orders of the commanding officer. By tradition and necessity the commander had complete control over all personnel under his supervision, and higher authority was extremely reluctant to disturb internal matters so long as major policies or directives were not violated. The local commander's first responsibility was for his own men, and any proposal to use a dental officer outside the organization, or for the benefit of other troops, was almost certain to meet with prompt and vigorous opposition. As a staff officer, on the other hand, the division dental surgeon generally had no authority to issue orders. He could make recommendations to dental officers and commanders, but neither was obligated to accept his counsel. If his advice on an important matter was rejected his only

---

[3] Rpt, General Board, ETO, Study 95, Medical service in the communications zone in the European Theater of Operations. HD: 334 (ETO).

recourse was to present his problem to the division commander through the division surgeon. If approved, an official order could be sent through channels to the dental officer concerned. Approval of an action opposed by high-ranking subordinate commanders was very difficult to obtain, however, and the division dental surgeon, in the grade of major, who attempted to have a dental officer temporarily released from an infantry regiment commanded by a senior colonel often faced a fight to the finish. At best the procedure of issuing a division order was too ponderous to be of much help in making the frequent minor adjustments necessary to meet a rapidly changing situation. The following account is typical of the problem sometimes encountered by dental staff officers:

In 1943 the dental surgeon of the Middle East theater found that the dental officer of a unit which had been cut to about 400 men was being given full-time duty in administrative work, principally as court-investigating officer. On the same post three dental officers of other organizations were vainly trying to meet the needs of several thousand men, including the personnel of the unit in question. The unit commander flatly refused to release his dental officer for duty in the post clinic, or even to place him on professional work with his own personnel. The next higher commander admitted the need for corrective action but refused to interfere in what he considered the internal administration of the subordinate unit. The theater commander, in turn, did not consider the utilization of a dental officer a sufficiently important matter to warrant reversing the decision of another senior commander. In this particular case it was eventually possible to have the dentist transferred to another unit on the grounds that the original organization had been reduced in strength to a point where assignment of a dental officer was no longer necessary, but even this step was attained with difficulty and at the expense of the ill-will of the commander concerned.[4]

Surgeons and line commanders, like dentists, were only human; in some cases they did not exercise perfect judgment in dealing with dental problems. Nevertheless, they cannot be blamed for the main defects of the division dental service. Both were only exercising the established rights of any commander, and both felt that they were showing only praiseworthy concern for the welfare of their men when they refused to release a dental officer for temporary duty where his services were more urgently needed. Only a complete revision of the division dental organization could avoid the difficulties inherent in an attempt to provide uniform dental care with a number of small, independent, unit dental services.

Another problem of the division dental surgeon was keeping all unit dental officers performing professional duties whenever possible. In a reinforced division each dentist might have to care for as many as 1,500 men, and even the minimum needs of such a population could be met only if each

---

[4] Personal experience of the author who was dental surgeon of the Middle East theater at the time these events took place.

dental officer devoted all his time to the duties for which he was trained. Yet the dentists of units in combat could not operate clinics under fire and for weeks at a time could render only emergency treatment or act as assistant battalion surgeons.

As the war progressed it became increasingly evident that a more efficient use of tactical dental officers was imperative. A unit which entered combat in good condition could go for some time with emergency dental care only, plus the sporadic attention that was available between periods of fighting, but lack of definitive treatment eventually resulted in reduction of combat efficiency due to excessive evacuations for dental causes.[5]

Almost every World War II division ultimately attempted some modification of its dental service in an effort to improve the efficiency of dental officers assigned to combat units. The War Department apparently did not wish to prescribe any rigid reorganization however, until the more promising suggestions had been tested under field conditions, and no official change was published until near the end of hostilities. Most improvements were therefore made on the personal initiative of progressive dental officers, with the help and advice of far-sighted surgeons and line commanders. The final result, which differed in almost every organization, depended upon the individual ideas of the dental surgeon and the support received from his superiors. In a few divisions where dental surgeons were given complete control of all dental personnel and facilities, a near-ideal type of service was possible. In one such division the dental service was organized as follows:[6]

The division dental surgeon kept the dental survey records showing the condition of the command and supervised the operation of all dental facilities. One dentist of the medical battalion acted as division prosthodontist and operated the dental laboratory. The remaining 10 dental officers were assigned to staff 2 clinics. Each of these clinics had its own electrical generator and tentage and could be employed alone if necessary. Both clinics might be set up near the clearing station, or either or both might be moved on short notice to some location where they were more urgently needed. On the rare occasions when all combat units were committed to action the clinics worked for service personnel and for replacements. Treatment for the latter was particularly important since many hundreds might arrive in a single day and many needed care before they were assigned to combat organizations. The advantages of this type of division dental service became most apparent, however, when an infantry regiment or other combat unit was withdrawn from action. When the command arrived at its designated rest area it found a clinic staffed by at least five dental officers. It was equipped with electric engines and lights and so organized as to use the special skills of all its personnel. With such a

---

[5] History of the Dental Division, Hq, ETO, 1 Sep through 31 Dec 44. HD.

[6] The dental service described is that of the 8th Div, 9th Army, ETO. Info furnished by Brig Gen James M. Epperly, former dental surgeon, 9th Army.

concentration of dental facilities it was possible to complete a great amount of work in a short time and no dental officer wasted his efforts in nonprofessional duties or tried to operate under hopelessly adverse conditions. If necessary, single dentists could, of course, be sent to individual units, but the improvement in dental care for the whole command which resulted from the procedure just outlined greatly lessened the need for emergency treatment even in the small organizations. Though the dental service remained under the ultimate control of a medical officer (the division surgeon) this experienced senior medical officer who was more interested in the dental welfare of the whole command than was the average regimental surgeon, saw to it that service was impartially rendered to all elements.

In divisions where similar plans were effected the reaction of both dental officers and line commanders was uniformly favorable. (One armored division disapproved the centralized dental service because it was believed that individual officers were given an incentive for better work when they were responsible for the same troops at all times, but this division had not actually tested the plan.) It was found that with centralization even the larger organizations received much better care than had been possible when their own dentists had tried unaided to meet the needs of their commands in the short intervals between actions, while the smaller units were able to get treatment on the same basis as the larger. An effective division prosthetic service was provided and dental officers worked under conditions which promoted maximum efficiency. Line commanders were relieved of the unfamiliar responsibility for the Dental Service of their commands and their traditional rights were not compromised since the dentist was now assigned directly to a medical unit.

The increased output attained by centralizing the division dental service and placing it under immediate dental control was surprising even to the sponsors of such plans. One division in Europe reported that during the first week of operation 5 dental officers in a central clinic produced 17 times as much work as they had when working with their individual units.[7] During periods of combat the output of 10 dental officers of this division had previously fallen to 40 percent of the theater average (combat and noncombat) and to only 20 percent of their own noncombat average. With inauguration of the central clinic in a rear area the same officers completed more than four times the theater average of work even during combat, and during the exceptionally unfavorable circumstances existing in December 1944 their output still exceeded the theater average by 70 percent.

By the end of 1944 the Dental Division felt that sufficient experience had accumulated to justify an effort to have a revision of the division dental service authorized in tables of organization. Three senior officers who had been dental surgeons of armies or major theaters were requested to submit a joint

---

[7] Annual Dental Rpt, 8th Div, ETO, 1944. HD.

ADMINISTRATION OF THE DENTAL SERVICE 295

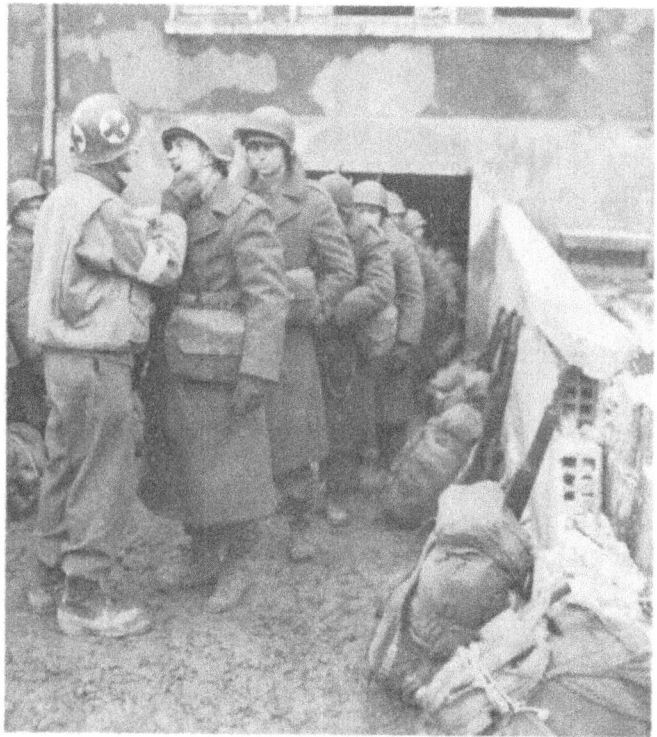

Figure 29. Dental Survey in European Theater, 1944.

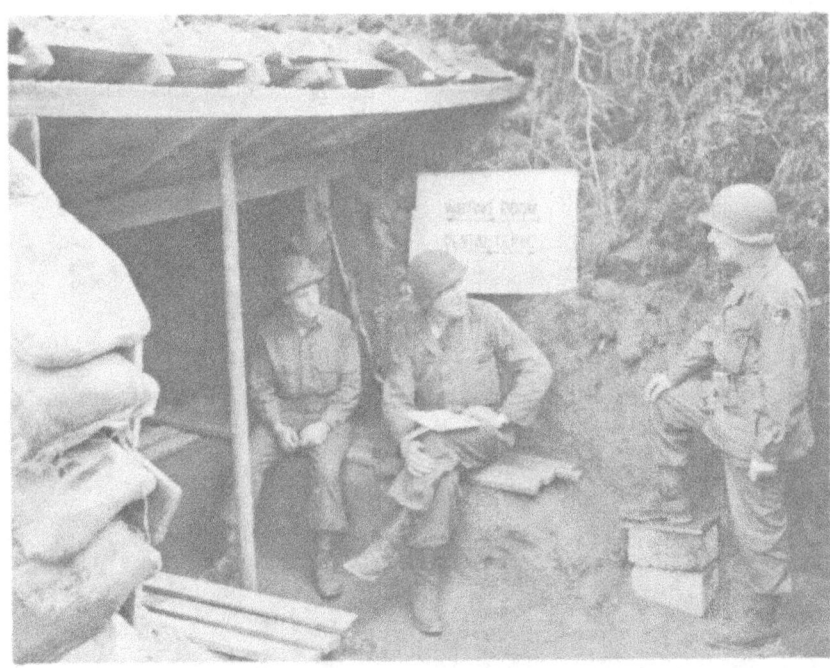

Figure 30. Waiting Room of Dental Clinic, 66th Infantry Division, France, 1945.

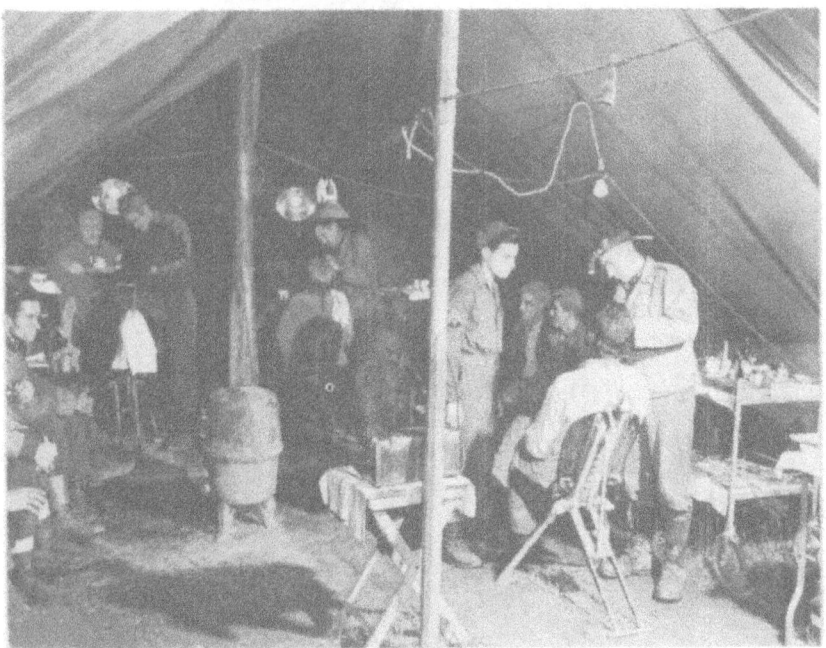

Figure 31. Dental Clinic, 9th Evacuation Hospital, France, 1944.

study of the dental service in the field. On 8 February 1945 they reported to the surgeon of the Army Ground Forces as follows:[8]

> Under the present method of assignment of dental officers to various units within the division the control and disposition of the division dental service by the division dental surgeon is greatly hampered. He may desire to utilize certain dental officers in other than their assigned units, and if the regimental or unit surgeon objects the dental surgeon is often overruled since the regimental or unit commander accepts the advice of his surgeon. . . . The unit surgeon's view is often selfish, being concerned only with his organization. For maximum efficiency the dental service of a division must be flexible, and if flexibility is obtained the dental officers can be busily engaged in constructive operational procedures under practically all conditions. . . . The dental needs of a division require the full and most efficient utilization of its dental personnel in dental capacities at all times. To secure this the following outline of a divisional dental service is offered:
>
> a. The division dental service to consist of a division *dental detachment directly under the division dental surgeon*, who in turn functions directly under the division surgeon.
>
> b. Detachment to consist of:
>
> | | |
> |---|---|
> | Division dental surgeon | 1 |
> | Prosthodontist | 1 |
> | General operators | 10 |
> | Total officers | 12 |
> | Clerk (for divisional dental surgeon) | 1 |
> | Technicians (067) | 2 |
> | Technicians (855) | 11 |
> | Total enlisted men | 14 |
>
> With this centralization of control the division dental surgeon can utilize personnel to maximum advantage by attaching officers or establishing clinics with units or in locations where the greatest amount of work can be accomplished. Normally five officers should be attached to forward units to provide emergency treatment and at the same time to accomplish as much definitive work as possible. These five would normally be distributed as follows: Each infantry regiment (1), division artillery (1), and engineer battalion (1). The remaining six officers (exclusive of the division dental surgeon) to be held in service areas where dental work can constantly be performed upon rear echelon troops and combat troops in reserve and in rest areas. These six may be utilized as one large clinic if the situation warrants, divided into two groups of three each, or three groups of two each. The division laboratory would normally be in conjunction with one of these rearward clinics. . . .
>
> The important and fundamental features to be stressed for a division dental service are: (1) Centralized control; (2) Maximum motorization possible.

Based on these recommendations, new tables of organization and equipment for the headquarters and headquarters company, medical battalion, were published on 1 June 1945.[9] This reorganization concentrated the entire division dental service in a "division dental section" in the medical battalion, consisting of a division dental surgeon in the grade of major, a division prosthodontist, and 10 general operators in the grades of lieutenant or captain.

---
[8] Memo, Maj Gen R. H. Mills for Gen F. A. Blesse, 8 Feb 45. SG: 444.4.
[9] T/O&E 8-16, 1 Jun

Thirteen enlisted assistants were authorized as follows: 1 sergeant (855) for supply and administration, 10 technicians grade 5 (855) as dental assistants, 1 technician grade 3 (067) in charge of the laboratory, and 1 technician grade 4 (067) as laboratory assistant and truck driver. The division dental section was also authorized a dental laboratory truck; one 2½-ton cargo truck with a 1-ton, 2-wheel trailer; six ½-ton trucks ("jeeps") with ½-ton, 2-wheel trailers; a 3-KVA generator; 11 Chests No. 60; a field kit for each officer; and enlisted man's kits for 11 of the dental technicians. It was provided that "normally 1 dental officer (general operator), and 1 technician, dental, (855), will be attached to the following units when in actual combat: each infantry regiment; engineer combat battalion."

World War II ended before the reorganization prescribed in T/O&E 8-16 could be put into effect, but previous experience with similar unofficial plans in individual divisions justified the belief that it would result in more adequate dental service for all personnel of units larger than regiments.

Even with the new centralized dental service there would undoubtedly be occasions when dental officers could not function in a professional capacity. In an invasion, for instance, dentists could be of most service as assistant surgeons during the period when the landing was being consolidated. Under such circumstances there was nothing to prevent the division surgeon, who had the dental detachment at his disposal, from using all or part of the dental personnel for nondental duties. But as soon as conditions permitted, the dental detachment could be reassembled to resume its primary function of preserving the dental health of the command.

DENTAL SERVICE OF A FIELD ARMY

Since the composition of a field army was determined by its mission rather than by fixed tables of organization, the number of dental officers assigned might vary within wide limits—from a minimum of about 100 to a maximum of many hundreds. (The Ninth Army had 650 officers at one time.)[10] Something less than half of the dentists of an army were assigned to the component divisions operating under the general supervision of division dental surgeons. The larger proportion, however, were assigned to hospitals and army units other than divisions, and the army dental surgeon was directly responsible for their activities, as well as for the general guidance of the division dental services.

Medical units assigned to an army were concerned primarily with the evacuation and care of casualties, and except for the provision of extremely limited prosthetic facilities their dentists could not be counted upon to render routine treatment for army personnel. Army medical units varied as widely

---

[10] Info furnished by Brig Gen James M. Epperly, former dental surgeon, 9th Army.

as did other elements, but a typical allotment (units with dental officers only) for an army of nine divisions would have been: [11]

Units	Numbers	Dental officers
Medical clearing companies	9	18
400-bed evacuation hospital	9	18
750-bed evacuation hospital	1	3
Auxiliary surgical group (Before April 1944)	1	7
Gas treatment battalion	1	3
Convalescent hospital	1	4
Field hospital	5	15
Medical depot company (After March 1944)	1	2
Total		70

In addition to the dentists assigned to army medical units, a large number of dental officers were on duty with the many service and combat elements allotted the command for the reinforcement of the basic infantry and armored divisions. The number of dentists so available was not constant, but generally exceeded the total of all dental officers with the combat divisions.

The problems of an army dental surgeon were essentially those of a division dental surgeon, on a larger scale. However, the difficulties of providing adequate dental care for the organization as a whole were increased in an army, partly because a larger number of troops were involved, but mainly because a much larger proportion of the army troops had no regularly assigned dentists. The principle of allotting dental officers directly to individual units had been based on the assumption that such distribution would provide for the majority of the troops in an area and that the relatively unimportant remainder could be taken care of by means of minor adjustments in the overall dental service. This assumption was partly justified in a division where the assignment of 7 dental officers to the 3 infantry regiments and the division artillery provided at least minimum dental care for four-fifths of the total strength of the command. But in an army the situation was reversed, and dentists assigned to individual army units provided dental care for only a very small proportion of the total strength. The nature and magnitude of this problem was more clearly revealed in a study carried out by the dental surgeon of the Ninth Army in Europe. His analysis of the dental service of a "type army" (3 corps of 2 infantry divisions and 1 armored division each) disclosed the following situation: [12]

Number of nondivisional troops with a type army	157,493
Number of dental officers assigned to nondivisional troops (including medical units)	205
Average number of troops per dental officer	768
Number of units *with* assigned dental officers	141 (23.3%)
Number of units *without* dental officers	463 (76.7%)

[11] T/O&E's for the organizations listed varied somewhat from time to time.
[12] See footnote 10, p. 298.

Number of troops *with* assigned dental officers_____ 48,225 (30.6%)
Number of troops *without* dental officers_____ 109,268 (69.4%)

It will be noted from this summary that the problem of an army dental surgeon resulted principally from inequities of distribution rather than from shortages of facilities. The overall ratio of 1 dentist for each 768 men was higher than in combat divisions, yet only 48,225 troops were cared for by their own assigned dentists. The remaining 109,268 had to receive dental attention from officers assigned to other units. In addition to the usual difficulties of persuading dentists to provide adequate treatment for the personnel of other units, the army dental surgeon was thus faced with the necessity of making, with every important change in the general tactical situation, new arrangements for the treatment of 100,000 or more men in 463 units.

The dental surgeon, Ninth Army, also emphasized another fact often overlooked; namely that the dental service of nondivision troops of an army far overshadowed that of the divisions themselves. There was a strong tendency to regard the divisions as the "core" of an army and to depreciate the importance of the "auxiliary" army troops, but the type army considered in the aforementioned summary required only 108 dental officers for the treatment of division troops while 205 were assigned to army units. Improvements in the Dental Services of divisions, important as they were, failed therefore to solve many of the overall problems of army dental services.

The striking advantages which resulted from concentrating all dental facilities of a division into a central detachment under the division dental surgeon suggested to some senior dental officers the possibility of applying the same principles to the problems of army dental services. Among the more interesting proposals along these lines was a plan submitted by the dental surgeon of the Mediterranean Theater of Operations.[13] This plan, which was designed to insure greater efficiency and a more equal distribution of dental service to all military personnel in theaters of operations, presented the following changes for eliminating the weaknesses of the system then in effect:

1. Removal of all dental officers from present individual assignments, except for those with hospitals, general dispensaries, and administrative headquarters.

2. Organization of dental detachments of 15 dental officers, 1 Medical Administrative Corps officer, and 24 enlisted assistants and technicians. Each detachment to have its own essential transportation and tentage and a mobile dental laboratory. The dental detachment to be organized and equipped so that it could function as one large clinic or as a number of smaller installations.

3. Each major force to be authorized dental detachments in the ratio of 1 detachment for each 15,000 men. Each detachment would be assigned to an appropriate area and the dental surgeon in charge would be responsible for utilizing his resources in the most efficient manner for the benefit of all troops in the area.

---

[13] Col Lynn H. Tingay, dental surg, MTO, Suggested plan for Dental Service in a theater of operations, 15 May 45. SG: 703.

During the war no such sweeping reorganization of an army dental service was attempted, however, and the coordinating activities of army dental surgeons were generally limited to relatively minor shifts of local facilities to meet changing situations.

Another persistent problem of the army dental surgeon, especially during the first years of the war, was the provision of an adequate prosthetic service. This was partly solved by the addition to combat divisions of prosthetic facilities, but it still did not provide the army dental surgeon with adequate facilities to care for special army troops. Of the army medical units, the 400-bed evacuation hospitals and the field hospitals had no laboratories; the larger evacuation hospitals were often not supplied in armies; and the convalescent hospitals, limited in number, were usually fully occupied with treating their own patients. The army dental surgeon might thus have only the three prosthetic teams of an auxiliary surgical group and a small number of prosthetic field chests from army medical battalions and clearing companies to render laboratory service for nondivision troops totalling more than 150,000 men. Though this situation was greatly improved by the arrival in quantity of the prosthetic trucks, it was still necessary to operate improvised (and unauthorized) laboratories in subordinate units (e. g. corps) and in such strategic locations as army replacement depots.

There is evidence in fact that even if the authorized ratio of 1 mobile prosthetic team for each 30,000 men had been attained in World War II, the full laboratory needs of armies and other major units would not have been met. From figures on the monthly requirements for replacements in the Fifth Army and from production records of the prosthetic teams, Colonel Lynn H. Tingay, former dental surgeon of the Mediterranean Theater of Operations, calculated that a single team with a division would meet about 75 percent of the prosthetic needs of the (approximately) 15,000 men of that unit.[14] This left a residue of 25 percent of all prosthetic service for divisions to be met by other means. On a similar basis, a single truck assigned to 30,000 army troops would be able to complete only about 35 percent of all needed dental prostheses, leaving 65 percent to be constructed by other installations. Colonel Tingay estimated that a "type" army (nine divisions) would need laboratory facilities for handling about 1,000 cases a month in excess of the combined capacity of the authorized prosthetic teams and army hospital laboratories. To meet this situation he recommended that "BI" teams ("dental prosthetic detachment, fixed," with 2 officers and 6 technicians) of the medical service organization be authorized for armies in the ratio of 1 team for each 100,000 men. Under favorable circumstances two or more teams could be grouped to afford the advantages of "production line" operation. Though it cannot be determined without further experimentation whether this or a mobile type of installation would be more

---

[14] Personal Ltr, Col Lynn H. Tingay to author, 13 Feb 47.

effective in meeting the prosthetic requirements of an army, most dental surgeons were agreed that some reinforcement was urgently needed.[15]

DENTAL SERVICE IN THE COMMUNICATIONS ZONE

The organization of a communication zone varied so widely according to the size and geography of the theater, and the nature of the principal mission to be accomplished, that its dental service could have no uniform structure. In particular, the dental surgeon might be directly responsible for all dental activities in the area, or he might act through two or more dental surgeons of subordinate "base commands." In general, however, communications zone dental facilities could be grouped under the following broad classifications:

1. Dental officers assigned directly to tactical commands. (In a communication zone, as in a combat zone, it was difficult to provide a uniform dental service with hundreds of individual officers concerned only with their own units. A detailed discussion of this problem has already been presented in connection with the dental services of the divisions and armies.)

2. Dental clinics and detachments established in connection with standard table of organization medical units.

3. Special dental facilities set up to meet unusual situations.

In the communications zone auxiliary dental care was provided by a number of medical organizations. In addition to those discussed in connection with an army dental service, the communications zone might have available any or all of the following, in numbers depending upon the strength of the theater:[16]

Units	Dental personnel Officer	Enlisted
1,000–2,000-bed general hospitals	5–10	9–13
25–900-bed station hospitals	1–4	1–7
Convalescent centers (3,000-bed)	5	9
Convalescent camps (1,000-bed)	3	6
Medical supply depots	1	
Medical dispensaries, aviation	1	1
Dental prosthetic detachments, mobile (1 for each 30,000 men)	1	3
Dental prosthetic detachments, fixed	2	6
Dental operating detachments, mobile (1 for each 25,000 men)	1	1
General dispensaries (serving 2,000–10,000 troops)	1–3	2–4
Dispensaries (serving 1,500–3,000 troops)	1	1
Medical detachments (assigned separate battalions)	1	1
Hospital centers (headquarters only)	1	
Maxillofacial detachments	1	1

The hospitals provided all types of dental care for their own patients; also treated the more serious oral surgical conditions of troops in nearby units. They had small laboratories and during the first part of the war it was

---

[15] (1) Personal interviews by author with senior dental surgeons. (2) See footnote 3, p. 291.
[16] The last eight installations listed were part of the Medical Service Organization, T/O&E 8–500, 18 Jan 45.

expected that these would provide an important part of the prosthetic service in theaters of operations. It will be pointed out, however, in the discussion of the overseas prosthetic service, that the demand for dental appliances soon became too large to be met by the hospital laboratories. Planned primarily to care for the sick and wounded, the hospitals did not have enough reserve capacity to supply dental service for large bodies of troops.

Of the smaller detachments, the "medical dispensary, aviation," and the "medical detachment" were assigned to separate bodies of troops having no regular dental officers, providing a service similar to that furnished by unit dentists. Before hostilities ended dental prosthetic detachments and dental operating detachments were available only in very small quantities and were generally used where more critically needed—in the combat zone. General dispensaries were employed only in connection with the more important headquarters, but with only three assigned dental officers the amount of dental care provided was woefully inadequate.[17] The dental officer with a hospital center was engaged in purely administrative duties. The functioning of the maxillofacial detachment will be discussed in connection with the evacuation of dental casualties. These smaller dental units met critical needs but they were specialized organizations designed to meet specific requirements for mobility or to provide care for definite bodies of troops who otherwise would be neglected. Even had they been available in the numbers authorized, the bulk of the communications zone dental service would still have been rendered by unit dentists and hospital clinics.

Standard dental facilities sometimes failed completely to meet the needs of large concentrations of troops in the communications zone. The fixed prosthetic team of 2 officers and 6 technicians, for instance, was not designed to supply large scale laboratory service for hundreds of thousands of men, and a 100-man laboratory had to be established in England. Similarly, the largest general dispensary had only 3 dental officers, yet 35 dentists were required just to care for military personnel in and around Paris.[18] Large clinics had to be supplied such installations as the replacement depot near Naples where 5,200 men arrived in one day.[19] Consequently the communications zone dental surgeon, who was also the theater dental surgeon in most instances, was required to improvise a considerable number of large clinics and laboratories not contemplated in tables of organization.

The theater dental surgeon had no reserve pool of dental personnel with which to establish these essential but nonstandard installations. Depending upon the urgency of the situation he had possible recourse to two alternatives:

1. If the need for the special facility could be adequately foreseen, the dental surgeon could submit for it a tentative table of organization. If

---
[17] See footnote 3, p. 291.
[18] Ibid.
[19] Rpt, Peninsular Base Sec, supp. to the Dental History, MTO. HD.

approved by the theater commander and the War Department, this table of organization became the authority for requisitioning necessary personnel from the Zone of Interior. The principal defect of this method was the time element for even under the most favorable circumstances several months were required to get the approval of all concerned and to complete the shipment of personnel to the theater. On the other hand, staff officers were slow to be convinced that a unit not contemplated in existing tables was actually necessary. The whole process of having a special table of organization authorized was so cumbersome that only one dental installation, a central dental laboratory, was so procured in the European theater during hostilities.

2. The theater dental surgeon might, with the consent of the theater commander, establish the needed installation with personnel already in the area. This procedure did not increase the total number of officers allotted to the theater, however, and it could be accomplished only by "robbing Peter to pay Paul"; men had to be "borrowed" from other organizations from which they could ill be spared.[20] Dental surgeons used devious methods to obtain the officers to staff such facilities with a minimum of disruption of the dental service. Most of the dentists drafted for such duty could be used for only a few weeks and the turnover of personnel was high. Constant supervision was needed to insure a steady flow of replacements and to provide qualified officers for the oral surgical and prosthetic services. Very little organization for efficiency was possible when key men might be lost at any time. Personnel from the smaller dental detachments were sometimes juggled to provide a reasonable approximation of the desired unit. In Europe, for instance, 6 fixed prosthetic detachments were used to establish a 36-man laboratory in Frankfurt.[21] Since only 2 of the 12 officers obtained were needed in the laboratory the other 10 were used to reinforce the badly overworked dental dispensary in the same city. Such subterfuges were countenanced because the results justified the means and no one was willing to inquire too closely into how they were obtained. The formation of these nonstandard, improvised units was necessary in the absence of any better plan, but the difficulties encountered emphasized the need for establishing approved tables of organization for all important installations which may be required in an overseas campaign.

Even more than an army dental surgeon, the theater dental surgeon was heavily burdened with the never-ending task of maneuvering minor, widely scattered, dental facilities to provide care for units with no dental officers and to make available the personnel needed to staff the large nonstandard clinics and laboratories. World War II experience indicated that the problems of a theater dental surgeon could be materially reduced, and the dental service improved, by two steps:

Make available to the theater dental surgeon a small pool of reserve per-

---

[20] See footnote 3, p. 291.
[21] Personal knowledge of author who was stationed in Frankfurt at the time.

sonnel to meet emergencies and add flexibility to the dental service. The dental surgeon of the European theater stated that "the one recommendation which this division cannot stress too strongly is that some provision be made for a pool of dental officers in theaters of operations." [22]

Remove dental officers from individual tactical units and assign them to dental detachments of 15 or more dentists, similar to those already discussed in connection with the dental service of an army. Each dental detachment, under an experienced officer, would, regardless of parent organization, be responsible for the care of all troops in its area. Detachments would be allotted throughout the communications zone on the basis of 1 unit for approximately 15,000 troops and according to the disposition of personnel each detachment would establish a dental laboratory and 1 to 4 or 5 clinics. The theater dental surgeon would make an equitable distribution of the detachments to meet overall needs but minor local adjustments would be made on the spot by the detachment commander who would also supervise the detailed functioning of his men. Such a reorganized dental service would have the following advantages: [23]

1. The provision of uniform treatment for large and small units would be simplified.

2. Dental officers would function under the immediate observation of an experienced officer rather than under the loose supervision of a line commander or a surgeon unfamiliar with the requirements for a good dental service. Line commanders would be relieved of the responsibility for the detailed operation of a highly technical activity having no relation to the primary mission of the organization.

3. To handle difficult conditions specially qualified men could be provided.

4. Dental officers would be relieved of individual responsibility for supplies, records, and other miscellaneous overhead, allowing them to devote more time to their proper duties.

5. Local adjustments of dental service could be made at once, on the spot, without the necessity for prolonged consultations with numerous individual commanders and dental officers.

It would also appear that the dental surgeon of a major theater would be able to discharge more effectively his responsibility for the quality of the dental treatment if given the assistance of one or more dental consultants. The

---

[22] History of the Dental Division, Hq, ETOUSA, from inception to 1 Sep 44. HD.

[23] This plan for the organization of the Dental Service has been proposed by several senior dental officers who occupied positions of responsibility during the war, particularly by Maj Gen Thomas L. Smith, Chief of the Dental Service, and by Brig Gen James M. Epperly, former dental surgeon, 9th Army, Europe. General Smith, however, has also suggested certain disadvantages of such a policy. In the invasion of France, purely dental units were given such a low priority for shipment that some would not have arrived in less than 3 months. It was found that dental installations could be moved to France in time to accomplish their mission only if attached to a combat command. One laboratory received a warning order for its move several weeks after it had already set up on the continent subsequent to having been informally attached to a line unit for the channel crossing. Application of the "cellular" type of dental organization would also necessitate some revision of plans for dental surveys, but satisfactory alternate schemes have already been worked out in some divisions and armies.

European theater had the services of an oral surgery consultant during the war but no full time consultant was on duty in any other theater headquarters. The administrative duties of a theater dental surgeon were sufficient to occupy most of his time, and in any event it would seem to be expecting too much of any one man to ask him to pass on the quality of the care given by specialists in three or more fields.

DENTAL SERVICE IN AN INVASION

Dental preparations for an invasion began long before the event with an intensified effort to put all men in the best possible condition. The dental officers of individual units brought surveys up to date, eliminated conditions which might cause men to become noneffective, and speeded up the tempo of routine treatment. At the same time dental surgeons of major commands reinforced unit dental officers with all available prosthetic and operative resources, and a special effort was made to complete essential replacements.

With the assembly of the invasion force in the vicinity of the ports of embarkation it was no longer possible to continue dental service on a large scale and emphasis shifted to the care of last minute emergencies. Since by this time the equipment of unit dentists had been packed, the bulk of dental care in the marshalling areas had to be furnished by installations not involved in the movement.

In the actual invasion and during the initial assault phase, the activities of dental officers differed with the type of action and resistance encountered but in general they served as assistant battalion surgeons or performed other nondental duties. In subsequent periods they usually continued in such capacity until dental equipment could be assembled for the resumption of normal dental activities. In the meantime, though the incidence of emergency dental cases was low, dental kits were utilized to care for those which did occur.

Lag in commencement of dental operations, as such, varied from several days to several weeks, and in some combat units fully 50 percent of the dental officers continued to be employed in a medical status for a number of months. In one such combat unit a dental officer remarked "I gave more plasma than I inserted fillings." [24]

The prolonged use of dental officers as auxiliary medical officers was widely condemned by most senior dental officers, but it cannot be denied that due to the exigencies of the first phases of an invasion, dental officers must be prepared to assume other duties until the situation has become partially stabilized. However, experience has shown that unless dental officers resume their normal functions at the earliest possible date any advantages gained by their emergency assistance will be offset by increased evacuations for dental reasons.[25]

---

[24] Rpt, 7th Army Sec, supp. to the Dental History, MTO. HD.
[25] See footnote 5, p. 293.

DENTAL SERVICE FOR REDEPLOYING TROOPS

With the end of hostilities in Europe the Dental Service was suddenly charged with the responsibility for surveying and completing essential dental treatment for thousands of men being redeployed to other combat areas. Due to the following circumstances this task involved unusual difficulties:

1. Personnel being processed in redeployment centers were available for a very short time only, and often arrived in waves which taxed the facilities provided for normal operation.

2. Redeployment centers were often established in areas where existing dental facilities were limited or nonexistent, so that clinics had to be built, equipment obtained, and personnel assembled before treatment could be started.

3. The general reshuffling of officers and men incidental to making up units for redeployment to the Far East affected dental personnel as well as combat troops and the confusion of the period multiplied the difficulty of obtaining sufficient dentists and technicians for operation of the necessary clinics and laboratories. No tables of organization were drawn up for these interim installations and personnel had to be borrowed from hospitals or other organizations, usually on a temporary duty status.

So that he could plan the clinics and supervise their construction or conversion the dental surgeon assigned to a redeployment center usually arrived about a week or two before operations were to begin. He then submitted requisitions for equipment and personally followed their progress through intermediate offices to insure rapid action. Dental personnel, supplies, and patients usually came in at about the same time. About half of the staff were obtained from the redeployment center complement and the remainder borrowed from organizations currently being processed. Basic equipment was normally the M. D. Chest No. 60 plus such civilian items as could be procured locally. Lights, cuspidors, and other improvised supplies were constructed and installed by engineer or ordnance detachments. Since prosthetic treatment made up a high proportion of all dental care rendered in redeployment centers a laboratory was essential, and in the absence of other trained personnel it was often staffed in part by qualified prisoners of war.

At the Florence Redeployment Center,[26] which had a maximum capacity of 25,000 men, provision for a 21-chair clinic was made. A single oral surgeon was able to handle all extractions but three officers were placed on prosthetic duty. One chair was devoted to examinations and one was used by the x-ray service—the remainder for routine operative procedures. The permanent staff numbered 16 officers and 36 enlisted men; the rest of the personnel required to operate the installations were obtained from transient units.

---

[26] History, Dental Clinic, Florence Redeployment Center, 10 Aug 45, inclosure to Supp. to Dental History, MTO. HD.

Dental officers on loan from other organizations had to be replaced at short intervals and dentists of the station complement had to be released for redeployment or return to the United States. Thus the turnover of personnel was constant and heavy. One of the principal duties of the dental surgeon was to estimate future requirements for his staff and arrange for necessary replacements.

When a unit arrived in a redeployment center the dental surgeon immediately contacted the organization commander and arranged for a dental survey if one was necessary. If the unit had an assigned dental officer he was directed to report to the central clinic for duty as long as he was in the camp. Men in Class I or I-D were called for early treatment, followed by as many less urgent cases as could be handled in the time available. All urgent treatment was completed and, except in periods of peak operation, a large proportion of minor defects were corrected as well, so that a high ratio of the men departing from a redeployment center were in Class IV. Since from 20,000 to 30,000 men might be processed in less than 2 months such a result could be achieved only with the most efficient organization and supervision.

The dental condition of men going through the redeployment centers varied widely according to whether or not they had been in extended combat and whether or not their units had had assigned dentists. In general, however, dental defects were not excessive. The following comparison of the classification of men redeployed through a center in Italy and men inducted at Camp Robinson (Arkansas) in 1942 shows that the dental condition of most men had been greatly improved during their Army service, even while in combat: [27] [28]

Class	Redeployment Center Florence Percentage	Training Center Camp Robinson Percentage
I	0.9	
I-D	2.7	26.5
II	19.5	29.3
III and IV	76.9	44.2

THE EVACUATION OF MAXILLOFACIAL CASUALTIES

Since maxillofacial casualties went immediately into the general chain of evacuation the dental service had no special responsibility for their management beyond cooperating in their treatment at medical installations en route. Methods of handling wounded men varied with geography, combat conditions, and transportation facilities, but a typical system might be described as follows:

1. Within a few minutes after receiving his wound the injured man was usually picked up by a "company aid man" of his own organization. This

---
[27] See footnote 26, p. 307.
[28] Health of the Army, vol. I, Report 1, 31 Jul 46, p. 8.

Medical Department soldier was trained in first aid and could stop bleeding or take other steps immediately necessary to save life but his principal function was to get the casualty into the hands of a supporting medical unit which would remove him from the combat area. The aid man stopped hemorrhage, applied a bandage, and directed the wounded man to the battalion aid station several hundred yards to the rear. If the patient could not walk he was carried by litter bearers sent forward from the same installation.

2. The battalion aid station was set up with field chests in the first available cover behind the "front line." Here the casualty was seen by a medical officer and possibly a dental officer as well, though the latter was more often located at the regimental aid station. Since the battalion aid station had meager facilities and poor protection from enemy fire the wounded man was held there only long enough to prepare him for further evacuation and to arrange his transportation to the rear. His bandages might be adjusted, he might be given plasma or a sedative if required, and an open airway was assured, but as soon as possible he was turned over to litter bearers sent forward from a collecting station which had been established by medical troops of the division medical battalion. The regimental aid station was usually bypassed at this point.

3. Division collecting stations were normally established within litter-carry distance of the battalion aid stations they served and, if possible, on a motor road passable to the rear. Two medical officers were available and with slightly more elaborate equipment they could attempt emergency procedures which were not practical at the battalion aid stations. However, the collecting station was still within easy range of hostile artillery and mortar fire and its primary mission was the assembly and evacuation of patients rather than treatment. In the absence of a dental officer at the collecting station the maxillofacial patient usually received only such general care as would minimize the danger of further transportation by ambulance to the clearing station.

4. Clearing stations were division medical installations which were normally established several miles behind the lines for the further assembly and treatment of patients from the collecting stations. Four medical officers and at least one dentist were in attendance and equipment included a small operating room and ward tents for the temporary care of patients who could not immediately be removed to a hospital. A clearing station had to be ready to move on short notice, however, and only the most urgent operational procedures were undertaken. A maxillofacial injury normally received little care at this point beyond the control of bleeding, treatment of shock, and possibly the temporary immobilization of fractured jaws with some type of bandage. As soon as possible the patient was removed by ambulance to an evacuation hospital.

5. Evacuation hospitals of 400 or 750 beds were army installations established beyond the range of ordinary artillery fire and within reach of reliable transportation to a major hospital in the communications zone. Though they were mobile and often operated under tentage they were true hospitals and had the equipment and personnel to institute general definitive treatment for casualties who had received emergency care in the installations already discussed. They possessed medical, surgical, and x-ray facilities, and the dental officers sometimes, though not always, had prosthetic chests in addition to the authorized dental operating chests. When casualties were heavy a special maxillofacial team might be attached. If such a team was available, the maxillofacial injury received conservative debridement, foreign bodies and unattached bone fragments were removed and fractured jaws immobilized with more permanent fixation than was afforded by bandages. Drainage was provided and prophylactic doses of penicillin or sulfa drugs administered, if indicated. In the hands of specially trained personnel this treatment added to the comfort of the patient and minimized disfigurement. In the absence of a maxillofacial team, however, extensive intervention at this point might do more harm than good, and evacuation hospitals were frequently instructed to limit their maxillofacial treatment under such circumstances to conservative measures to prevent infection and the application of new bandages and temporary fixation.[29]

6. As soon as it was safe for a patient with a maxillofacial injury to leave an evacuation hospital, he was usually transferred by train, plane, ambulance, or ship to a general hospital in the communications zone. Here he was put in the care of a team which included a plastic surgeon, an oral surgeon, an anesthetist, and specially trained assistants. His wound was thoroughly cleaned and nonviable tissue and bone removed; permanent fixation was applied; drainage was provided and infection, if any, controlled; eventually the wound was closed in a way which would best facilitate future plastic repair. If the injury was not too serious the patient might be retained at this point until he could be returned to duty. In most instances, however, the severe nature of maxillofacial wounds and the probable need for future plastic operations made it advisable to return the patient to the Zone of Interior when he could be transported without danger. Maxillofacial patients were given a high priority for air evacuation, and in a single 5-month period in 1945, 4,907 casualties with head and neck injuries were returned by air from overseas areas.[30]

Circumstances often made it necessary to modify the "type" procedure described. In the invasion of a Pacific island, for instance, a wounded man might be taken directly from the beach to a ship having medical facilities on board and transported to a general hospital in a rear area without passing through any of the installations mentioned. Patients from a battalion aid

---

[29] See footnote 10, p. 298.
[30] Leibowitz, S.: Air evacuation of sick and wounded. Mil. Surgeon 99 : 7, Jul 1946.

station were sometimes taken directly to an evacuation hospital if there was sufficient cover for ambulances to reach the aid station without being fired upon, while if there was no cover at all patients might have to be treated in a battalion aid station or a collecting station until nightfall or until the enemy was driven from the immediate area. In general, however, the following cardinal principles were observed: the patient was removed from the combat area with all practical speed with only the most urgent treatment given en route, and definitive care, especially that which involved removal of tissue or bone, was delayed until he could be put in the hands of qualified plastic and oral surgeons.

THE MOBILE DENTAL OPERATING TRUCK OVERSEAS [31]

The need for a mobile operating truck overseas was based on the following general considerations:

Any practical means of bringing convenient base equipment into the combat zone could be expected to increase materially the efficiency of dentists with tactical units.

Many small units had no regular dental officers and depended upon itinerant facilities for their dental care. Officers assigned to such duty required equipment which was both efficient in operation and readily transportable, with time lost for packing and unpacking supplies reduced to a minimum.

Requests for mobile operating trucks were received from overseas units early in World War II, but development was exceedingly slow and delivery in quantity did not start until the spring of 1945.

Since the official model of the operating truck did not arrive overseas until shortly before the end of hostilities, reports on its functioning were meager, though uniformly favorable.[32] However, more elaborate reports are available on the many improvised operating trucks placed in operation before the arrival of the standard vehicle.

In the absence of an official model, almost every theater managed to assemble a considerable number of improvised dental operating trucks of widely varying characteristics. In many cases these were built by small organizations with captured and makeshift equipment, but in Italy the Fifth Army went so far as to authorize the construction of dental trailers on standard bodies in the ratio of five trailers for each infantry division.[33] The following reports are typical of a large number received:

Fifth Army. As in the case of the mobile prosthetic trucks, the mobile operating trucks could function under any conditions, and by seeking out the

---

[31] For a description of the mobile operating truck see chapter V. The history of the development of this item has been told in Johnson, J. B., and Wilson, G. H.: History of wartime research and development of medical field equipment. HD.

[32] Ibid.

[33] Rpt, 5th Army Sec, supp. to Dental History, MTO. HD.

patient saved an inestimable number of man-hours which would otherwise have been consumed by patients travelling to a point where their needs could be met.[34]

Twelfth Air Force. In May 1943 it became increasingly evident that a great deal of operating efficiency at the chair was being lost due to the time required to set up and tear down the dental equipment before and after an organizational move. At this time efforts were directed toward construction of a number of complete dental offices in covered trucks or trailers which were to remain in operative condition during an overland move.

> One such unit was constructed at the direction of the surgeon of the Twelfth Air Force in the 809th Engineer Aviation Battalion. At the same time another mobile unit was being manufactured by . . . the 560th Signal Air Warning Battalion. These two units proved so successful in giving dental attention to outlying stations and facilitating the service as a whole that coordinated efforts were continued along this line. . . . Through the individual efforts of the organization dental officers and with the cooperation of the Ordnance Section of both the Twelfth Air Force and the Twelfth Air Force Service Command, nine mobile dental units were in operation 1 February 1944.[35]

There could be no doubt of the superior convenience of the mobile operating truck over the dental facilities available in the M. D. Chest No. 60, and there was every reason to believe that similar vehicles would henceforth be considered essential to the dental service overseas and in maneuver areas in the United States. However, in determining the extent to which mobile units would eventually supplant dental field chests several other factors had to be considered. In the first place, the operating trucks were not a substitute for large, conveniently equipped clinics, wherever the latter were practical. Further, the mobile units cost about $9,000 each, while the Chest 60 cost only a little over $300. Obviously it would be necessary to determine whether or not manpower and materials would be available for the construction of several thousand operating trucks in a time of national emergency before this item could be adopted as standard equipment for any large proportion of the dentists with the field forces. Also, the mobile units were not adapted for use in jungle areas or on small Pacific islands where a chest which could be carried by hand might actually be more mobile than a truck.

It is highly probable that future experimentation with mobile units will find means to reduce materially both the cost and the weight of the dental operating truck, possibly by installing lighter equipment in a trailer or in a smaller self-propelled vehicle. In 1945 the Director of the Dental Division recommended further study along these lines.[36]

---

[34] See footnote 33, p. 311.
[35] Rpt, 12th AF Sec, supp. to Dental History, MTO. HD.
[36] Final Rpt for ASF, Logistics in World War II. HD.

THE PROSTHETIC SERVICE OVERSEAS

World War I

The more rigid physical requirements which were in effect during most of the First World War prevented the induction of such large numbers of dental cripples as were accepted for full military duty in World War II. Also, the early end of World War I brought demobilization of the Armed Forces before the full effect of meager overseas prosthetic facilities could be felt. As a result, the provision of prosthetic dental appliances for the personnel of the American Expeditionary Forces in 1918 and 1919 was a comparatively minor problem. Only 13,140 new dentures and repairs were completed in France from July 1917 through May 1919. Of these only 2 percent were full dentures.[37] Only 1 soldier out of each 150 men in the AEF was provided any denture service overseas.

In World War I, laboratory equipment was initially furnished abroad only in base hospitals, evacuation hospitals, and in certain large clinics in the principal centers of population. Installations which were called central dental laboratories were established in base sections and depot division areas but these laboratories functioned mainly for the camps in which they were operating, usually taking impressions as well as completing the fabrication of cases. No official laboratories were set up specifically to process appliances from impressions taken within the smaller organizations. No prosthetic facilities were provided in the combat divisions and men in those commands who needed dental replacements had to be sent to a hospital or to one of the large clinics in the communications zone.

It was soon apparent that there was urgent need for prosthetic equipment within combat units to avoid unnecessary evacuation of personnel. A man sent to a base hospital for construction of dentures might be lost to his organization for as long as a man hospitalized with a moderately serious wound, and the mere fact that a soldier had to leave the combat zone for any type of prosthetic treatment encouraged the willful destruction of dental appliances and increased the demand for replacements which could not be considered essential. The experience of one division dental surgeon graphically illustrates the situation which sometimes arose. This officer was called to investigate a report that due to absences for construction of dental appliances the strength of one company of an infantry regiment was being dangerously reduced. He found that the trouble had started several days before when a single officer had been authorized to go to Paris for construction of a needed replacement. The following day several persons with more or less legitimate requirements had requested the same privilege. On the third day approximately a dozen had reported for this purpose, and on the fourth 20 men, many of whom were merely hopeful, asked

---

[37] The Medical Department of the United States Army in the World War. Washington, Government Printing Office, 1927, vol II, p. 121.

to be sent to Paris. It was necessary to limit further evacuations from that company to cases approved by the division dental surgeon.[38] As a result of such experiences, which were repeated in less exaggerated form in many divisions of the AEF, a special prosthetic chest weighing about 200 pounds was assembled and issued to each division as it entered the final phase of combat training.[39] This chest was used to establish a laboratory in the division field hospital where it effectually prevented the evacuation of troops for dental care. Other changes in the overseas prosthetic service during World War I were of minor importance.

World War II

With the experience of World War I in mind the Dental Division was careful to make what was considered ample provision for prosthetic facilities in theaters of operations. Tables of organization in effect at the start of World War II authorized dental laboratories in many convenient installations in the communications zone and as far forward into the combat zone as they could safely be operated.

In rear areas small permanent laboratories were provided in all general hospitals and in all station hospitals of more than 50-bed capacity; later they were also supplied in convalescent camps and convalescent centers.

Though central dental laboratories were not specifically prescribed for overseas use, it was anticipated that they could be obtained on special tables of organization when required.

In the combat zone, fixed or semifixed laboratories were of course impractical, but the portable equipment contained in the M. D. Chests Nos. 61 and 62 was provided all convalescent hospitals, evacuation hospitals, and field hospitals. Portable laboratory equipment was also carried by the medical battalion assigned to each division. The field sets, with their hand-operated lathes and lack of protection from the elements, were not suitable for large scale production but they brought laboratory facilities within easy reach of the fighting man. The Dental Division also expected to obtain modern laboratory trucks for the use of prosthetic teams in the combat zone,[40] and after July 1942 three mobile units were authorized, in theory at least, for each of the auxiliary surgical groups supposed to be assigned to field armies. In spite of these facilities, however, the provision of prosthetic replacements overseas proved to be one of the major problems of the Dental Service during the first years of the war.

Difficulties in providing adequate prosthetic care overseas resulted mainly from the fact that demands for dental appliances greatly exceeded all calcu-

---

[38] Personal experience of Maj Gen Thomas L. Smith who was dental surgeon of the 80th Infantry Division, AEF.
[39] See footnote 37, p. 313.
[40] Fairbank, L. C.: Prosthetic dental service for the Army in peace and war. J. Am. Dent. A. 28: 801, May 1941.

lations. In contrast with the total of 13,140 dentures constructed in France during the First World War, 845,000 prosthetic cases were completed for military personnel outside the United States in the 4 years from 1942 through 1945; an additional 20,000 appliances were constructed for civilians and prisoners of war.[41] The following prosthetic operations of various types were completed for each 1,000 men overseas during the 3-year period 1943–45:[42]

Year	Full dentures	Partial dentures	Repairs	Total
1943	10.0	28.1	19.9	58.0
1944	12.3	37.9	29.4	79.6
1945	9.2	40.3	33.6	83.1
Yearly average	10.5	37.2	29.6	77.4

Theater reports in 1944 placed the proportion of overseas personnel wearing dentures at about 10 percent.[43] [44] [45] [46]

In every area the dental laboratories were pushed to the limit of their capacity. The Dental Division reported that 7.2 prosthetic operations were completed for each 1,000 men overseas in the single month of August 1944.[47] The Fifth Army in Italy found that 9 men per 1,000 required prosthetic treatment every month.[48] The First Army in France reported that "the construction, reconstruction, and repair of dental prostheses is the main dental problem that we have had to contend with."[49] A single prosthetic team on a Pacific island (Saipan) constructed 300 dentures a month,[50] and on the Anzio beachhead, where 1 dental officer was killed, 5 wounded, and 1 captured, laboratories in tents protected by sand bags completed 373 cases under constant shelling and bombing during March 1944.[51]

The unexpectedly large requirements for prosthetic treatment overseas may be attributed to a number of factors. Early in the war it was necessary to ship personnel to foreign areas before essential dental care could be completed, and these men often needed replacements on arrival in the theater. Many cases were started in the United States but not completed before departure of the patient, and nearly all of the dentures made under these circumstances were either lost in shipment or reached the individual after so many months that they were useless. In the rush to get troops ready for duty abroad prosthetic appliances were unavoidably placed too soon after extraction and the dental surgeon of the European theater reported in 1943 that 10 percent of

---
[41] Data compiled by author from reports in the files of the Dental Division, SGO, 1947.
[42] Ibid.
[43] ETMD Rpt, SWPA, 6 Jul 44. HD: 350.05.
[44] Quarterly Rpt of Dental Activities, Hq Base Section No 3, SWPA, 20 Apr 44. HD.
[45] Medical History 1312th Engineer General Service Regiment, SWPA, May–Jul 1944 (4 Jul 44). HD.
[46] Quarterly Dental History, Hq Base E, SWPA, 23 Jul 44. HD.
[47] Memo, Maj Gen R. H. Mills for Technical Div, SGO, 18 Nov 44. SG: 400.34.
[48] See footnote 33, p. 311.
[49] Dental History, 1st Army, 18 Oct 43 to 30 Jun 44. HD.
[50] Annual Rpt, 148th GH (Saipan), 1945, p. 24. HD.
[51] Cowan, E. V. W.: North African Theater. Mil. Surgeon 96: 142, Feb 1945.

the men who received prosthetic treatment shortly before shipment were unable to wear their appliances on arrival in England.[52] The lack of prosthetic facilities in forward units early in the war also encouraged carelessness in the handling of dentures since loss or willful destruction of an appliance might lead to evacuation from a combat area.

All of these factors were secondary, however, to the simple fact that an unexpectedly large number of men who required dental appliances had been taken into the Army, thus increasing the demand for both initial and maintenance treatment far beyond what had been anticipated. Many of these dental cripples had already been supplied replacements when they arrived overseas, but dentures are necessarily fragile and require occasional reconstruction to compensate for gradual changes in the oral structures. Others, borderline cases, needed appliances after the loss of only one or two additional teeth. The Fifth Army reported:[53]

> It is of interest to note how quickly prosthetic needs appear in newly arrived divisions (85th, 88th, and 91st) even though these divisions' troops embarked for overseas duty with all dental requirements fulfilled. Also of significance is the rate of new dentures and the rate of denture repairs within veteran divisions (1st Armored, 34th, 36th, and 45th).

When nearly 500,000 men overseas were wearing one or more dentures it is not surprising that over 800,000 cases were completed during 4 years of field operations. Prosthetic requirements overseas, though not as great as in the large camps receiving recent inductees in the United States, were somewhat greater than for noncombat troops living under relatively stable conditions, but the bulk of the prosthetic treatment rendered overseas was routine in nature and would have been necessary wherever an equal number of men had been on duty.

The situation resulting from the unexpected demand for prosthetic service overseas was further complicated by the removal, early in the war, of all portable laboratory equipment from medical battalions and regiments, from the 400-bed evacuation hospitals, and the field hospitals. Very little correspondence has been found to explain this important action, and it was apparently based largely on informal agreements. As nearly as can be determined the Army Ground Forces and the Dental Division, the two agencies most concerned, were actuated by entirely different motives. The AGF had streamlined the division and was anxious to keep noncombatant personnel and equipment in the combat zone to a minimum. The Dental Division, on the other hand, certainly had no intention of leaving the forward areas without prosthetic service, but it was equally anxious to substitute laboratory trucks for the less efficient portable outfits and it appears to have concurred in the proposed action in the belief that the trucks would be able to provide an even better service by the time the field chests were removed.[54] This optimism was later proved premature since

---

[52] Personal Ltr, Col William D. White to Maj Gen R. H. Mills, 22 Oct 43. HD: 703 (ETO).
[53] See footnote 33, p. 311.
[54] Memo, Col Rex McK. McDowell for Insp Br, Plans Div, SGO, 15 Jan 44. SG: 703.

development of the trucks lagged and delivery did not start until the summer of 1944.

In any event, the Dental Division recommended in November 1942 that the field laboratory chests be removed from all medical battalions.[55] No further correspondence has been found on this recommendation but it is apparent that oral approval was granted and the portable sets were removed not only from the medical battalions but also from the smaller evacuation hospitals. Changes in equipment lists were made very informally at this time, often by undated pencilled notations; it is therefore not clear exactly when the field chests were eliminated, but by 7 September 1943 the Dental Division noted that "with the exception of the 750-bed evacuation hospitals and the convalescent hospitals the prosthetic service in an army area is provided only by the prosthetic teams, of which there are three in the auxiliary surgical group."[56]

Removal of Chests 61 and 62 from the medical battalions and small combat zone hospitals left the divisions with no prosthetic service whatever and drastically reduced the facilities of the armies. Even with the 3 prosthetic teams which had been added to the auxiliary surgical group, an army of 10 divisions, with 3 evacuation hospitals and 1 field hospital, suffered a net loss of 11 field laboratories. The mobile laboratories of the auxiliary surgical group were expected to function with more efficiency than the equipment carried in chests, but the trucks were not available until well into 1944, a year after the field chests were eliminated.

The hospitals of the communications zone were already busy providing prosthetic treatment for their areas and they could increase their output only to a limited extent. Also, since patients had to be sent from many miles away, hospitals had to devote beds needed for the care of the wounded to men who required only a place to sleep and eat while their appliances were being constructed. At one time in 1943, 250 prosthetic patients occupied beds in general hospitals of the Mediterranean Base Section.[57] In March 1943 the dental surgeon of the North African theater reported:[58]

> At present there are thirty-five patients occupying beds in the 21st General Hospital, awaiting denture prostheses as part of their medical treatment. The 64th Station Hospital is servicing an engineer regiment of the 6th Corps. This regiment is soon to move east and has over 50 denture cases awaiting treatment. . . . The 7th Station Hospital is constantly being asked by organizations within a radius of 80 miles to hospitalize men for full or partial denture work, and at present is dated up to the first day of May, 1943.

The necessity for evacuating prosthetic patients from combat areas also resulted in great loss of manpower. The dental surgeon of the China-Burma-India theater reported that it often took a month for a man to be shipped to a

---
[55] Memo, Col Rex McK. McDowell for Supply Serv, SGO, 3 Nov 42. SG: 400.34-1.
[56] Memo, Brig Gen R. H. Mills for Oprs Serv, SGO, 7 Sep 43. SG: 322.15-16.
[57] See footnote 51, p. 315.
[58] Ltr, Col E. W. Cowan to Surg. NATOUSA, 13 Mar 43, sub: Dental needs in the theater of operations, incl to personal ltr, Col William D. White to Brig Gen R. H. Mills, 7 Apr 43. HD: 703 (ETO).

hospital, have his work completed, and return to his unit.[59] The dental surgeon of the North African theater stated that one of his biggest problems was to prevent the evacuation of men from combat areas for prosthetic treatment.[60] When hospitals were flooded with wounded any patients not requiring immediate care to save life were sent to the rear as rapidly as possible to make room for the more seriously injured, and under these circumstances the evacuation of a prosthetic case might go to fantastic lengths. One man who reported for repair of a denture in Sicily eventually arrived in North Africa after passing through four hospitals with such speed that he was never seen by a dentist.[61] Even when prosthetic cases could be handled on an outpatient basis results were not too good since either the patient or the hospital might be moved before the denture could be completed.

The situation resulting from the drastic reduction in prosthetic capacity in forward units soon led the theaters to take independent and unofficial action to restore at least part of the lost facilities. The European and North African theaters issued field chests to evacuation hospitals and medical battalions on their own responsibility.[62][63] The Southwest Pacific theater issued them to field hospitals as well.[64] In general, in every important theater the portable laboratories were restored at least to the medical battalions with divisions. Most theaters went further and anticipated the arrival of approved laboratory trucks by improvising models of their own.

The Dental Division did not modify its original stand on removal of field laboratories from the divisions and combat zone hospitals but it did give tacit approval to the action of the theaters as an emergency measure by approving requisitions for enough Chests 61 and 62 to allow issue of the equipment in excess of the quantities authorized by tables of organization. In February 1944 the Dental Division briefly considered restoration of the portable laboratories to the medical battalions,[65] but in May of the same year stated "it is the opinion of the Dental Division that sufficient dental laboratory facilities will be available when the mobile dental laboratories are supplied to the units in the number called for by T/O's."[66] Since the mobile units were slow in arriving, Army Ground Forces suggested in November 1944 that the portable chests be returned to evacuation hospitals.[67] By this time, however, laboratory trucks were finally en route to the theaters and the Dental Division disapproved the recommendation of Army Ground Forces

---

[59] Ltr, Col Dell S. Gray to CofS, Hq, USAF, CBI, 30 Jan 44, sub: Report of theater dental surgeon on trip to Calcutta, 8–22 Jun 44. On file as incl to ltr, Dell S. Gray to Col Rex McK. McDowell, 1 Jul 44. HD: 333 (Dental) CBI.
[60] Interv, author with Col Lynn H. Tingay. Report of dental activities in the North African Theater of Operations, 29 Dec 44. HD: 00.71 (NATOUSA).
[61] History of the Army Dental Corps (MTO) 1943–44. HD.
[62] See footnote 5, p. 293.
[63] Chief Surg, NATO, Ltr 1, 6 Jan 44. HD: 314. (NATO).
[64] Annual Rpt, Chief Surg, SWPA, 1944. HD.
[65] Memo, Col Rex McK. McDowell for Col J. B. Mason, 4 Feb 44. SG: 444.4–1.
[66] Memo, Maj Gen R. H. Mills for Oprs Serv, SGO, 18 May 44. SG: 444.4–1.
[67] Memo, Maj Gen R. H. Mills for Insp Br, Oprs Serv, SGO, 4 Nov 44. SG: 400.34.

and restated its position that the laboratory trucks were the real answer to the prosthetic problem in the combat zone.[68] By the end of 1944 the improvised laboratory trucks and the field chests which had been issued in excess of tables of organization, plus the newly arrived mobile units, had the prosthetic situation well in hand. Further recommendations of the Dental Division were concerned principally with utilization of the laboratory trucks.

It cannot be said how many of the 865,000 prosthetic cases completed overseas were constructed with the portable sets or improvised laboratory trucks but the number was certainly important. The First Infantry Division, alone, completed 1,945 appliances in 1 year.[69] During 1944 a total of 15,288 cases was constructed by units of the Fifth Army, and 3,503 new dentures and 2,081 repairs were completed within combat divisions of that Army in the same period.[70] The unhappy results of removal of the divisional prosthetic service, and the amount of work which was accomplished after some facilities had been restored, left no doubt that dental laboratories were essential in the forward areas.

The importance of an adequate prosthetic service as a morale factor was unexpectedly demonstrated by an embarrassing experience in the North African theater in 1943. This theater was established at a time when earlier physical standards had been drastically lowered, men were still being shipped

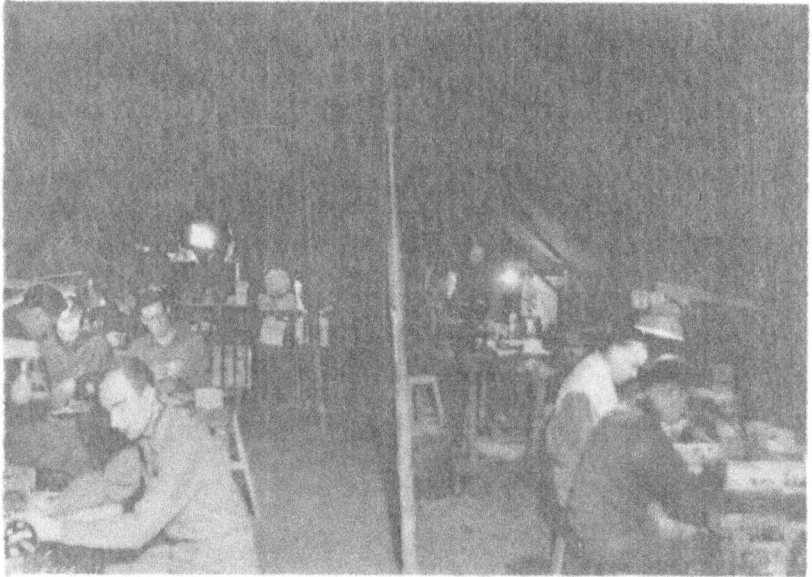

Figure 32. Dental Laboratory, 602d Clearing Company. Italy, 1944.

---

[68] See footnote 47, p. 315.
[69] Annual Dental Rpt (1944), 1st Division, 25 Jan 45. HD.
[70] See footnote 33, p. 311.

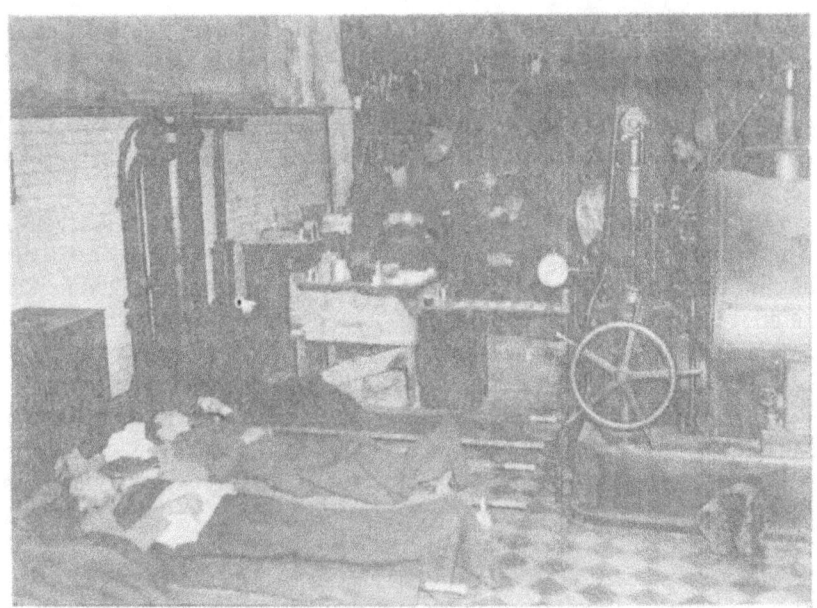

Figure 33. Small Prosthetic Laboratory in the Field. France, 1944.

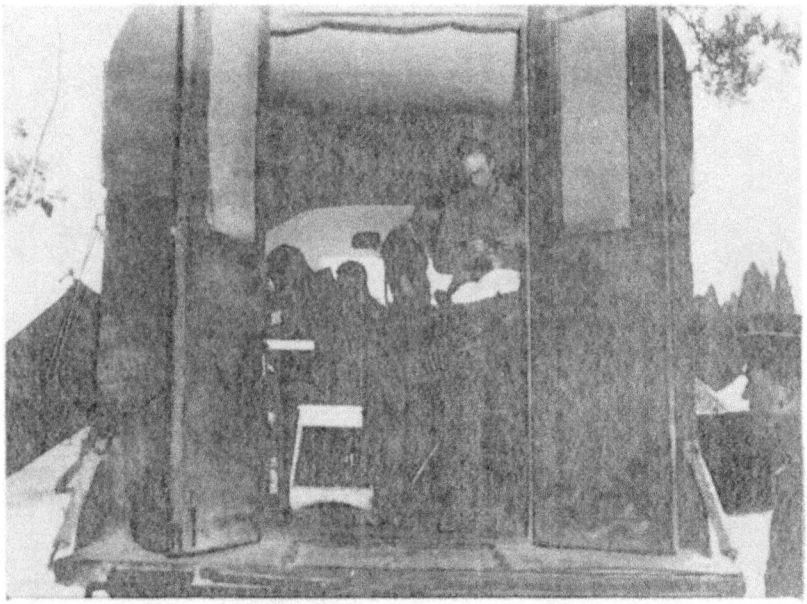

Figure 34. Improvised Prosthetic Truck with the Fifth Army. Italy, 1944.

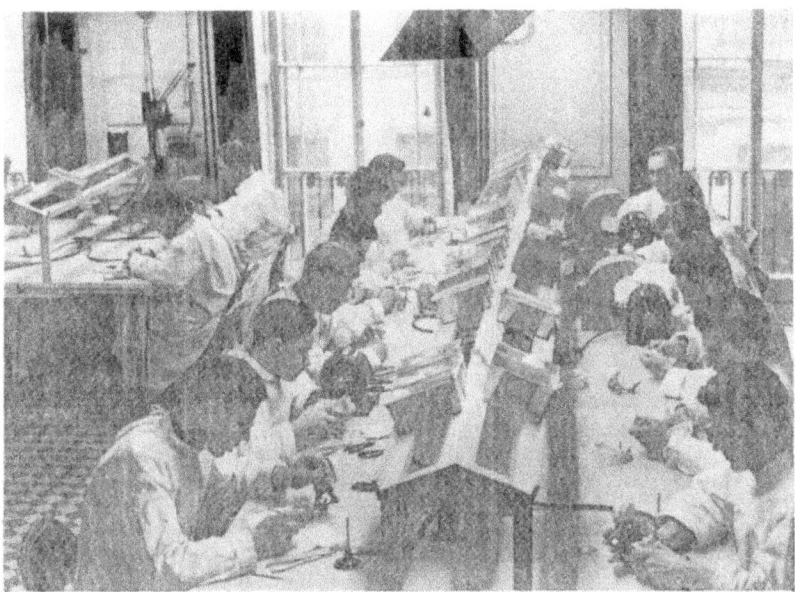

Figure 35. Gold and Clasp Room, Central Dental Laboratory No. 1. London, 1943.

overseas before completion of their dental work, and the portable laboratories had just been removed from a large number of combat zone medical organizations. Consequently the prosthetic service in North Africa was at a low ebb in 1943. General Eisenhower had asked that mail censors tabulate the complaints noted in soldiers' letters, and to the astonishment of all concerned the Dental Service took first prize with "gripes" relative to the inability of getting dental replacements.[71] The fact that troops getting their first taste of action were more voluble about difficulties in getting dentures than about defects of food or the discomforts of combat showed that the prosthetic service was almost as important to morale as to health.

Utilization of the Mobile Prosthetic Trucks

Long before the first laboratory trucks (described in Chapter V) were delivered overseas considerable difficulty had been encountered in finding organizations to which the prosthetic teams could conveniently be assigned. Since the mobile laboratories had to move from unit to unit and from area to area on short notice they could not be assigned permanently to the small individual commands which they served. They were initially too few in number to be assigned even to divisions. They could have been given to field armies in the combat zone, but large headquarters frequently protested at having their staff personnel involved in the detailed administration of minor units. It was

---

[71] See footnote 51, p. 315.

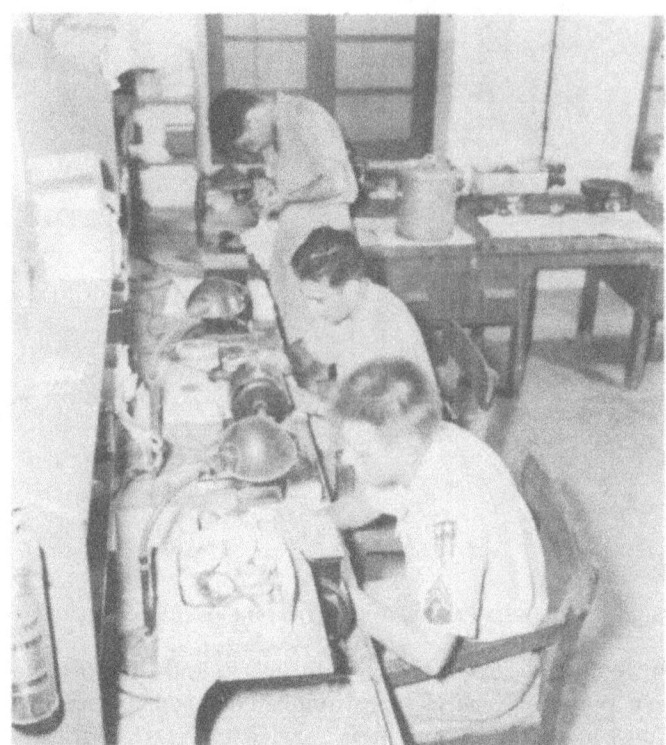

Figure 36. Dental Laboratory of the 181st General Hospital. India, 1944.

felt in the Dental Division that until the value of the trucks had been proved the Army Ground Forces, which had to approve any change in the organization of combat units, would vigorously oppose any proposal to add them to the tables of organization of any large line unit. To avoid controversy with Army Ground Forces the Dental Division therefore recommended that the mobile laboratories be added to a medical unit, the organization of which was a responsibility of the Medical Department.[72]

Obviously the prosthetic teams, whose functions were unrelated to most medical activities, could not conveniently be added to hospitals or most other large medical units. The auxiliary surgical group, however, was itself a catchall, composite, organization of just such semi-independent, highly specialized, medical units, and the prosthetic teams could be incorporated in its tables of organization without materially disrupting its operations. In July 1942, therefore, almost 2 years before the trucks became available in quantity, 3 prosthetic teams and laboratory trucks were added to a new table of organ-

---

[72] Personal interview between author and Colonel Beverly Epps who was on duty in the Dental Division, SGO, during most of the war.

ization for this unit.[73] M. D. Chests Nos. 61 and 62 were substituted for the trucks pending arrival of the latter. It had been planned originally that one auxiliary surgical group would be assigned to each army, but no specific allotment had been authorized. By 7 September 1943 estimates of the number of auxiliary surgical groups to be organized had been reduced to a total of 5, and in addition The Surgeon General was recommending that only 2 prosthetic teams be included in each group. The total of 10 prosthetic teams which would have been provided overseas by 5 auxiliary groups was only a fraction of the number urgently needed and the Dental Division recommended that the teams be deleted from the surgical groups and added to the general headquarters of a theater in the ratio of one for each division or equivalent number of troops.[74] The Surgeon General disapproved this recommendation on the grounds that since the tables of organization of a general headquarters was the concern of Army Ground Forces, the latter should be requested to initiate the change. The Surgeon General also recommended that the Dental Division plan on supplying prosthetic trucks overseas in the ratio of 2 for each 3 divisions, but added the ambiguous statement that they should be shipped only on request of the theaters concerned in a ratio not to exceed *one per division*.[75] The Dental Division then asked the surgeon, Army Ground Forces, to approve a table of organization embodying the recommended modifications, but no action was taken on this request.[76] It is known that general headquarters of the European theater opposed the assignment of incidental units to its overhead and it is probable that this attitude was reflected in Army Ground Forces headquarters in Washington.[77]

Early in 1944 the proposed reorganization of two medical installations made it possible to continue the assignment of the prosthetic teams, as before, to medical units. On 17 March 1944 a new T/O 8–667, Medical Depot Company, provided for 2 prosthetic teams in that organization, which was expected to serve about 75,000 troops.[78] On 23 April 1944, the auxiliary surgical group was absorbed into a new "medical service organization" which included prosthetic trucks "as needed."[79] In a memorandum to the Operations Service, SGO, on 4 February 1944, the Dental Division stated that the prosthetic teams in the medical service organization would be able to provide mobile prosthetic service in the communications zone and that the teams with the medical depot companies would do the same for the combat zone.[80]

Neither assignment worked out as planned, however. A change in the tables of organization for the medical depot company in August 1944 provided

---

[73] T/O 8–571, 13 Jul 42.
[74] See footnote 56, p. 317.
[75] Memo, Col Arthur B. Welsh for Dental Div, SGO, 11 Sep 43. SG: 322.3–1.
[76] Memo, Brig Gen R. H. Mills for Surg, AGF, 13 Sep 43. SG: 322.3–1.
[77] Info from Maj Gen Thomas L. Smith, former dental surgeon, ETO.
[78] T/O 8–667, 17 Mar 44.
[79] T/O&E 8–500, 23 Apr 44.
[80] See footnote 65, p. 318.

that 1 unit would serve 125,000 troops instead of 75,000, leaving only 1 prosthetic team for each 62,500 personnel.[81] The authorization of prosthetic teams in the medical service organization "as needed" also proved too vague and was generally not interpreted to provide an adequate number of trucks in the communications zone. Because of the prospective reduction in the number of prosthetic teams in the combat zone, incident to the change in the medical depot company, the Dental Division recommended in November 1944 that the trucks be made available directly to armies in the ratio of 1 mobile unit for each 30,000 men.[82] Though this proposal was not put into effect, approximately the same result was attained on 18 January 1945 when the number of teams assigned to the medical service organization was increased to "one for each 30,000 troops," apparently anticipating that the needs of both the combat zone and the communications zone would henceforth be met from this unit.[83] Finally, when the division dental service was reorganized in June 1945, one prosthetic team was authorized for direct assignment to the dental detachment of each division.[84] The previous allotment of trucks to the medical service organization was not rescinded at this time, however, and at the end of hostilities the prosthetic teams were authorized, in theory at least, both in the ratio of 1 for each division, in the dental detachment, and 1 for each 30,000 total strength of a theater, in the medical service organizations. It is probable that correction of this duplication was delay pending expected changes in the organization of the Army following the war.

The actual utilization of the prosthetic teams overseas was highly complex and followed no definite pattern. Flexibility of operation, which was essential to meet unexpected situations, often necessitated wide and unorthodox variations from the plan contemplated in tables of organization. In the European theater, for instance, three teams were assigned to a central dental laboratory where they were available on short notice for use in any area. These three teams were given blanket orders every month to proceed to any part of the theater "to carry out the orders of the theater commander." The theater dental surgeon, in turn, could move the teams at any time by a telephonic order, giving him a small reserve pool of prosthetic personnel and equipment to meet emergency situations. Other teams were assigned to the base sections where they operated under the base section dental surgeons. Several teams were assigned to the communications zone for replacement of units which might be lost to combat organizations, but these teams were temporarily loaned to army replacement depots which were overburdened with work for new men; eventually they were turned over to the armies. Other teams were assigned to the combat armies, either directly or as part of medical depot companies. The army units in the European theater were utilized in various ways. Some were

---

[81] T/O&E 8-667, C 1, 11 Aug 44.
[82] See footnote 47, p. 315.
[83] T/O&E 8-500, 18 Jan 45.
[84] See footnote 9, p. 297.

kept under army control; others were in turn attached directly to divisions. Some had their overhead functions carried out by a parent organization; others were nearly independent, relying on the units to which they were attached for little more than rations and housing. About the only generalizations which can be drawn are that the teams were seldom assigned to the auxiliary surgical groups or the medical depot companies of which they were ostensibly a part, and control was generally retained in one of the higher headquarters where the dental surgeon could utilize the limited number of teams in the best interests of the whole command. The official assignment of laboratory trucks to individual divisions, under T/O 8–16, was not directed until June 1945, near the end of hostilities.[85]

Evaluation of the Mobile Prosthetic Trucks. Reports from every theater confirmed the value of the prosthetic trucks. During the fighting in France the First Infantry Division, for instance, had made it a practice to set up the Chests 61 and 62 only when it appeared that no move would be necessary within 3 days. When the division reached Belgium it obtained a mobile laboratory and thereafter the prosthetic clinic operated whenever it could count on a single day in any given location.[86] The Ninth Infantry Division reported "prosthetic dental chests cannot be used efficiently in bivouacs of short duration. A mobile dental laboratory is essential to meet the prosthetic needs of a division."[87] A general board which made a study of medical activities in Europe at the end of the war found that:[88]

> A large number of mobile laboratories and operating units are required in warfare involving rapid movement, and when attached to divisions provide uninterrupted dental care and eliminate the evacuation of troops from divisional areas. It has been found that mobile dental units can offer the maximum service to forward units. The extreme value of the mobile type of prosthetic unit was proved beyond all question once the lines had become extended beyond the point at which semifixed installations were effective.

The Director of the Dental Division stated in 1945:[89]

> The mobile dental laboratory is a most useful, efficient and economical mechanism for the rendering of prosthetic laboratory work in Army areas, in the communications zone, on maneuvers in the continental United States, and in certain isolated stations in the United States.

In spite of the success of the mobile dental laboratories, however, it would be a mistake to regard them as the final, universal answer to all prosthetic problems, even in the field. They brought modern equipment to the combat zone where it was badly needed, but in other areas, where mobility was of less importance, the prosthetic trucks could not equal the efficiency of larger, fixed

---

[85] Data on the use of the dental prosthetic trucks were seldom a matter of record. Information given here has been assembled by the author by means of interviews with senior dental surgeons.
[86] See footnote 69, p. 319.
[87] Annual Rpt, 9th Division, ETO, 1943, 21 Jan 44. HD.
[88] Interviews, The General Board, USFET Medical Section, ETO, vol IV. HD: 334.
[89] See footnote 36, p. 312.

or semifixed installations operating day after day under relatively stable conditions. It is difficult to obtain figures on the output of the prosthetic teams, but 5 mobile units of the First Army completed an average of about 1.5 cases per technician per working day during 5 months in 1944 and 1945, compared with an average for large laboratories of about 2.5 cases per technician per working day.[90] The mobile units were admittedly crowded, and since the equipment was tied to its means of transportation, operations had to be suspended when the truck was used to carry water or supplies, or when normal maintenance was required. Time was lost in moves and several days might elapse after a change of location before all troops in the vicinity could be notified that prosthetic services were available.

In divisions the need for mobility outweighed all other considerations. The prosthetic laboratory had to be ready to move on short notice and to function when no more than 24 hours could be spent in any given location. Time lost in packing and unpacking equipment with every move would have offset any advantage of setting up in more spacious quarters even if permanent buildings had been available. Dental surgeons were therefore generally agreed that only a completely mobile unit, with built-in equipment, could meet the prosthetic needs of a division with reasonable efficiency. For similar reasons it was necessary that armies, and even higher headquarters, should have at least a few prosthetic teams which could be used to meet emergencies or for assignment with small commands which for any reason could not use the central dental laboratories. But while the mobile dental laboratories probably did more to improve the prosthetic service than any other wartime development, they were not a substitute for the larger fixed laboratories wherever the latter could be used.

The prosthetic trucks also had certain limitations under special conditions. On small island areas, for instance, usefulness of the mobile units was limited by lack of roads, and in addition the trucks were usually given a low priority in an invasion. For some time after a beachhead was established prosthetic service had to be rendered from field chests.[91]

The mobile units themselves might be expected to undergo modification from time to time, though at the end of the war the line which future development would take was not clear. One important defect, the fact that operations had to be suspended whenever the truck was moved, could of course be eliminated by mounting the equipment in a trailer, but it was feared that this change would make it easier for commanders of units to which the laboratories were attached to appropriate the trucks, leaving the prosthetic teams worse off than before. A truck and trailer combination would also be less able to negotiate unfavorable terrain. It was further noted that whenever a prosthetic team could expect to be in a given location for any considerable length of time, as much of the equipment as possible was usually unloaded from the truck and

---

[90] See footnote 10, p. 298.
[91] See footnote 36, p. 312.

set up in any available permanent shelter. It was therefore suggested that prosthetic teams assigned in the rear of the combat zone or in other areas where frequent movement was less essential, should be supplied cargo trucks and equipment designed for use in a building or tentage. The necessity for supplying a highly mobile prosthetic service well forward in the combat zone was proved beyond all doubt, but the means by which it would be rendered would probably need to be reexamined periodically in the light of changing conditions of warfare.

Central Dental Laboratories

It has been seen that the prosthetic needs of divisions and comparable combat units could be met only by small, mobile laboratories functioning in the immediate vicinity of the troops they served. Only a relatively small proportion of the personnel in a theater were assigned to combat commands, however; the remainder obtained replacements from some more permanent type of installation. Hospitals of the communications zone were authorized small dental laboratories but these were inadequate to meet the demands of large surrounding areas. The largest general hospital was allotted only two technicians and the largest station hospital had but one. Further, these dispersed installations could not be organized for maximum efficiency. This could be attained only when large numbers of skilled technicians repeated over and over the limited operations in which they were most proficient. As a result the hospital laboratories were unable to meet the enormous demands for prosthetic service in a theater of operations.[92]

In the continental United States the bulk of routine dental laboratory service was provided by large central dental laboratories organized to function on a "production line" basis, but this type of installation had not been specifically authorized in tables of organization for overseas use. Failure to provide for central dental laboratories outside the United States was probably due in part to the fact that the magnitude of the prosthetic problem had been underestimated but there is reason to believe that other factors were also taken into consideration. First, the requirements of different theaters would obviously vary greatly and no single organization could meet the needs of every area. Also, a central dental laboratory must have rapid, dependable communications with all parts of the area it serves, and in the more backward regions, where United States troops first saw service, existing transportation facilities were often meager. The question of establishing central dental laboratories was therefore left to the individual theaters which could recommend special tables of organization to meet their own needs.

Central dental laboratories eventually proved practical and necessary in most of the major theaters. Considerable delay was encountered in getting

---

[92] See footnote 3, p. 291.

them in operation, however. Until a theater had been at least partially organized and the direction of its future development determined, the dental surgeon could not know how many troops would have to be served nor where he would have to concentrate his facilities. After these questions had been answered, he still had to get his tentative table of organization approved in his own headquarters and by the War Department, then wait for many months while personnel and equipment were assembled and shipped. As a result most central dental laboratories were staffed with men taken from hospitals or other dental installations. By this means a limited number of technicians were utilized with the greatest efficiency and laboratory service was provided for all on an equal basis, though hospital laboratories were robbed of needed personnel. The experience of the dental surgeon of the European theater, which was fairly typical, was described as follows:[93]

> It is to be noted that no provisions were ever made as far as I can find out for Tables of Organization for central dental laboratories in any theater of war. During the past few months I have often wondered why. My first official act on arriving in this theater was to have a cable sent to the Chief Surgeon requesting one central dental laboratory complete, for which there was both a T/O and a T/BA at the time. My reply was to requisition both personnel and equipment from here. This occurred on or about 1 July 1942, and those instructions were promptly carried out. Last week, after a delay of 15 months a few of these items requisitioned at that time arrived at one of our depots, but at this time have not yet arrived at the laboratories. In mentioning this it brings out a point which I wish to emphasize, that is the great delays which occur in wartime. I am wondering if it would be better to organize these units at home and send them forward with equipment and trained personnel like any other unit, rather than try to put them together in a new theater piece by piece. . . . The equipment which we now have in these laboratories has all been diverted from the hospitals for which it was intended.

An adequate central dental laboratory system, with nearly 150 technicians, was eventually established in England, but the fact that these facilities were not available for many months seriously hampered the prosthetic service and delayed the treatment of men being prepared for the invasion of France.

The General Board, United States Forces, European theater, also reported:[94]

> There were sufficient dental personnel in units operating under approved tables of organization in the communications zone, European Theater of Operations, to perform the mission of the separate units. However, the dental personnel in these units were not able to provide for an adequate overall communications zone dental service, particularly at the larger headquarters and in cities such as London and Paris. Fairly adequate dental service was eventually provided by organizing non-tables of organization laboratories and clinics. There was a definite shortage of dental officers to provide this additional service and it was only accomplished at the expense of taking dental officers and technicians out of general hospitals, dispensaries and other medical units under communications zone control . . . thereby reducing the efficiency of the

---

[93] See footnote 52, p. 316.
[94] See footnote 3, p. 291.

dental service of these units. A great amount of improvisation was required as a result of failure to provide for adequate personnel and equipment in sufficient time to make the indicated service possible.

It would seem that considerable difficulty and delay would be eliminated if central dental laboratories for overseas use were established by tables of organization. Laboratories of the sizes required could then be requisitioned as units and shipped from the United States complete, ready to function on arrival.

Hospital Laboratories

During the war very few official changes were made in the authorized personnel or equipment of hospital laboratories. Unofficially, both personnel and equipment often had to be augmented to meet special situations. General hospitals of 1,000 beds or over were authorized two dental laboratory technicians; hospitals of less than 1,000 beds were authorized only a single technician or none at all. Since a single officer can keep approximately 5 technicians occupied it is obvious that the 1 or 2 men assigned to a hospital laboratory could not complete all the cases started by even one officer on full time prosthetic duty. When, as frequently happened, a hospital in an isolated location had to provide prosthetic service for all surrounding commands, its efforts to keep ahead of the flood of cases were doomed from the start even when it neglected the care of its own patients. Under these circumstances the theater dental surgeon had to attach up to a dozen men to the hospital laboratory which then acted as a subcentral laboratory for the area. Since, initially, the theater dental surgeon had no reservoir of personnel for such duties, they were usually taken from other units which needed them only slightly less urgently. Later in the war fixed prosthetic teams of a medical service organization were sometimes used for this purpose.

In the combat zone the 750-bed evacuation hospitals which were at one time responsible for almost all the prosthetic service in army areas, were particularly ill-equipped to handle such a task. When the installation was functioning in combat the 3 dentists and 3 assistants were fully occupied with other duties, so that the dental laboratory chests were sometimes unopened for long periods of time. Almost all the dental officers interviewed by the European General Board recommended the addition of laboratory personnel to the tables of organization for the 750-bed evacuation hospital and restoration of the Chests 61 and 62 to the 400-bed hospital.[95] It is believed, however, that the opinions of most of these officers were based on their experiences during the period when the evacuation hospitals were vainly trying to provide all combat zone prosthetic service; the assignment of mobile prosthetic teams to divisions late in the war materially reduced the need for extensive laboratory facilities within evacuation hospitals and both the mission and organization of these units

---

[95] See footnote 88, p. 325.

seemed to indicate that they should not be expected to render any great volume of routine prosthetic treatment.

The experience of World War II demonstrated conclusively that: the laboratory personnel of the larger communications zone hospitals must be increased slightly if the dental service for hospital patients is to be adequately maintained, and hospital laboratories cannot provide prosthetic service for surrounding commands without extensive reinforcement of wartime tables of organization.

Summary

In the continental United States, with its rapid communications and large concentrations of troops, there was no question of the superior efficiency of large central dental laboratories staffed by experts and outfitted with the most modern equipment. In many overseas areas, however, a compromise had to be made between the efficiency of the large establishments and the convenience of the smaller, dispersed installations. The mobile prosthetic teams provided an acceptable solution of the laboratory problems of divisions and similar organizations though some dental surgeons felt that the teams could function better if their equipment were carried in a weapons carrier or light truck. In the rear areas of the communications zone, at least in those theaters where communications were not a major problem, it was generally agreed that the bulk of the prosthetic service should be rendered by central laboratories operating under stable conditions. Hospital laboratories could complete cases for their own patients and render occasional emergency care for other personnel and, if effectively reinforced, might act as subcentral laboratories in isolated locations, but they should not be expected to provide "mass production" facilities for the routine treatment of large commands. The need for approved tables of organization for overseas central dental laboratories was evident.

There was less agreement on the most effective prosthetic service for army areas in the rear of the combat zone where neither the mobile teams nor the central laboratories seemed to meet all requirements. Some army dental surgeons felt that extreme mobility was still essential even in regions where contact with the enemy was relatively improbable and recommended that field armies be provided enough of the prosthetic trucks and teams to care for all army troops. Others felt that while some mobility was essential it was not necessary to use built-in equipment with consequent limitation on space, and that communications in an army area were sufficient to allow some concentration of laboratory facilities into more efficient units. After a study of his prosthetic organization [96] one army dental surgeon expressed the following views:

> 1. While the prosthetic teams (preferably with demountable equipment mounted in light trucks) may be able to meet most of the laboratory needs of divisions, provision must also be made for the care of army troops, which in a type army have approxi-

---
[96] See footnote 10, p. 298.

mately the same total strength as the troops in the divisions and corps. About nine prosthetic teams are required to provide prosthetic care for the divisions of a type army and approximately equal facilities would be needed for army troops.

2. Instead of using nine separate prosthetic teams for army troops a more efficient service would result if the 27 technicians of these teams were grouped into a single "prosthetic detachment." This prosthetic detachment would have for the army prosthetic service the same advantages of centralization and control that the new division dental detachment offered for the division Dental Service. The detachment would have to be organized along cellular lines so that it could operate either as a large laboratory or as two or more smaller laboratories of not less than six men each. Equipment would be demountable and sufficiently mobile to be moved by trucks when required, but the army laboratories would be located so as to require changes of position as infrequently as possible. Transportation needs would be reduced since only rarely would the whole laboratory have to be moved at one time. Since equipment would not be mounted in the trucks, these would be available for carrying supplies, picking up and delivering cases, or other necessary routine duties.

None of the many opinions quoted on the army prosthetic service was expected to offer the final solution of the problem, and it may be that no single plan would be uniformly applicable. It is possible, for instance, that the scheme for an army prosthetic detachment and a centralized army laboratory would have worked effectively in Europe where the road net was extensive, but it might have proved less satisfactory in the Pacific jungles. The significant point at this time is that while the needs of the divisions and the base areas were being satisfactorily met at the end of the war there was a fairly general feeling that the prosthetic service of the field army should be given further attention.

CHAPTER IX

Demobilization of Dental Corps Personnel

WORLD WAR I

Following World War I, demobilization of Dental Corps personnel was rapid and relatively uncomplicated. Those overseas had to be returned to the United States, and some dentists were retained to care for the 120,000 casualties under treatment in general hospitals when the armistice was signed,[1][2] but reduction of the Army to a skeleton force soon after hostilities ended greatly simplified planning for the postwar period. Since no dental officer had to serve very long after the end of the war each man could be discharged as his unit was disbanded or as he became surplus to its needs. No elaborate plans for interchanging dentists between organizations or even between geographical areas on the basis of length of service, dependency, et cetera, were necessary. Under the policy of "down the gangplank and out," dental officers in units with a low priority for disbandment had to serve a little longer than those in more fortunate commands, but since all nonvolunteers could be ordered released by 1 October 1919, no man had to serve as much as a year beyond the armistice against his will.[3] From 11 November 1918 through June 1920 the Dental Corps was reduced as follows:[4]

Date	Strength of the Dental Corps	Regular Army	Temporary officers
11 November 1918	4,510	227	4,283
1 July 1919	2,219	218	2,001
30 September 1919	773	209	564
1 January 1920	369	202	[1] 167
30 June 1920	322	196	[1] 126

[1] All volunteers.

WORLD WAR II

Demobilization From V-E Day to V-J Day

The early losses of physicians and dentists at the close of World War I had, at times, seriously hampered the medical service. With this in mind, The

---

[1] Annual Report of The Surgeon General, U. S. Army, 1919. Washington, Government Printing Office, 1919.
[2] The Medical Department of the United States Army in the World War. Washington, Government Printing Office, 1923, vol. I, p. 159.
[3] Annual Report of The Surgeon General, U. S. Army, 1920. Washington, Government Printing Office, 1920.
[4] Ibid.

Surgeon General pointed out as early as August 1943 [5] and later in April 1944 [6] that demobilization of Medical Department officers would not only fail to precede that of other branches, but would lag behind if the needs of the sick were to be met and separation examinations carried out.

With the end of the war in Europe, pressure for the release of medical and dental officers increased rapidly. Within 1 month after V-E Day a Senate resolution was submitted calling for an investigation of "hoarding of physicians and dentists" by the Army,[7] and this action was just one symptom of the general expectation that Medical Department personnel would be discharged in large numbers as soon as Germany was defeated. The Surgeon General, however, consistently discouraged this attitude for the following reasons:

1. The war was not ended; it was to a great extent merely transferred to the Pacific area. Many units in Europe would be held for occupation duties; others would be sent to the Pacific either directly or after furloughs and retraining in the United States.

2. Except in Europe The Surgeon General had no excess of Medical Department personnel. On the other hand, shipping priority went to units being transferred to combat areas, and other categories had to wait. In July 1945 it was reported that there were 6,000 surplus medical officers in Europe, but that current shipping schedules would return only 30 percent of them to the United States before the end of October.[8] As early as September 1944 The Surgeon General had asked for the early shipment of Medical Department personnel after the end of hostilities in Europe,[9] and in June 1945 the War Department had directed such return,[10] but a force which had been building up for 3 years could not be moved in a few weeks. Also, some time was required to screen Medical Department personnel on duty in Europe to determine which should be sent to the Pacific, which held for occupation duties, and which returned to the United States. Meanwhile, units awaiting return had to be supplied medical care.

3. Shipping shortages had precluded the regular rotation of personnel between overseas theaters and the Zone of Interior. Now that units were passing through the United States en route to the Pacific it was necessary to replace men with the most overseas service with Zone of Interior personnel who had not had foreign duty. But each such exchange required 2 extra officers for a period of 2 months or more. The officer returning to the Zone of Interior had to be given leave and travel time before he reported to his new post; the officer

---

[5] Memo, Col R. W. Bliss for Dir Spec Planning Div, WDGS, 16 Aug 43, sub: Demobilization planning. SG: 370.01-2.

[6] Memo, Brig Gen R. W. Bliss for Dir Spec Planning Div, WDGS, 27 Apr 44, sub: Demobilization planning. SG: 370.01-2.

[7] S. Res. 184, 79th Cong, 12 Jun 45.

[8] Memo, Eli Ginzberg, Dir Resources Anal Div SGO, for SG, 5 Jul 45, sub: Redeployment policy. SG: 370.01.

[9] Memo, Maj Gen LeRoy Lutes for SG, 19 Jan 45, sub: Priority return of medical personnel from inactive theaters after V-E Day. SG: 370.01.

[10] Radiogram 16876, 14 Jun 45; cited in footnote 8, above.

replacing him had to be granted leave and travel time before he left for overseas; a third officer had to be assigned to provide care in the absence of the other two. The Surgeon General estimated that the necessity for reshuffling personnel to meet the needs of the Pacific theater would delay the separation of surplus European theater officers by nearly 5 months.[11] From 20 June through 15 August 1945, 4,000 medical officers were exchanged between units.[12]

4. Casualties in Army hospitals had to be provided attention, and separation and redeployment centers had to be staffed, regardless of the end of the war in Europe.

Based on these considerations, General Kirk predicted in July 1945 that there would be no large scale separation of Medical Department personnel before the end of the year.[13]

During this period the situation was further complicated by the necessity for a general reconsideration of all personnel assignments. The fact that a man with 18 months' service was surplus in Europe did not justify his release from active duty if men with 36 months' service were still being held in the Pacific, and it was essential that there be established a basis for the equitable discharge or reassignment of all Medical Department personnel regardless of current place of duty. This was accomplished by an "adjusted service rating" (ASR) scored on the following credits:[14]

Each month of service since 1 September 1940	1 point
Each month of overseas service (in addition to points for total service)	1 point
Each combat decoration	5 points
Each child under 18 (maximum of 3)	12 points

(ASR scores were first calculated as of 12 May 1945; they were later adjusted as of 2 September 1945.)

On the basis of the ASR, personnel overseas were divided into the following categories:[15]

1. Men with the fewest points were put in units bound directly for the Pacific.

2. Men with slightly more points were put in units bound for the Pacific after a stopover for furloughs and training in the United States.

3. Men in the median ASR categories were returned to the United States for assignment to a strategic reserve for duty in the Pacific when and if needed.

4. Men in the moderately high point categories were held in Europe for occupation duties until eligible for release from the Army.

---

[11] Official announcement on redeployment and separation of Medical Department officers. J. Am. Dent. A. 32: 1177–1182, Sep 1945.

[12] Memo, Maj George L. Gleeson, Chief Oprs Br Pers Serv SGO, for SG, sub: Quarterly report of activities, Operations Branch, Personnel Service, for period 10 Jun 45 through 30 Sep 45. HD: 319.1–2 (F/Y 1946).

[13] No large release of dental officers before end of 1945. J. Am. Dent. A. 32: 908, Jul 1945.

[14] RR 1–1, 25 Jan 46.

[15] Medical Department Redeployment and Separation Policy as revised 6 Aug 45. HD: 314.

5. Highest point men were to be returned to the United States for immediate discharge.

On arrival from overseas any dental officer who was either over 50 years of age, or had an ASR over 100, was discharged.[16] Officers on duty in the United States were supposed to be discharged on the same basis, but ASF had to hold temporarily dentists with less than 110 points and refused to release any for age. A dental officer who: (1) was 40 years of age, (2) had 75 points, or (3) had 6 months of overseas service, was withdrawn from any unit on the way to the Pacific and replaced by one currently on duty in the United States. This "withdrawal score" was slightly lower than that for medical officers which required either age 45 or 12 months of overseas service. Officers who desired to remain on duty and who were wanted by the Army could voluntarily forego the privilege of separation. The fact that few dentists were expected to be discharged immediately is indicated by the estimate of the Resources Analysis Division of the Surgeon General's Office that under the criteria discussed only 31 men would be released in the United States and about 250 or 300 in Europe. Separation of men over 50 in the Zone of Interior was not recommended to start until September or October.[17]

Beginning on V-E Day, a special effort was made to have certain instructors released to resume their positions in dental colleges. The Procurement and Assignment Service notified the deans to name any five key men on their faculties whom they particularly needed. Names submitted were forwarded to The Surgeon General who in turn asked the theaters to return these men for discharge as soon as possible.[18] This program continued from V-E Day until the end of 1945 but was overtaken by the general demobilization following V-J Day. The total separated under it is not known; 18 dental officers were discharged as essential to national health or interest, and 20 more were discharged as key men in government or industry. Instructors might have fallen in either group as well as in other administrative categories. It is probable that many instructors were released in the normal, accelerated demobilization which followed V-J Day before their discharges could be accomplished under The Surgeon General's program. As late as 11 September 1945, for instance, overseas commanders were asked to release 19 dental instructors,[19] and most of these must have been nearly eligible for release on other criteria by the time these requests could be carried out.

---

[16] See footnote 15, p. 334.

[17] Memo, Eli Ginzberg for Dir Dental Div SGO, 17 Jul 45, sub: Separation of Dental Corps officers. HD: 314.

[18] Info given Dr. John McMinn, HD, by Lt Col William Piper, Mil Pers Div SGO. No documentary evidence on this point has been discovered.

[19] Ltr, Col Robert J. Carpenter, Exec Off SGO, to CGs of various overseas theaters, 11 Sep 45, sub: Separation of Medical Department personnel essential to medical and dental schools. SG: 210.8.

It will be noted in Table 16 that during the months of May, June, July, and August 1945, 610 dental officers were discharged from the Army.[20]

TABLE 16. DEMOBILIZATION OF DENTAL CORPS OFFICERS BY MONTHS, MAY 1945–JUNE 1947

Date	Number separated		Date	Number separated	
	Each month	Cumulative total		Each month	Cumulative total
1945			*1946*—Continued		
May	50	50	June	675	11,500
June	105	155	July	600	12,100
July	295	450	August	440	12,540
August	160	610	September	635	13,175
September	415	1,025	October	275	13,450
October	1,505	2,530	November	400	13,850
November	1,430	3,960	December	350	14,200
December	1,225	5,185	*1947*		
1946			January	200	14,400
January	2,190	7,375	February	125	14,525
February	1,575	8,950	March	75	14,600
March	800	9,750	April	125	14,725
April	540	10,290	May	125	¹ 14,850
May	535	10,825	June	150	¹ 15,000

¹ Estimated.

The release of any large number of dental laboratory technicians immediately following V-E Day also proved impractical. In September 1944 The Surgeon General, foreseeing a moderate shortage of such personnel, had recommended that they be retained by Zone of Interior service commands until declared surplus by the surgeon.[21] At first it was not expected that the shortage would be sufficiently severe to warrant transferring technicians from commands where they were surplus to others where they might be needed, but on 7 June 1945 the War Department directed that certain enlisted men, including dental technicians, be transferred to new commands when declared surplus in their own units. However, organizations receiving these men were to use them only in their special duties, and they were to be released as soon as replacements could be obtained; assignment overseas of technicians otherwise eligible for

---

[20] Table 16 assembled from data given the author on 13 Feb 48 by the Strength Accounting Br, AGO. It should be noted that the AGO did not process separations until the end of terminal leave which was often several months after the last day of active duty. However, in the demobilization of Dental Corps officers, as shown in Table 16, the date indicates the actual month in which the officers were lost to the effective, administrative strength of the SGO.

[21] Memo, Col J. R. Hudnall, Chief Pers Serv SGO, for Col G. M. Powell, Dir Spec Planning Div SGO, 5 Sep 44, sub: Demobilization of enlisted personnel. SG: 370.01.

discharge was prohibited.[22] By 31 August 1945 it was possible to direct that no dental technician would be transferred to another command when he became surplus in his own.[23]

Demobilization after V-J Day

(See Table 16 for separations by months)

The composition of the Dental Corps on V-J Day in respect to priority for discharge is not known. On V-E Day, however, there were approximately 14,700 dentists on duty, distributed as follows:[24]

Regular Army	250
Volunteers for extended service	750
ASTP graduates	1,900
AUS officers desiring early separation	11,800

Most of the ASTP graduates listed were ineligible for separation until long after V-J Day so it can be assumed that the majority of the 610 dental officers discharged between V-E Day and V-J Day came from the category of AUS officers desiring early separation, leaving about 11,190 men in this group at the end of hostilities. Procurement from civil practice had practically ceased in December 1943, and over 9,000 dentists had come on active duty before the end of 1942, so that by V-J Day almost all non-ASTP AUS officers had had over 1½ years of service and a large proportion of them had been in the Army more than 2½ years. The release of such a number of high point men in the proper priority, according to length of service and dependents, and without jeopardizing the provision of essential care for an Army which at the end of 1945 still numbered over 4 million men, was certain to involve knotty problems.

It has been seen that prior to V-J Day dentists returning from overseas were separated only if they had 100 points or were over 50 years of age; in the United States they could be released only if they had 110 points. On 8 September 1945 new separation criteria for both the Medical and Dental Corps provided that field grade officers (colonels, lieutenant colonels, majors) with 100 points, and company grade officers (captains, lieutenants) with 85 points, could be released. On the same day the Resources Analysis Division, SGO, recommended that the criteria for medical and dental officers be further reduced to 80 points, and that additionally, any man 48 years of age or over, or who had been in the Army on 7 December 1941, should be released. On 12 September 1945 this recommendation was approved and published.[25] Medical and dental officers thus enjoyed, temporarily, more favorable separation criteria than those of most other branches who were still required to have ASR's of 100 points for officers of field grade, and 85 points for men of company grade.

---

[22] WD Memo 615-45, 7 Jun 45.
[23] WD Memo 615-45, 31 Aug 45.
[24] Memo, Isaac Cogan, Chief, Resources Anal Div SGO for Chief, Dental Consultants Div SGO, 8 Oct 46, sub: Basic data for Dental Corps. SG: 322.0531.
[25] Teletype, SG to CGs all SvCs, 12 Sep 45. SG: 210.8.

On 14 September 1945 The Surgeon General promised to release 10,000 dental officers by the end of June 1946.[26] A few days later it was stated that 3,500 dentists would be separated by 25 December 1945. An additional number of dental officers became eligible for separation when ASR scores were recomputed on 2 September to include credit for service subsequent to V-E Day. On 17 September 1945 it was announced that no dentist would be sent overseas if he was 40 years of age or had 45 points.[27]

On 22 September War Department Circular 290 emphasized and liberalized somewhat the provisions of WD Circular 485, 29 December 1944, concerning release of officers not eligible for separation on point scores.[28] Specifically, it authorized separation of the following:

1. Officers who were surplus to the needs of the Army, and who could not be economically trained in new positions, if they had served a reasonable period.

2. Individuals presenting documentary evidence that they would be more useful to the nation in a civilian capacity.

3. Individuals who had suffered undue hardship by reason of military service.

4. Officers over 50 years of age, at their own request.

On 1 October 1945 separation criteria for male officers of most branches were reduced to a straight 75 points but medical and dental criteria remained unchanged, thus for the first time placing this group at a slight disadvantage. On 6 October the War Department notified all commands that civilian needs for Medical Department personnel were critical and directed them to be alert for the uneconomical use of physicians, dentists, and nurses. Persons found surplus were to be released without delay; overseas personnel were to be returned by the fastest transportation, and Medical Department officers processed expeditiously through separation centers.[29] On 16 October, The Adjutant General asked Zone of Interior commands to release physicians and dentists with at least 2 years' service at any time they became surplus, regardless of points.[30] Such cases were to be referred to The Surgeon General for final decision, but telephone communication was authorized. On 18 October The Surgeon General complained that Medical Department officers eligible for release were still being held as essential, and emphasized that such action was permissible only in very exceptional cases.[31]

On 20 October separation criteria for medical and dental officers were again dropped below those of the line branches when either an ASR of 70 points, or 45 months of total service, were specified.[32] On 1 December 1945 separation criteria for line branches were dropped to 73 points and the maxi-

---

[26] Army to release more medical officers. J. Am. Dent. A. 32: 1321, Oct 1945.
[27] Limited number of dental officers to go overseas. J. Am. Dent. A. 32: 1474, Nov-Dec 1945.
[28] WD Cir 290, 22 Sep 45.
[29] WD Cir 307, 6 Oct 45.
[30] Teletype, TAG to CGs all SvCs, 16 Oct 45. SG: 210.8.
[31] Teletype, Brig Gen R. W. Bliss to CGs all SvCs, 18 Oct 45. SG: 210.8.
[32] Teletype, TAG to CGs all SvCs, 19 Oct 45. SG: 210.8.

mum service requirement for medical and dental officers simultaneously reduced to 42 months, though the ASR remained at 70 points. Former ASTP students received credit only for time served after receiving their commissions and were required to put in at least 36 months regardless of points.

On 7 December 1945 all previous agreements to volunteer for additional periods of service were cancelled. By that time it was possible to give temporary officers more complete information on the possibility of entering the Regular Army, the length of time they could expect to serve on foreign service, et cetera, and it was felt that they should be given an opportunity to revise their earlier commitments and plan their future on a more stable basis than had been practical immediately following the war. All officers were at this time required to sign statements placing them in one of the following categories: [33]

> Category I—Elect to remain on active duty for an unlimited period.
> Category II—Elect to remain on active duty until 30 June 1947.
> Category III—Elect to remain on active duty until 31 December 1946.
> Category IV—Elect to remain on active duty for a specified period agreed upon between the officer and his commanding officer, but not less than 60 days after the date of signing.
> Category V—Desire separation as soon as possible.

On 31 December 1945 new criteria became effective under which physicians and dentists could be separated if they were 45 years of age, had 42 months of service, or an ASR of 65 points. Line officers were required to have either 70 points or 48 months total service. Somewhat more than 5,000 dental officers were separated between V-E Day and 31 December 1945 (see Table 16).

During the period from V-E Day to the end of 1945 the demobilization program of the Army in general and of the Medical Department in particular was the target of considerable criticism from Congress, the medical professions, and from laymen.[34] Such criticism will be covered in detail in other sections of the Medical Department history, and will be discussed here only in relation to the Dental Corps.

On 1 October 1945 the American Dental Association reported that it had received many complaints on the slow release of dental officers.[35] At that time this organization stated that it was not in a position to say whether the Armed Forces were justified in their separation policies, and limited its comments to pointing out the need for the earliest possible release of medical personnel. On 21 November 1945 the Secretary of War notified the Chief of Staff that he had received criticism of delays in releasing medical and dental officers, and that a threatened senatorial investigation had been called off only on his promise to investigate and take necessary corrective measures.[36] He directed The Surgeon

---

[33] WD Cir 366, 7 Dec 45.
[34] S. 134, 79th Cong., introduced 12 Jun 45; S. 1355, 79th Cong., introduced 6 Sep 45; S. J. Res. 97, 79th Cong., introduced 24 Sep 45; H. R. 4425, 79th Cong., introduced 18 Oct 45.
[35] Release of dental officers from the armed services. J. Am. Dent. A. 32: 1292–1293, Oct 1945.
[36] Memo, SecWar for CofS, 21 Nov 45. SG: 210.8.

General and the General Staff to conduct a study to determine how many officers could be released and how they could be separated with the least delay. A mission of senior officers was to be sent to the overseas theaters and Medical Department personnel were to be shipped to the Zone of Interior as soon as declared surplus, even ahead of other, higher point officers.

On 1 January 1946 the ADA published a bitter editorial criticism of dental demobilization claiming that the Army and Navy had, at the very least, been "ultraconservative and discriminatory," that hundreds of dentists were standing idle while their professional skills rusted, and that there had been no apparent effort to discharge dentists in the same ratio as enlisted men.[37]

There is some statistical justification for claims that dental demobilization lagged behind that of the Army as a whole. The ratio of dental officers to total strength went from 1.74 per 1,000 troops on V-E Day to a maximum of 2.23 per 1,000 in December 1945, and did not return to the V-E Day average until the middle of 1946.[38] However, other factors must be considered in this connection. Procurement had been allowed to lag for several months before the end of the war in Europe and the number of dentists on duty in May 1945 was about 500 less than the authorized figure. If dentists had been discharged in the same ratio as enlisted men, it would have been impossible to maintain a ratio of at least 2 per 1,000; dental officers would be the first to insist that such a ratio was necessary to render effective care. Dentists were needed to provide treatment for patients remaining in Army hospitals, and to examine and treat men being processed in separation centers. Further, the loss of time of dental officers during demobilization was high. Thus, although delayed demobilization of dental officers from V-E Day to the middle of 1946 did result in the ratio exceeding the normal proportion over a period of 6 months, in only 2 months did it exceed the 2 per 1,000 ratio by as much as 5 percent.

The Army as a whole had set for itself a demobilization program which no senior officer would guarantee could be met. In the face of that situation The Surgeon General had two choices: He might delay the separation of Medical Department personnel slightly until it was clear that the Army would actually be reduced as planned, or he might gamble on the demobilization program being carried out according to schedule and release every officer who could be spared. In the first case he risked criticism for holding officers a month or two longer than necessary; in the second he risked a breakdown of the medical service if shipping shortages or other circumstances delayed general demobilization. If a gamble had to be taken The Surgeon General apparently preferred to be sure that the troops would receive adequate medical care.[39] The

---

[37] The right to gripe: the fifth freedom. J. Am. Dent. A. 33: 118–122, Jan 1946.

[38] Ratios calculated by the author from data on the effective, administrative strength of the Dental Corps. This information, furnished by the Resources Anal Div, SGO, does not include officers on a terminal leave status. See footnote 20 for explanation of effective, administrative strength.

[39] Info given to author by Mr. John D. Rice, Resources Anal Div SGO, 19 Feb 48.

fact that the Army demobilization schedule was not only met but exceeded did not impair the wisdom of that decision.

Claims that dental officers were not always fully employed probably arose most often from the fact that the flow of troops through separation centers could not be constant. At times there was more work than could be handled; at others there was little to do. But personnel in these centers could not be juggled from day to day to meet changing demands.

The slight extent to which the separation of dental officers was delayed in 1945 as compared with the Army as a whole, is shown by an analysis of the situation existing in December 1945 when the excess of dentists was at its maximum. In that month there were 2.23 dental officers for each 1,000 men, but if those who were separated just a month later had been discharged in December the ratio of dentists would have fallen to 1.7 per 1,000, or considerably less than the number actually needed. It is thus apparent that even when the situation was most unfavorable, dental officers could not have been separated more than a few weeks earlier without causing a shortage of personnel to staff essential dental installations.

It is significant in this connection that after repeated hearings on the "hoarding" of Medical Department personnel, in which the matter was thoroughly discussed before congressional committees, none of the proposed legislation to force faster demobilization was passed.

By the first of January 1946, the Dental Service was faced with a rapidly developing shortage of officers. On 21 January a representative of the Military Personnel Division, SGO, pointed out that procurement to meet postwar needs was very uncertain and that unless replacements could be obtained it would soon be necessary to hold the remaining dentists to provide essential care for the troops.[40] He advised The Adjutant General that a new objective of 750 men would have to be established without delay if a "serious public relations problem" was to be avoided. This recommendation was approved,[41] but in the absence of the ASTP and without the stimulus of patriotism in time of combat, only 15 dentists were obtained by the first of May. Nevertheless, a new change in criteria, effective 1 February, reduced the separation requirements for both medical and dental officers to age 45, 60 points, or 39 months total service.[42] On 15 February, it was further announced that physicians and dentists who were declared surplus in any Zone of Interior command and who were within 4 months of being eligible for discharge would be released immediately.[43] On 23 April The Surgeon General recommended that the separation criteria, for medical officers only, be reduced to 30 months total service (other

---

[40] Ltr, Col Robert J. Carpenter to TAG, 21 Jan 46, sub: Procurement objective for appointment in the Army of the United States (Dental Corps). SG: 210.8.
[41] See Chapter III.
[42] WD radiogram 42485, 30 Jan 46.
[43] ASF Cir 40, 15 Feb 46.

requirements remaining unchanged).[44] This request was approved and the new standards were published effective 1 May.[45] Probably no action of the War Department caused greater unrest among dental officers than this maintenance of separate criteria for the Dental Corps, especially since it had been announced in March that male officers of the nonmedical branches would be released with 24 months' service after the end of August. However, it has since been shown in the discussion of medicodental relations in chapter I that no discrimination was intended, and that the termination of the dental ASTP, which precipitated this action, had been based on what were considered good and sufficient reasons.

In May and June 1946 arrangements were made to obtain 800 dental officers from the Navy, and another 1,500 through Selective Service (see chapter III, p. 74), and on 27 May it was announced that dentists would be released after 36 months of service.[46] On 1 September it was directed that dentists, including former ASTP students, would be separated after 30 months of service and finally, on 1 November 1946, dental officers were ordered released after 24 months of service under the same criteria as applied to male officers of most other branches.[47]

By October 1946 all of the 11,800 V-E Day nonvolunteers (excluding ASTP graduates) and 1,200 of the ASTP graduates had been separated.[48] At the end of 1946, 14,200 dental officers, of 14,700 on duty at the end of the war in Europe, had returned to private practice, and it appeared that the last nonvolunteer officer who had been in the Army on V-E Day would be released by the end of February 1947.[49] After February 1947 the active duty Dental Corps consisted only of the Regular Army, former ASTP students, officers on loan from the Navy, and those who had signed voluntary agreements to serve after they became eligible for discharge.

After 11 January 1946 any temporary officer who had served in the grade of first lieutenant for 18 months, in that of captain or major for 24 months, or lieutenant colonel for 30 months, with 50 percent additional credit for overseas service, was eligible for a promotion of one grade on separation if he had an efficiency index of 40 or above. This regulation also applied to any temporary officer with an efficiency index of 40 or over who had served at least 24 months without any promotion.[50]

Regulations in effect on V-J Day provided that until they could be replaced or declared surplus dental laboratory technicians could be retained within their current commands after becoming eligible for discharge on points.

---

[44] Memo, Brig Gen. R. W. Bliss for ACofS G-1, 23 Apr 46, sub: Demobilization of Medical Corps officers. SG: 210.8.
[45] WD radiogram 37758, 1 May 46.
[46] WD radiogram 44675, 27 May 46.
[47] WD radiogram 21743, 15 Oct 46.
[48] See footnote 24, p. 337.
[49] Ibid.
[50] WD Cir 10, 11 Jan 46.

There was no change in this policy until the end of 1945 when it was directed that no dental technician would be held for more than 6 months after he was eligible for release under existing criteria.[51] In February 1946 dental technicians were removed from the "scarce" category and it was directed that all men with 45 points or 30 months of service would be discharged by 30 April, and that all technicians with 40 points or 24 months of service would be separated, or en route to the United States for release, by 30 June 1946.[52]

Summary

The principal conclusions to be drawn from Army experience during the demobilization period are the following:

Pressure from civilian communities for the return of dentists after the fighting stops will generally be strong. The Armed Forces will be able to hold dental officers beyond the end of a war only when it can be shown that a clear and urgent need exists for their services.

Gradual replacement of dental personnel during a long conflict is highly desirable to permit the release of older men with the longest service and men who are less efficient than the average. Unless some "turnover" is maintained the Dental Corps will approach the end of hostilities with a high proportion of officers with such extensive service that public opinion will force their release regardless of the need for their services.

Voluntary procurement cannot be relied upon to furnish replacements for officers being demobilized after a war has ended if any sizeable force is to be maintained.

---

[51] WD Cir 382, 21 Dec 45.
[52] WD Cir 51, 20 Feb 46.

Index

AAF. *See* Army Air Forces.
ADA. *See* American Dental Association.
Adjusted service rating: 334, 337, 338, 339. *See also* Demobilization.
Adjutant General, The: 88, 89, 90, 94, 133, 135, 154, 155, 211
    applications for original appointment in Dental Corps, instructions concerning: 54
    charge for destroyed dental appliances, comment on: 234
    DC-2 clinic in general hospitals of 250 beds or more, approval of: 278
    DC-3 clinic for camps of 3,000 to 6,000 men, approval of: 260
    dental officers, evaluation of professional qualifications: 107
    limitation on dental attendance for temporary personnel, disapproval of: 211
    mandatory tables of organization for ZI dental services, disapproval of: 45–46
    maxillofacial hospitals, designation of: 273
    maximum utilization of Dental Corps officers, instructions concerning: 286
    Medical Officer Recruiting Boards, addition of dental officers, instructions for: 54
    on legislation for Dental Corps, transmittal of SecWar's views to The Surgeon General: 4
    procurement for Dental Corps
        discontinuance of: 61
        objectives, suggested review of: 60
    release of physicians and dentists in ZI, request for: 338
    use of tactical unit dentists in ZI camp clinics, instructions concerning: 285
Adjutant General's Office, the: 155, 211
Administration of the Dental Service
    in a theater of operations: 34. *See also* Communications Zone dental service; Division dental service; Field Army dental service; Redeployment center dental service; Tactical units dental service.
    in Army Ground Forces: 33

Administration of the Dental Service—Con.
    in camps and stations, ZI: 32. *See also* Replacement depot dental service; Replacement training center dental service; Separation center dental service; General hospital dental service; Station hospital dental service.
    in Corps Areas (later service commands): 30
    in The Surgeon General's Office: 27–28
    reorganization of the Army, 1942, effect on: 28
AEF. *See* American Expeditionary Forces.
AGF. *See* Army Ground Forces.
AGO. *See* Adjutant General's Office, the.
Air Surgeon's Office, Dental Section
    establishment: 31
    function: 32
Alaska: 215
"Amalgam line." *See* Morale.
"Amalgam mills." *See* Morale.
American Dental Association
    ASTP, comment on: 141
    Committee on Dental Education: 7
    Committee on Dental Preparedness: 227
    Committee on Legislation: 17, 18
    demobilization program, views on: 11, 340
    dental treatment, comment on: 214
    ethical status, role in determination of: 85, 95–96
    induction of dentists and dental students as enlisted men, objection to: 86
    Military Preparedness Committee: 70
    National Health Program Committee: 227
    objectives for improvement of the Dental Service: 15–20
        advanced rank for Director of Dental Division: 15–16
        "autonomy" for Dental Service: 17–18
    PAS, views on: 82
    personnel survey, findings of: 41, 78
    procurement, role in: 83–86
    procurement program, views on: 104
    professional status, role in determination of: 85

American Dental Association—Continued
  promotion policies, comment on: 113
  rehabilitation prior to induction, comment on: 227. *See also* Dental rehabilitation prior to induction.
  Selective Service deferment restriction (1944), protest of: 132
American Dental Trade Association: 169
American Expeditionary Forces: 174, 193, 313, 314
American Medical Association: 228
Ames, John R.
  appointment to Dental Corps after act of 1911: 3
Anzio beachhead: 315
Armed Forces Institute of Pathology. *See* Schools.
Armies
  Fifth: 311, 315, 316, 319
  First: 315, 326
  Ninth: 293, 298, 299, 300
  Seventh: 233, 306
Army Air Forces: 10, 32, 33, 34, 64, 90, 100, 106, 107, 112, 184, 196, 288. *See also* Air Surgeon's Office, Dental Section.
Army and Navy Munitions Board: 168
Army Dental Corps. *See* Dental Corps, Army.
Army Dental School: 119, 120, 125, 126, 128, 156, 157, 160
Army Ground Forces: 33, 90, 288, 297, 316, 318, 322, 323
Army Ground Forces Replacement Depot No. 1, Fort George G. Meade, Md.: 234
Army Medical Bulletin: 212
Army Medical Center: *See* Schools.
Army Medical School: *See* Schools.
Army-Navy General Hospital: 121, 159
Army-Navy Medical Procurement Office: 173
Army of the United States: 62
  as temporary emergency force: 64
  new appointments in, need for: 54
  officers called to active duty: 48–51
Army Regulations
  changes in: 19
  40–15, Dental Service, provisions for administration of: 10, 16, 20, 21, 22, 31, 151, 152
  40–510, treatment rendered, provisions for: 9n, 33n, 205n, 231, 232n, 283n

Army Service Forces: 23, 28, 45, 56, 58, 88, 94, 107, 154, 172, 288
Army Service Forces Replacement Depot, Camp Reynolds, Pennsylvania: 234
Army Specialized Training Program: 55, 56, 57, 58, 59, 61, 66, 67, 74, 86, 87, 88, 89, 91, 104, 116, 136–145, 149, 151, 342
  activation: 138
  cost: 140
  curriculum, preprofessional: 137
  curtailment: 138–140
  demobilization criteria affected by termination: 11–12, 342
  discontinuation of, factors involved: 11–12, 56–58, 342
  discussion of: 141–151
  enrollment in: 138
  enrollment in dental schools, effect on: 142
  graduates
    commissioned by Navy: 58
    lack of vacancies for: 47, 56, 58
    release of to private practice, 1944: 57, 66, 144
  morale of other military personnel, effect of: 143–144
  procurement: 55
  results: 140
  schools participating: 138
  students release of: 61
  termination: 11, 88, 140
  undergraduates: 136
Army transports, dental service on: 275–277
  base outfits recommended for: 277
  M. D. chest 60,
    provided for: 276
    unsuitability of: 276
  necessity for: 275
Artificial eye, acrylic, role of the Dental Service in the development of: 235–237
ASR. *See* Adjusted service rating.
Association of Dental Manufacturers of America: 168
Association of Military Dental Surgeons: 4
  journal of: 6
ASTP. *See* Army Specialized Training Program.
Attrition. *See also* Combat casualties; Demobilization; Release from active duty:
  acceleration of, 1944: 47

INDEX 347

Attrition—Continued
  December 1941–June 1945: 86
  estimated: 45
  low rate: 56, 110
AUS. *See* Army of the United States.
Australia: 175, 230, 289, 290
Authorized dental treatment. *See* Treatment, dental aspects of.
Auxiliary dental personnel. *See also* Hygienists, civilian.
  allotment authorized by tables of organization: 302
  allotment recommended for
    camps, ZI: 46
    dental clinics, ZI: 46–47
    station hospitals: 46
  assignment of: 151–152
  assistants, chair: 158. *See also* Occupational classification.
  authorization for: 151
  care of equipment, instructions on: 162, 176
  civilians, utilization of: 159–160
  discussion of: 162–164
  grades, compared with medical service personnel: 152
  laboratory technicians. *See also* Occupational classification.
    demobilization of: 336, 342–343
    effective utilization of: 155
    shortage of: 153–155
  morale: 152
  on-the-job training: 162
  prosthetic supply clerks: 158, 171
  training program: 156–158
    curriculum: 156
    duration of course: 156
    enrollment per month: 157
    results of: 157
  WAC personnel
    for duty as dental assistants
      disadvantages of: 159
      recommendation for: 158–159
    training of: 159
Awards: 117

Beaumont General Hospital: 121, 159
Bernheim, Julien R.
  appointment to Dental Corps after act of 1911: 3
  assignment in Dental Division, SGO: 22
Blesse, Gen. F. A.: 297n

Bliss, Brig. Gen. R. W.: 45, 58, 60, 183, 184, 333, 338, 342. *See also* Surgeon General, The.
Boak, Siebert D.
  appointment to Dental Corps after act of 1911: 3
Borden General Hospital: 238
Brauer, Col. John C.: vii, 136, 153, 219
British Army: 167, 175
Brooke Army Medical Center. *See* Schools.
Brooke General Hospital: 159
Bronze Star: 117
Brown, Dr. Homer C.
  chairman, Legislative Committee, National Dental Association: 4, 6
Brown, Col. Pearson W.: vii, 97
Buhler, Dr. John E.: 142
  Secretary-Treasurer of the American Assoc. of Dental Schools: 141–142
Bureau of Standards: 170
Burs. *See* Supplies.

Camalier, C. W.
  chairman of War Service Committee, ADA: 70n, 76, 101, 130
Camp Crowder, Missouri: 236
Camp Greenleaf, Fort Oglethorpe, Georgia: 118
Camp Pickett, Virginia: 158
Camp Reynolds, Pennsylvania: 234. *See also* Replacement depot dental service.
Camp Robinson, Ark.: 206. *See also* Redeployment center dental service.
Canadian Dental Service: 18–19
Carpenter, Alden
  appointment to Dental Corps after act of 1911: 3
Carpenter, Col. Robert J.: 10, 57, 335, 341
Casaday, George H.
  appointment to Dental Corps after act of 1911: 3
CBI. *See* China-Burma-India theater.
Central dental laboratories (CDL). *See also* Laboratories.
  Army Medical Center, Walter Reed General Hospital: 217
  Beaumont General Hospital: 217
  Corozal, Panama Canal Zone: 217
  Fitzsimons General Hospital: 217
  Fort Clayton, Panama Canal Zone: 217
  Letterman General Hospital: 217

Central dental laboratories (CDL)—Con.
  Station Hospital, Fort Sam Houston, Texas: 217
Chair assistants. *See* Auxiliary dental personnel.
Chambers, William H.
  appointment to Dental Corps after act of 1911: 3
Chiefs of Dental Division, SGO: 22
China-Burma-India theater: 99, 177, 192, 194, 317, 318
Civilian Conservation Corps: 64
Civilian dentists, authorization for use of to procure emergency dental care: 232
Civilian professional men, tentative plan for draft of: 53
Classification, dental. *See* Treatment, dental, aspects of.
Clay, Maj. Gen. Lucius D.: 172n
Clinic facilities, ZI. *See also* Prosthetic facilities, Zone of Interior.
  cost of: 261
  description of
    DC-1: 257
    DC-2: 257
    DC-3: 260
    DC-4: 260
    DC-5: 261
    DC-6: 261
Combat activities: 117
Combat casualties: 86, 117
Command and General Staff School. *See* Schools.
Commission on Physical Rehabilitation. *See* Dental rehabilitation prior to induction.
Commissions. *See* Dental Corps, Army.
Committee to Study the Medical Department: 165
Communications Zone dental service. *See also* Tables of organization medical units.
  dental surgeon, responsibility of: 302
  facilities: 303
  improvements, recommended for: 304–306
  organization: 302
  personnel: 303–304
Confederate Army: 1
Conscription
  of dentists
    Confederate Army: 1
    proposed, World War II: 74

Conscription—Continued
  of physicians: 56, 73
Consultants: 127, 214, 222, 306
Contract dental surgeons
  assignment: 2
  authorization for employment: 2
  number authorized for employment: 2
  number employed, 1901–1911: 3
Corozal, Panama Canal Zone: 217
Cowan, Col. E. V. W.: 166, 317
Craven, Col. Robert C.: 44
Criteria, dental, for overseas service: 229–232. *See also* Standards for military service, dental.
  definite standards established: 230, 232
  lack of definite standards for, 1942–43: 230
  report on personnel arriving overseas: 230, 232

Daniels, Col. Thomas C.: 276
Dargusch, Brig. Gen. Carlton S.: 228
Demobilization
  criteria
    changes in: 337, 338, 339, 341
    criticism of: 11, 61, 339, 342. *See also* Army Specialized Training Program; Release from active duty.
  establishment of: 334
  following V-J Day: 337–343
  following World War I: 332
  Medical Department personnel, policy for: 333–335
  "hoarding": 333, 341
  pressure for release of: 61, 333, 343
  period from V-E to V-J Day: 332–337
  statistics, May 1945–June 1947: 336
Denit, Brig. Gen. Guy B.: 11
Dental Advisory Committee. *See* Selective Service.
Dental Bulletin: 285
Dental Corps, Army. *See also* Legislation pertaining to Dental Corps.
  age distribution, V-E Day: 94
  appointments in, after act of 1911: 3
  commissioned 1944: 59
  components, strength of, V-E Day: 62
  composition of, 1945, by
    age: 105
    component: 105
    race: 105
    specialty: 106

Dental Corps, Army—Continued
  development, progress of to World War II. *See* Legislation pertaining to Dental Corps.
  enrollment, 1938: 48
  establishment of: 2
  grades
    distribution of: 10, 35–36
    general officer: 11, 16, 112, 115
    initial appointment: 97, 109
  procurement objectives. *See* Procurement, officer personnel.
  standards for commission in
    ethical: 94–96
    physical: 92–94
    professional: 94–96
  status, during World War II: 16–21
  strength
    at the time of the Armistice, World War I: 35
    expansion, during World War II: v
    increased ratio: 340
    in 1940: 52
    maximum, World War II: 56, 59, 106
    reduction in, 1918–1920: 332
  vacancies, lack of in 1944: 56, 58
Dental Corps ratio to Army strength
  Director of Dental Division, SGO, comment on: 37
  goal of Chief of Dental Division, SGO: 43–44
  goal of The Surgeon General: 43–44
  increase of for tactical units, recommendation for: 27, 288
  in replacement training centers, 1944: 265
  in ZI, 1942–44: 264–65
  need for evaluation of: 41
  period between World War I and II: 35, 36, 37, 287
  V-E Day: 60
  World War I: 35
  World War II: 43–47
Dental Division, SGO
  maximum strength: 28
  organization during World War II: 22–30
  organization prior to World War II: 22
  redesignation of: 29
Dental field chests. *See* Field equipment.
Dental journals, status of Dental Corps, comment on. *See* Medicodental relations.

Dental rehabilitation prior to induction
  ADA
    comment on: 227
    cooperation of: 226
    recommendations for: 227
  Commission on Physical Rehabilitation (FSA), plans for: 226–227
  Dental Advisory Committee, Selective Service: 226
  Selective Service System, test program
    inauguration of: 228
    results of: 229
  Wartime Health and Education, Senate Subcommittee, report on: 229
  World War I: 225
Dental Service, formation and organization of: 2
Dental service in Confederate armies: 1
Dentistry, military status of
  during Revolutionary War period: 1
  in Confederate Army: 1
Dentures, excessive loss or destruction of: 232–235, 313
  Army Ground Forces, report on: 233
  North African theater, report on: 233
  property accountability, recommendation for: 235
  record of dental appliances in individual service records, recommendations for: 233
  Seventh Army, Mediterranean Area, report on: 233
  War Department directives for listing of dentures: 233
  when lost through carelessness or intent
    charge for, question concerning: 234
    courtmartial action, recommendation for: 234
    legality of, opinion of Legal Division: 235
Deshon General Hospital: 238
DeWitt, Brig. Gen. Wallace: 277
Dietz, Maj. Victor: 236
Diseases, dental, incidence of. *See* Statistics.
Distinguished Service Medal: 117
Director of the Dental Division, SGO: 13, 16, 31, 33, 37, 46, 71, 113, 114, 167, 175, 200, 210, 213, 225, 231, 257, 262, 280, 281, 325
  advice against termination of ASTP: 139, 144
  authority, extent of: 23, 27

Director of the Dental Division, SGO—Con.
  dental laboratory technicians, insure assignment to Medical Department, request for: 154
  dental representation in other divisions of SGO, recommendations for: 29–30
  duties: 22–23
  effectiveness of ASTP, comment on: 142–143, 151
  lack of a permanent corps of enlisted men, comment on: 15
  occupational classification, comment on: 108
  PAS, comment on: 82
Dental Laboratory Institute of America, survey of laboratory manpower: 154
Directors of Dental Division, SGO: 22
Divisions
  1st Armored: 316
  34th Armored: 316
  36th Armored: 316
  45th Armored: 316
  1st Infantry: 319, 325
  9th Infantry: 325
  41st Infantry: 289
  66th Infantry: 296
Division dental service
  dental surgeon, responsibilities of: 291–293
  organization: 290
  personnel authorized: 290–291
  reorganization
    comment: 294–297
    prescribed by TO&E: 297–298
    recommended: 293

Eanes, Richard H.
  Assistant Executive Officer, Selective Service: 81
Education. *See also* Schools.
  dental students
    deferment directives: 130–131
    deferment legislation for: 129
    deferment through reserve commissions: *See* Medical Administrative Corps, Reserve.
    military status of: 129
    predental students, limited deferment of: 132
Efficiency reports: 9, 14, 20
Eisenhower, Gen. Dwight D.: 321
England: 165, 175, 215, 276, 328

Epperly, Brig. Gen. James M.: 74, 102, 293, 298, 305
Epps, Col. Beverly: 322
Equipment and Supplies. *See* Equipment; Field equipment; Supplies.
Equipment. *See also* Field equipment; Supplies.
  cart, ward, dental: 197
  experience gained, World War II: 197–198
  for communications zone
    fixed installations: 178
    semifixed installations: 178
  for Zone of Interior installations: 178, 179
  handpieces, shortages of: 167
  heavy clinical, requirement for: 166
  nonstandard impression chests: 196
  procurement
    overseas, World War I: 174
    overseas, World War II: 175, 178
  repair of: 176
  shipment overseas
    removal of restrictions: 179
    restrictions on: 178
    without authorized field chests: 166, 171, 276
  shortages of: 165–168
  substitution of: 177
  used, program for purchase of: 171–174
Erpf, Capt. Stanley F.: 236, 237
Ethical standards for commission: 94
ETO. *See* European Theater of Operations.
Europe: 117, 165, 167, 175, 233n, 294, 299, 304, 307, 325, 331, 333, 334, 342
European Theater of Operations: 165, 167, 179, 192, 194, 236, 291, 293, 295, 305, 315, 318, 324, 328, 334
Evacuation
  dental causes: 99, 293, 317
  maxillofacial casualties, "type" procedure for: 308–311
    modification of: 310–311
    principles observed: 311
  treatment provided in the chain of
    at battalion aid station: 309
    at clearing station: 309
    at collecting station: 309
    at evacuation hospital: 310
    initial: 309

INDEX

Fairbank, Leigh C.: 23, 24, 27, 32, 37, 44, 69, 70, 123, 165, 170, 190, 200, 207, 257, 280, 314. *See also* Director of Dental Division.
    assignment, Dental Division, SGO: 22
Far East: 307. *See also* Pacific.
Federal Security Agency (FSA): 133, 226
Fedor, Maj. Ernest J.: 44, 57, 58, 59, 68, 73, 75, 81, 88, 136, 178
Female dentists: 102
Female civilian assistants. *See* Auxiliary dental personnel.
Field Army dental service. *See also* Table of organization medical units.
    dental surgeon, responsibility of: 299
    personnel allotment: 298–300
    prosthetic service, problems concerning: 301–302
    reorganization of, proposal submitted by dental surgeon, MTO: 300
    study of, ETO: 299–300
Field equipment. *See also* Mobile dental laboratory; Mobile dental operating truck.
    Army Air Forces operating chest: 184
    field chest, prosthetic
        M.D. 61: 184–185
        M.D. 62: 184–185
        World War I: 184
    kit
        assistant's: 186
        maxillofacial: 188
        officer's: 186
        utilization of: 306
    operating, M. D. chest No. 60
        addition to
            electric dental engine: 182
            miscellaneous: 183–184
            operating lamp: 183
            reduction in weight: 183
        World War I: 180
        World War II: 180
    pack chests "A" and "B": 186
    prosthetic, M. D. chest Nos. 61, 62
        change in: 185
        defects of: 190
        medical organizations
            issued to: 185, 314
            removed from: 317
        World War I: 184
        World War II: 184
Fifth Army: 311, 315, 316, 319, 320

First Army: 315, 326
Fitts, Lt. Col. Francis M.: 54, 93, 136, 144
Fitzsimons General Hospital: 121, 156, 159, 217
Florence Redeployment Center, MTO. *See* Redeployment center dental service.
Fort Bragg: 283
Fort Clayton: 217
Fort Dix, N. J.: 206n, 270, 271
Fort Huachuca, Ariz.: 159
Fort Knox, Ky.: 280. *See also* Replacement training center dental service.
Fort George G. Meade, Md.: 206, 234
Fort Monmouth, N. J. *See* Separation center dental service.
Fort Riley, Kans.: 283
Fort Sill, Okla.: 206
France: 296, 313, 315, 320, 325
Frankfurt: 304
Freeman, Dr. Charles W., Dean, Northwestern Univ. Dental School: 12, 66
Futterman, Dr. M. J., Chairman, National Victory Committee, Allied Dental Council, N. Y.: 95

General Board, U. S. Forces, European Theater of Operations
    mobile dental laboratory, comment on: 325
    personnel for prosthetic service, comment on: 328
    quality of dental service, comment on: 291
General hospital dental service, ZI: 273–274
Graham, George D.
    appointment to Dental Corps after act of 1911: 3
Grant, Brig. Gen. David N. W.: 32, 165
Gray, Col. Dell S.: 318
Greece: 117
Gulf Coast Air Corps Training Center. *See* Schools, military.
Gunckel, George I.
    appointment to Dental Corps after act of 1911: 3
Hall, Lt. Col. Durward G.: 45, 58, 60, 138, 139
Handpieces. *See* Equipment.
Harper, Col. Neal: 120
Hawley, Brig. Gen. Paul R.: 175

Health and Medical Committee: 226
Hearing-aid adapter, acrylic, role of the Dental Service in the development of: 237–238
Heavy clinical equipment. *See* Equipment.
Hemberger, Lt. Col. Arthur J.: 238
Hershey, Gen. Lewis B.: 228
Hess, John H.
  appointment to Dental Corps after act of 1911: 3
Hillman, Brig. Gen. C. C.: 172
Hoff General Hospital. *See* Hospitals.
Hospital laboratories. *See* Laboratories.
Hospital ships, dental service on
  equipment: 274
  facilities: 274
  personnel: 274
Hospitals
  named
    Army-Navy General: 121, 159
    Beaumont General: 121, 159, 217
    Brooke General: 159
    Darnall General: 126
    Fitzsimons General: 121, 156, 159, 217
    Fort Sam Houston, Station: 121, 125, 217
    Hoff General: 238
    Letterman General: 121, 217
    Thomas M. England General: 236
    Valley Forge General: 236
    Wakeman General: 159
    Walter Reed General: 120, 121, 125, 217, 238
  numbered
    2d Field: 290
    7th Station: 317
    9th Evacuation: 296
    21st General: 317
    30th General: 236
    64th Station: 317
    181st General: 322
Hospitals designated as specialized maxillofacial centers: 273
Hudnall, Lt. Col. J. R.: 90, 93, 139, 336
Huebner, Brig. Gen., AGF: 175
Hygienists, civilian
  commissions, recommendations for: 161
  conditions outlined for employment of: 160
  difficulties of procurement: 161–162
  pay of: 160
  status: 161
  status in Navy: 162

Iceland: 288
Ingalls, Raymond E.
  appointment to Dental Corps after act of 1911: 3
Instructors
  deferment of: 145
  program for release of: 335

Japan: 61
Johnson, Lt. J. B., co-author, "History of wartime research and development of medical field equipment": 188, 193, 194, 311
Judge Advocate General, The
  destroyed dental appliances, ruling on: 235
  promotion, ruling on: 113

Kennebeck, Col. George R.: 31, 162, 165, 184
Kirk, Maj. Gen. Norman T.: 14, 74, 161, 334. *See also* Surgeon General, The.

Laboratories
  camp: 280–281
  central dental laboratories
    overseas: 327–329
    Zone of Interior: 217, 281
  civilian, use of: 283
  hospital: 329
  output: 281, 282, 283
Laflamme, Frank L. K.
  appointment to Dental Corps after act of 1911: 3
  assignment, Dental Division, SGO: 22
Lauderdale, Clarence E.
  appointment to Dental Corps after act of 1911: 3
Lend—lease: 167
Legion of Merit: 117, 237
Legislation pertaining to Dental Corps
  act of 1911, command restriction, removal of, 1945: 21
  Adjutant General, views on: 4
  brigadier general, authorization for rank of, 1938: 22n
  enacted prior to World War I
    1901: 2
    1908: 2
    1911: 2
  grades and percentages of grades allowed for, 1917: 6n
  peacetime promotion schedule, establishment of, 1920: 6n

Legislation pertaining to Dental Corps—Continued
  retirement credits, establishment of, 1938: 6
  strength authorized, 1920: 6, 37
  strength increases, 1936, 1938, 1939: 6
  strength, reduction of, 1921, 1922: 6
Leslie, Samuel H.
  appointment to Dental Corps after act of 1911: 3
Letterman General Hospital: 121, 217
Liaison
  ADA: 55, 85, 95
  PAS: 79
Logan, Col. William H. G.: 118
  assignment, Dental Division, SGO: 22
Long, Charles J.
  appointment to Dental Corps after act of 1911: 3
Lott, F. M.: 18
Love, Col. Albert G.: 36, 67
Love, Col. Walter D.: 262, 280
Lull, Brig. Gen. George F.: 44, 61, 81, 114, 169.

Magee, Maj. Gen. James C.: 84, 113, 133, 134, 135
Manpower requirements, methods for determination.
  civilian experience: 36
  estimated need for dental treatment: 37–41.
  for tactical units: 45
  for Zone of Interior: 45–47
  pre-World War II military experience: 36–37.
  theoretical versus actual: 41
    impracticability of meeting theoretical needs: 38–40.
    mobilization rate, effect on: 38
Marshall, Gen. George C.: 134
Marshall, Dr. John S.
  appointment to Dental Corps after act of 1911: 3.
  contribution to military dental service: 2
  enlisted assistants, comment on: 151
Mason, George L.
  appointment to Dental Corps after act of 1911: 3.
Mason, Col. J. B.: 318
Maxillofacial and plastic training. *See* Training.

Maxillofacial care, hospitals designated for: 273
Maxillofacial casualties. *See* Evacuation.
McAfee, Gen. Larry B.: 45, 52, 68, 159, 161, 211
McAlister, John A.
  appointment to Dental Corps after act of 1911: 3
McCracken, Col. G. A.: 238
McCurdy, Howard A.
  first dental casualty to lose his life: 117
McDowell, Brig. Gen. Rex McK.: 99, 115, 162, 183, 192, 208, 222, 233, 276, 277, 316, 317
McNutt, Paul V.: 133, 135
  economical use of limited medical personnel, recommendations for: 53
M. D. Chests 60, 61, 62. *See* Field equipment.
Medical Administrative Corps: 21
Medical Administrative Corps Reserve
  commission in, to insure deferment: 133
  commissions in
    granting of new, discontinuance of: 136
    granting of new, request for: 61
  procurement source: 67
  students holding inactive commissions in
    available for active duty: 55, 56
    number placed on active duty: 136
  transfer to, of medical, dental or veterinary students holding a reserve commission in another branch: 133
Medical Corps: 6, 10, 11, 12, 16, 18, 20, 21, 66, 72, 109, 112, 113, 114
Medical Department: 2, 11, 16, 18, 23, 28, 30, 53, 55, 68, 69, 72, 82, 84, 92, 100, 108, 112, 115, 339
Medical Department Equipment Laboratory: 194
Medical Department Redeployment and Separation Policy. *See* Demobilization.
Medical Field Service School. *See* Schools.
Medical Officer Recruiting Boards: 77, 79, 80, 92
  dental applications for original appointments, instructions concerning: 54, 55, 82, 93, 94
  dental representatives
    added to: 54, 82
    removed from: 55
  establishment: 54, 96
  purpose: 54, 82

Medicodental relations
    ADA, Committee on Dental Education, views of: 7
    Director of the Dental Division, views of: 13
    discrimination: 7, 11, 12
    failure to consult dental surgeons on matters affecting dental service: 13
    lack of effective control of dental personnel: 14
    medical interference in dental administration, extent of: 15
    professional interference: 15
    professional journals, comments in
        Journal of American Dental Association: 7, 8, 11, 12, 14
        Oral Hygiene: 7, 9, 12
    promotion opportunities as compared with Medical Corps: 10, 112
    Surgeon General, views of: 9, 10, 13–14
Mediterranean Base Section: 317
Mediterranean Theater of Operations: 117, 233, 300, 301
Merritt, Dr. Arthur H., President, ADA: 84
Middle East Theater: 113, 165, 167, 175, 292
Military District of Washington: 90
Military Personnel Division: 30, 54, 57, 58, 59, 60, 75, 91, 98
Miller, Rep. Louis E.: 132
Mills, Robert H.: 13, 14, 15, 20, 25, 58, 60, 61, 68, 75, 90, 95, 99, 102, 115, 117, 123, 162, 165, 166, 167, 174, 175, 177, 178, 179, 211, 219, 224, 225, 230, 231, 261, 262, 280, 281, 297, 315, 317, 318, 323. *See also* Director of Dental Division.
    appointment to Dental Corps after act of 1911: 3
    assignment Dental Division, SGO: 23, 44
Mission and capabilities of the Dental Service: 204–207
    dental health
        maintenance of: v
        restoration of: v
Mobile dental laboratory: 188–193
    allotment authorized for overseas theaters: 192
    description of: 190
    evaluation of: 325–327
    improvised models, overseas: 190–192

Mobile dental laboratory—Continued
    number ordered for distribution overseas: 192
    report on: 190–192
    utilization of: 321–325
Mobile dental operating truck
    accepted as standard item: 194
    allotment authorized for overseas theaters: 194
    comparison with M. D. Chest No. 60: 312
    "dental ambulances," World War I: 193
    description of: 194
    Director of Dental Division, comment on: 195
    request for: 311
Mobilization. *See also* Procurement, officer personnel.
    monthly progress of
        AUS: 48–62
        National Guard: 48–62
        Regular Army: 48–62
        Reserve: 48–62
Mobilization Regulations (MR) 1–9. *See* Standards for military service, dental.
Mockbee, Col. James B.: 12
Morale: 115. *See also* Medicodental relations.
    "amalgam line": 264
    "amalgam mills": 116
    ASTP graduate personnel, proposed release of: 57, 116, 144
    unfavorable assignments: 116
    unfavorable promotion status: 113
    work quotas: 116
Mordecai, Lt. Col. Alfred, "History of the Procurement and Assignment Service for physicians, dentists, veterinarians, sanitary engineers, and nurses, War Manpower Commission:" 53, 76
MTO. *See* Mediterranean Theater of Operations.
Murray, Sen. James E.: 69, 70, 129

National Defense Act, 3 June 1916: 4, 113
National Dental Association. *See also* American Dental Association.
    Dental Corps, interest in improved status: 5–6
    legislative committee: 4
    legislative measures sponsored: 1, 4
National Guard: 63
    commissioned dental officers, 1917, 1918: 5

INDEX 355

National Guard—Continued
  Dental Corps organized in, 1916: 5
  number called to active duty: 48-51
  procurement, role in: 48
National Roster of Scientific and Specialized Personnel: 78
NATO. *See* North African Theater of Operations.
Navy Dental Corps: 16, 19, 35
Navy V-12 program: 149
New Guinea: 289. *See also* Pacific.
New York Port of Embarkation: 171, 276
Ninth Army: 293, 298, 299, 300
Nonprofessional use of dental officers. *See* Personnel, officer.
North African Theater of Operations: 166, 192, 194, 233, 317, 318, 319

Occupational classification
  enlisted
    chair assistants: 155
    technicians: 155
  officers: 106, 107-108
  standards, lack of: 97, 108
Occupational deferment of dentists. *See* Selective Service.
Office, Chief of Transportation: 90
Office of Defense Health and Welfare Service: 76, 133
Office of Production Management (OPM): 130
Office of The Air Surgeon: 31, 32
Office of The Surgeon General. *See* Surgeon General's Office, the.
Officer Procurement Service: 56, 80, 81, 82, 83
Officers Reserve Corps. *See also* Reserve.
  commissioned dental officers, 1917, 1918: 5
  establishment, 1916: 5
Oliver, Col. Robert T.
  appointment to Dental Corps after act of 1911: 3
  assignment, Dental Division, SGO: 22
  general hospital designated in honor of: 3
OPS. *See* Officer Procurement Service.
Order of the British Empire: 117
Organization of the Army Dental Corps prior to World War II: 1-7
Organized Reserve. *See* Reserve.

Pacific: 192, 194
  island: 310, 312, 315

Pacific—Continued
  landing: 117
  Southwest: 230, 232, 318
Palestine: 175
Panama: 64
PAS. *See* Procurement and Assignment Service for Physicians, Dentists, and Veterinarians.
Patterson, Robert F.
  appointment to Dental Corps after act of 1911: 3
Patterson, Robert P., Under Secretary of War: 134
Paul, Gen. Willard S., Acting Chief of Staff: 144
Pearl Harbor: 53, 66, 97
Pepper, Sen. Claude: 70, 102
Personnel, enlisted. *See* Auxiliary dental personnel.
Personnel, officer. *See also* Mobilization; Procurement, officer personnel.
  allotment authorized by tables of organization: 111, 299, 302
  allotment recommended for
    camps, ZI: 46
    dental clinics, ZI: 46-47
    station hospitals: 46
  assignment, by type of unit: 107
    overseas: 106
    ZI: 106
  commissioned during 1944: 59
  conservation of: 91
  estimated number to serve with Corps, World War II: 61-62
  nonprofessional use of: 14, 98-100
    as auxiliary medical officers, comment on: 99, 306
    restriction on: 286
  number on active duty, 1941: 53
  postwar, anticipated shortage of: 60, 91
  requirements for. *See* Manpower requirements, methods for determination.
  uneconomical use of as enlisted soldiers: 70
  use of at camps and stations: 284-285
Persons authorized to receive dental care. *See* Treatment, dental, aspects of.
Pharmacy Corps: 21
Physical standards for commission: 92
Preparation for overseas movement, 1943: 206. *See also* Criteria, dental, for overseas service.

Preparedness League of American Dentists: 118, 193, 225
President of the United States: 5
  empowered to call to active duty, with or without consent, any member of the Reserve or National Guard, 1940: 52
  "salvage" program to rehabilitate individuals rejected for dental defects: 228. *See also* Dental rehabilitation prior to induction.
Procurement and Assignment Service for Physicians, Dentists, and Veterinarians: 55, 56, 65, 72, 91, 97
  effectiveness of: 80–82
  initial recommendation for: 53
  instructors in dental schools, survey of: 145
  organization: 76
  personnel survey
    findings: 41–42
    recommendations: 42–43
  procurement functions: 77–79
Procurement, equipment and supplies. *See* Equipment; Supplies.
Procurement, officer personnel. *See also* Mobilization.
  ceiling: 45, 58
  discontinuance of: 56, 61
  grades
    as an aid in procurement: 97–98
    authorized: 96
    offered: 97
  improvement in: 74
  lack of vacancies, 1944, problem of: 56, 58
  methods
    ADA: 83–86
    Medical Officer Recruiting Boards: 80–82
    Officer Procurement Service: 83
    PAS: 76–82
    Selective Service: 67–76
  objectives for
    1942: 53–54, 92, 94, 96
    1943: 55–56, 142
    1945: 60
  postwar: 102
    draft of dentists: 74, 342
    from the Navy: 342
  program, summary: 103–104
  ratio objectives
    analysis: 45
    weaknesses: 40–41

Procurement, etc.—Continued
  ratios authorized: 35, 36–37
  replacement pools: 53, 125
  requirements, table of organization units: 45
  sources of
    ASTP: 55, 60, 67, 138
    civil: 67–86, 91
    enlisted reserve: 67
    inducted dentists: 60
    Medical Administrative Corps Reserve: 56, 60, 67, 133, 136
    National Guard: 62, 63
    Organized Reserve: 48–53, 63–66
    Regular Army: 62
  survey (projected to the end of 1943)
    defects of: 42–43
    maximum number available from civilian practice: 41
    PAS findings: 42
    PAS recommendations: 43
  voluntary program, lag in: 61, 72
  World War I: 35, 41
Professional standards for commission: 94
Promotion
  Dental and Medical Corps, comparison of: 10, 112
  Director of Dental Division, SGO, comment on: 113, 115
  eligibility for, in World War II: 110
  general officer: 114
  in ZI: 110–111
  Judge Advocate General, ruling on: 113
  lack of opportunity for: 110
  morale factor: 113
  overseas: 111–112
    increased opportunity: 114
  peacetime schedule, establishment of: 6, 109
  regulations, suspension of: 109
  service required for
    Regular Army: 109
    Reserve: 109
Prosthetic facilities, ZI
  laboratories
    camp: 278–281
    civilian, use of: 283–284
    station: 278–281
  laboratory service, operation of: 281–283
  need for expansion, World War II: 278–280
  prior to World War II: 278

INDEX 357

Prosthetic service. *See also* Dentures, excessive loss or destruction of.
  professional standards: 221–222
  requirements for, as revealed by wartime experience: 219–220
Prosthetic service, overseas
  World War I
    equipment: 313–314
    prostheses constructed: 313
    requirement for: 313
  World War II
    equipment: 314, 316–318
    facilities: 314
    morale factor: 319–320
    prostheses constructed: 315. *See also* Statistics.
    removal of chests 61 and 62, effect on: 317–319
Prosthetic service, policies for provision of: 211–212
  central dental laboratories, establishment of: 217
  during World War I: 216
  period between World Wars I and II: 216–218
  prior to World War I: 216
  World War II: 218–219
Prosthetic supply clerks. *See* Auxiliary dental personnel.
Prosthetic teams: 301, 323
Publications. *See* Training aids.
Public Health Service, United States (USPHS): 227
  personnel survey, aid in: 41
Purple Heart: 117

"Quota" dentistry: 117, 223–225

Redeployment center dental service
  dental condition of redeploying troops: 308
    comparison of with inductees (Camp Robinson, Ark.): 308
  equipment and facilities: 307
  organization of (Florence Redeployment Center, MTO): 307
Regular Army Dental Corps. *See* Dental Corps, Army.
Release from active duty. *See also* Demobilization.
  administrative discharges: 87
  create vacancies for younger men: 59, 89
  dental defects: 255

Release from active duty—Continued
  essential to national health: 91
  hardship: 91
    War Department Circular 485, 1944: 91
  limited service: 87
  no suitable assignment: 88, 94
  physical disqualification: 87
  quotas for: 90
Relocation program for civilian dentists
  abandoned: 101
  applications, number received for: 101
  experience gained: 102
  funds appropriated
    by Congress: 101
    local community: 101
  initiated: 101
  overall utilization of dental manpower, effected by: 101
  payment to volunteers: 101
  purpose: 101
Renfrow, Col. Louis H., Selective Service System: 75
Replacement depot dental service
  description of operations (Camp Reynolds, Pa.): 265–266
  details of operation: 265
  function of: 265
  personnel allotment: 265
  treatment rendered: 265
Replacement training center dental service
  description of operation (Ft. Knox, Ky.): 262–263
  function of: 262
  personnel allotment: 262–265
  treatment rendered: 264
Reserve
  age, limitation for initial active duty, 1940: 64
  call to active duty, lieutenant colonels and colonels: 54
  commissions, suspension of: 52
  disadvantages of membership in: 66
  enrollment
    1938: 63
    1941: 51–52, 63, 121–122
  establishment of: 5
  evaluation of: 65–66
  grade distribution, 1941: 63
  number called to active duty, 1939–46: 48–51, 64, 122
  number on active duty, 1941: 52
  procurement for: 51, 63

Reserve—Continued
  procurement, role in: 48
  release from active duty, suspension of: 53
  release of ASTP graduates, criticism of: 66
Reserve Officers' Training Corps. *See also* Training.
  termination of: 48
Reynolds, Brig. Gen. Russel B.: 89, 90, 139, 231
Rhoades, Rex H.: 22
  appointment to Dental Corps after act of 1911: 3
Robinson, J. B., President, ADA: 113, 168
ROTC. *See* Reserve Officers' Training Corps.
Ryan, Edward P. R.
  appointment to Dental Corps after act of 1911: 3

Saipan: 315. *See also* Pacific.
San Francisco Port of Embarkation: 276
Sanitary Corps: 21
Scherer, Dr. W. H., President, ADA: 11n
Schools, civilian. *See also* Training.
  Columbia University, N. Y.: 126
  dental registration
    1932 through 1940: 146
    1941 through 1945: 146
  freshman enrollment, 1945: 147
  Harvard University, Cambridge, Mass.: 126
  Howard University, Washington, D. C.: 138
  Mayo Foundation, Minn.: 126
  Meharry Medical School, Nashville, Tenn.: 138
  Northwestern University, Chicago: 118
  Tulane University, New Orleans: 126
  University of Pennsylvania (Thomas W. Evans Institute), Philadelphia: 118, 126
  Washington University, St. Louis: 118, 126
Schools, military. *See also* Training.
  Army Dental School: 119, 120, 125, 126, 128, 156, 157, 160
  Armed Forces Institute of Pathology: 120, 128
  Army Medical Center: 126
  Army Medical School: 120, 125
  Brooke Army Medical Center: 124

Schools, military—Continued
  Central Dental Laboratory: 120
  Command and General Staff: 120, 121
  Dental Research Laboratory: 120
  Gulf Coast Air Corps Training Center: 125
  Medical Field Service School, Carlisle Barracks: 14, 119, 120, 121, 123, 124, 125
  War College: 121
Schwichtenberg, Col. A. H.: 275
Scott, Harold O.
  appointment to Dental Corps after act of 1911: 3
Scott, Minot E.
  appointment to Dental Corps after act of 1911: 3
Secretary of War: 4, 23, 35, 44, 94, 102, 209, 228, 339
Selective Service: 52, 58, 65, 77, 129. *See also* Dental rehabilitation prior to induction.
  deferment directives for
    general: 131
    preprofessional students: 132
    professional students: 130–131, 132
  Dental Advisory Committee: 226
  draft of dentists: 74
  induction boards, dentists appointed to: 203
  induction of dentists, criticism of: 68
  occupational deferment of dentists, consideration of: 71
  prerogatives of: 53, 70
  procurement policies: 67–76
Separation center dental service. *See also* Treatment, dental, aspects of.
  personnel allotment: 267
  policies for provision of dental care: 266–267
  prosthetic replacements, extensive need for: 270–271
  system of operation (Ft. Monmouth, N. J.): 268–270
Separation criteria. *See* Demobilization.
Services of Supply (SOS): 28, 54
Seventh Army: 306
SGO. *See* Surgeon Generals' Office, the.
Sheppard, Hon. Morris: 69, 129
Shook, Col. C. F.: 172
Silver Star: 117
Skull plates, role of Dental Service in development of: 238

Smith, Brig. Gen. Thomas L.: 23, 26, 99, 173, 228, 233, 235, 305, 314, 323
   assignment Dental Division, SGO: 23
Soldier's Medal: 117
South Pacific Base Command: 192, 194
Southwest Pacific theater: 179, 192, 194, 230, 318
Sparkman, Hon. John J.: 102
Specialty classification. *See* Occupational classification.
Stallman, George E.
   appointment to Dental Corps after act of 1911: 3
Standards for military service, dental. *See also* Dental Corps, Army.
   airborne duty: 203
   cadets: 203
   changes in: 201–202
   divers: 203
   for overseas service: 229–232
   lowering: 202, 211
   mobilization regulations
     disqualifications under: 200–201
       rate, 1942: 203
       rate, 1943: 203
     revision of: 202–203
   peacetime: 199
   Regular Army: 203
   rejections, causes for: 201
   voluntary enlistment in National Guard: 201
Station hospital dental service, overseas. *See* Communications Zone dental service.
Station hospital dental service, ZI: 271–272
Station Hospital, Fort Sam Houston: 121, 125
Statistics
   dental diagnoses, 1938–45
     cellulitis of dental origin: 239
     fractured mandible: 240
     fractured maxillae: 241
     osteomyelitis of oral structures: 242
     Vincent's stomatitis: 243
   dental diseases, incidence of, 1942–45
     cellulitis, dental origin: 244
     osteomyelitis, oral structures: 246
     Vincent's stomatitis: 245
   output per dental officer (five principal operations), 1 Jan 1942–31 Aug 1945: 256
   output per laboratory technician, 1943–44: 283

Statistics—Continued
   protheses constructed
     bridges: 223, 252
     dentures: 223
       full: 249
       partial: 250
   prosthetic operations per 1,000 men per year: 219–220
   repairs: 223, 251
   treatment, cash value of: 255
   treatment rendered, 1 Jan 42–31 Aug 45
     extractions: 248
     fillings: 247
     prophylaxes: 254
     teeth replaced: 253
Stimson, Henry L.: 69, 129
Stone, Frank P.
   appointment to Dental Corps after act of 1911: 3
   assignment to Dental Division, SGO: 22
Students, dental, deferment of. *See* Education; Selective Service.
Supplies
   burs
     collection of, from civilian sources: 168
     Medical Supplies Commission, report on civilian purchase of: 168
     requirement of, 1943, compared with average prewar demand: 168
     War Production Board report on status of, 1943: 166
   conservation of: 176
   dental items, simplification of: 169
   distribution, improvement in: 170
   effects of climate: 177
   experience gained in World War II: 197–198
   local procurement
     overseas: 175
     Zone of Interior: 174
   methods to assure effective utilization: 169
   packing, general principles for: 177
   porcelain teeth, storage, and issue: 170
   shipping, general principles for: 177
   shortages: 165–168
   storage and issue of: 170–171
   substitution of: 177
Supply Division, SGO: 167
   dental officer assigned to: 30, 170
   surplus burs, comment on: 168

Surgeon General, The: 2, 9, 35, 43, 44, 45, 48, 51, 52, 54, 55, 56, 59, 60, 64, 67, 73, 77, 79, 80, 81, 82, 83, 84, 85, 88, 89, 90, 91, 92, 93, 94, 96, 97, 99, 107, 118, 133, 134, 135, 138, 139, 144, 151, 155, 169, 170, 172, 173, 176, 193, 211, 214, 216, 225, 227, 230, 232, 234, 238, 266, 277, 278, 288, 323, 335, 336, 338
- administrative action for improvement of dental service: 16
- authority, extent of: 10, 23, 28–29, 33
- demobilization of Medical Department officers, on progress of: 333–334, 340–341
- exemption from military service through Reserve commissions, views on: 53, 70
- female civilian assistants, conditions specified for hire: 159–160
- increased responsibility for dental surgeons, interest in: 19
- inducted professional personnel, commissions recommended for: 68
- nonprofessional use of dental officers, action concerning: 14
- on legislative action to increase efficiency of the Dental Corps: 4, 6
- promotion announcement: 16
- promotion efforts in behalf of dental officers: 11
- release from active duty of "limited service" personnel, recommendations for: 57–58
- subordinated status of Dental Corps, disapproval of: 13–14
- wasteful use of physicians and dentists as enlisted soldiers, views on: 70

Surgeon General's Office, the: 22, 29, 30, 45, 61, 66, 79, 82, 96, 194

Surgeons, dental. *See also* Contract dental surgeons.
- first lieutenants appointed after act of 1911: 3

Table of Organization and Equipment 8–16, 1 June 1945. *See* Division dental service.

Table of organization medical units, overseas
- auxiliary surgical group: 299, 301
- clearing company: 299, 301
- convalescent camp: 302
- convalescent center: 302

Table of organization medical units, overseas—Continued
- detachments
  - dental operating, mobile: 302
  - dental prosthetic, fixed: 301, 302, 304
  - dental prosthetic, mobile: 302
  - maxillofacial: 302, 303
  - medical: 302, 303
- dispensaries, medical
  - aviation: 302, 303
  - general: 302
- gas treatment battalion: 299
- hospitals
  - centers: 302, 303
  - convalescent: 299
  - evacuation: 299
  - field: 299
  - general: 302
  - station: 302
- medical depot company: 299
- medical supply depot: 302

Tactical units dental service: 287–289

Technical Manuals
- TM 8–255. *See* Separation center, dental service.
- TM 8–638. *See* Auxiliary dental personnel.
- TM 12–406. *See* Occupational classification.

Technicians. *See* Auxiliary dental personnel.

Thomas M. England General Hospital. *See* Hospitals.

Tignor, Edwin P.
- appointment to Dental Corps after act of 1911: 3

Tingay, Col. Lynn H.: 300, 301, 318

Training. *See also* Training aids.
- consultants: 127
- during World War II
  - basic, Medical Department replacement pools: 125
  - basic, Medical Field Service Schools duration: 124
    - number graduated: 125
  - maxillofacial and plastic
    - civilian institutions: 126
    - hospitals: 126
  - professional, Army Dental School: 125
  - refresher courses, Army hospitals: 126
  - unit: 126
- enlisted personnel. *See* Auxiliary dental personnel.

INDEX

Training—Continued
  officers, Regular Army, prior to World War II
    advanced graduate course, Army Dental School
      duration: 120
      number graduated: 120
    advanced officers' course, Medical Field Service School
      duration: 120
      number graduated: 120
    basic graduate course, Army Dental School
      duration: 119
      enrollment: 119
    dental internship: 121
    extension courses: 121
    instruction in civilian institutions: 120
    nonmedical service schools: 120
    officers' basic course, Medical Field Service School
      duration: 119
      number graduated: 120
  officers, Reserve, prior to World War II
    extension courses: 122
    ROTC: 122
    summer camps: 123
  World War I
    field service school, Camp Greenleaf, Ga.: 118–119
    Preparedness League of American Dentists: 118
    Surgery of the Head, SGO, section established: 118
Training aids
  film strips: 127
  moving pictures: 127
  publications
    Atlas of Dental and Oral Pathology: 128
    Dental Bulletin, supplement to the Medical Bulletin: 128
    technical manuals: 128
Treatment, amount rendered. *See* Statistics.
Treatment, dental, aspects of. *See also* Dental rehabilitation prior to induction.
  before and during an invasion: 306
  cash value of. *See* Statistics.
  classification, precedence for: 205–206
  consultants, report on: 214
  criticism of: 213–216

Treatment, dental, aspects of—Continued
  enlisted personnel, attitude of: 214–216
  extent of: 210
  for General George Washington: 1
  limitations on: 211, 212
  persons entitled to
    civilian dependents: 207
    civilian employees: 209
    military: 207
    Red Cross: 209
  policy for: 211
  quality rendered: 212
  refusal of: 223
  rehabilitation requirements
    for inductees: 266
    for separatees: 266–267
Twelfth Air Force: 312

Undergraduate dental education. *See* Army Specialized Training Program; Education; Selective Service.
United States Public Health Service (USPHS): 76, 79

Vail, Col. Walter D.: vii
Valley Forge General Hospital: 236
Veterans Administration: 97, 237, 255
  dentists commissioned: 56
Veterinary Corps: 21
Voorhees, Hugh G.
  appointment to Dental Corps after act of 1911: 3

WAC. *See* Women's Army Corps.
WAC personnel. *See* Auxiliary dental personnel.
Wakeman General Hospital: 159
Walter Reed General Hospital: 120, 121, 125, 238
  Army Dental School: 119, 120, 125, 126, 128, 156, 157, 160
War College. *See* Schools.
War Department: 2, 10, 11, 18, 20, 35, 56, 57, 69, 70, 72, 73, 87, 88, 100, 102, 281, 336
War Department Circular
  No. 85, 1943. *See* Criteria, dental, for overseas service.
  No. 32, 1945. *See* Dentures, excessive loss or destruction of.
War Manpower Commission (WMC): 41, 55, 72, 73, 76, 131, 132

War Production Board
  burs, report on: 166
  general limitation order, 1942: 169
  general limitation order, 1943: 170
Washington, General George: 1
Westerman, Cmdr. J. V., USN: 75
Weible, Brig. Gen. Walter L.: 230, 231
White, Maj. Gen. M. G.: 58, 87, 139
White, Col. William D.: 165, 166, 167, 276, 316
Wilson, Lt. Graves H., co-author, "History of wartime research and development of medical field equipment:" 188, 193, 194, 311
Wing, Franklin F.
  appointment to Dental Corps after act of 1911: 3

Wirtz, Maj. Milton: 236
Wolven, Frank H.
  appointment to Dental Corps after act of 1911: 3
Women's Army Corps: 161

Yates, Capt. Richard E., "The procurement and distribution of medical supplies in the Zone of Interior during World War II": 165

Zone of Interior (ZI): 45, 46, 47, 86, 90, 100, 110, 111, 114, 154, 174, 178, 265, 271, 272, 273, 333, 335, 336, 338, 340, 341

www.ingramcontent.com/pod-product-compliance
Lightning Source LLC
Chambersburg PA
CBHW082106230426
43671CB00015B/2616